SILENT MYOCARDIAL ISCHEMIA

SILENT MYOCARDIAL ISCHEMIA

SHLOMO STERN MD FACC FESC

Emeritus Professor and Head
Department of Cardiology
Bikur Cholim Hospital
Jerusalem
Israel

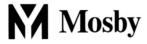 Mosby

St. Louis Baltimore Boston Carlsbad Chicago Naples New York Philadelphia Portland
London Madrid Mexico City Singapore Sydney Tokyo Toronto Wiesbaden

MARTIN DUNITZ

© Martin Dunitz Ltd 1998

First published in the United Kingdom in 1998 by
Martin Dunitz Ltd
The Livery House
7–9 Pratt Street
London NW1 0AE

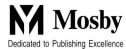 **Mosby**

Dedicated to Publishing Excellence

A Times Mirror Company

Distributed in the U.S.A. and Canada by

Mosby–year Book	Times Mirror Professional Publishing Ltd.
11830 Westline Industrial Drive	130 Flaska Drive
St. Louis, Missouri 63146	Markham, Ontario L6G 1B8

A CIP catalogue record for this book is available from the British Library

ISBN 1-85317-381-9

Composition by Scribe Design, Gillingham, Kent
Printed and bound in Great Britain by
Biddles Ltd, Guildford and King's Lynn

Contents

Contributors

Thomas von Arnim MD
Professor, Ludwig-Maximilians Universitat
Munchen and Chefarzt, Medizinische
Abteilung, Krankenhaus Rotes Kreuz,
Nymphenberger Strasse 163, D-80634
Munchen, Germany

Antonio Bayés de Luna MD
Professor of Cardiology, Autonomous
University Barcelona and Chief of the
Cardiology Department, Hospital de Sant Pau,
SAM Claret 167, 08025 Barcelona, Spain

George A Beller MD
Ruth C Heede Professor of Cardiology, Chief
of the Cardiovascular Division and Vice
Chairman of the Department of Medicine,
University of Virginia Health Sciences Center,
Box 158, Charlottesville, VA 22908, USA

Barry D Bertolet MD FACC
Division of Cardiology, Box 100277, JHMHC,
University of Florida, Gainesville, FL 32610,
USA

Christopher S Brown MD FACC
Division of Cardiology, Box 100277, JHMHC,
University of Florida, Gainesville, FL 32610,
USA

Dennis A Calnon MD
Clinical Fellow, Cardiovascular Division,
University of Virginia Health Sciences Center,
Box 158, Charlottesville, VA 22908, USA

Enrique V Carbajal MD FACC
UCSF School of Medicine, Department of
Medicine, Veterans Administration Medical
Center, 2615 East Clinton Avenue, Fresno, CA
93703, USA

Peter F Cohn MD
Professor of Medicine and Chief of
Cardiology, State University of New York,
Health Sciences Center, Stony Brook, NY
11794-8171, USA

C Richard Conti MD FACC
Chief of Cardiology, Division of Cardiology,
Box 100277, JHMHC, University of Florida,
Gainesville, FL 32610, USA

**Prakash C Deedwania MD MBBS FACC
FCCP FACP**
Chief, Cardiology Section, UCSF School of
Medicine, San Francisco and Chief,
Cardiology Section, Veterans Administration
Medical Center, 2615 East Clinton Avenue,
Fresno, CA 93703, USA

Serge G L G Degré MD PhD FESC FACA
Professor of Cardiology, Université Libre,
Bruxelles and Head of the Department of
Cardiology, Hopital Acadimique Erasme, 808
Route de Lennik, B1070 Brussels, Belgium

Myrvin H Ellestad MD FACC
Professor of Medicine and Cardiology and
Director of Research, Memorial Heart
Institute, Long Beach Memorial Medical
Center, 2801 Atlantic Avenue, Long Beach,
CA 90801, USA

John S Gottdiener MD FACC
Professor of Medicine and Director,
Echocardiography Laboratory, Division of
Cardiology, Georgetown University Medical
Center, 3800 Reservoir Road NW, Washington,
DC 20007, USA

William B Kannel MD MPH FACC
Professor of Medicine and Public Health, BU
Framingham Heart Study, 5 Thurber Street,
Framingham, MA 01701, USA

Willem J Kop MD PhD
Research Assistant Professor of Medical and
Clinical Psychology, Uniformed Services
University of the Health Sciences, 4301 Jones
Bridge Road, Bethesda, MD 20814, USA

David S Krantz MD PhD
Professor of Medical and Clinical Psychology,
Uniformed Services University of the Health
Sciences, 4301 Jones Bridge Road, Bethesda,
MD 20814, USA and Professor of Psychiatry
and Medicine, Georgetown University Medical
Center, Washington, DC 20007,
USA

David Mulcahy MD MRCPI FESC
Consultant Cardiologist, Department of
Cardiology, The Adelaide Hospital, Peter
Street, Dublin 8, Republic of Ireland

Carl J Pepine MD FACC
Professor of Medicine and Co-Director,
Division of Cardiovascular Medicine, College
of Medicine, University of Florida, Gainesville,
FL 32610, USA

Arshed A Quyyumi MD FACC
Senior Investigator, Cardiology Branch NHLBI,
Building 10, Room 7B15, 10 Center Drive,
MSC-1650, Bethesda, MD 20892-1650, USA

Andrew P Selwyn MD FACC
Cardiovascular Division, Brigham and
Women's Hospital, 75 Francis Street, Boston,
MA 02115-6195, USA

Bramah N Singh MD DPhil FRCP FACC
Professor of Medicine and Staff Cardiologist,
West Los Angeles VAMC UCLA School of
Medicine, Cardiology Section, 11301 Wilshire
Boulevard, Los Angeles, CA 90073, USA

Shlomo Stern MD FACC FESC
Emeritus Professor of Medicine and Head of
the Department of Cardiology, Bikur Cholim
Hospital, 5 Strauss Street, Jerusalem 91004,
Israel

Peter H Stone MD FACC
Cardiovascular Division, Brigham and
Women's Hospital, 75 Francis Street, Boston,
MA 02115-6195, USA

Xavier Viñolas MD
Department de Cardiologia I Circurgia
Cardiaca, Hospital de Sant Pau, SAM Claret
167, 08025, Barcelona, Spain

Donald A Weiner MD
Professor of Medicine, Boston University
School of Medicine and Director, Exercise
Laboratory, Boston Medical Center, 88 East
Newton Street, Boston, MA 02114, USA

DEDICATION

For my grandchildren
Leigh, Nikka, Omer and Noya

Introduction

Even in ancient times, at the dawn of modern medicine, pain was recognized as a most significant sign, leading the person suffering pain to focus his attention and telling him that something in his body is not functioning properly. This same sign guided his healer, showing him where to concentrate efforts to restore health. During the second half of the eighteenth century, Heberden recognized 'pain in the breast' or angina pectoris as an independent entity. Although he characterized this syndrome without relating it to the heart, his description has remained valid for centuries, even after the connection between chest pain and disease of the coronary arteries became evident. This association, pain and atherosclerotic narrowing of the coronary arteries, became not only firm but also inseparable: no one suspected the presence of coronary artery disease, or its synonym 'angina pectoris', in a person not experiencing pain in the left chest.

The medical world was taken by surprise in the early 1970s when continuous ambulatory monitoring of the electrocardiogram during daily activities demonstrated the presence of transient ST depressions in patients with coronary artery disease, without the examinee complaining of chest pain. Was this myocardial ischemia without pain or was some other mechanism at play? This problem puzzled investigators for a few years, until convincing evidence accumulated proving the ischemic nature of these asymptomatic episodes.

But why the surprise? Why be amazed by the phenomenon of 'silent ischemia' during everyday activity, when it was already understood for many years that more than half of patients have no pain during the period of ST depression in a positive exercise test; even myocardial infarction occurs without pain. Yes, these were known facts, but still this knowledge did not penetrate and nothing made us aware of the significance and even dangers of asymptomatic myocardial ischemia or 'angina pectoris sine angina'.

In this book we have assembled up-to-date knowledge on silent myocardial ischemia and the Editor was fortunate to have many pioneers of this topic as authors. The thousands of references cited, many published during the year of the appearance of this book, demonstrate how important this subject is today. The Editor has tried to avoid repetitions, but obviously this could not always be done. Even some contradictory views can be detected in the book, but this is also understandable, as we tried to collect balanced opinions and to provide the widest spectrum of information available in a field where knowledge is expanding steadily.

The publisher should be praised for his part in producing a high-quality publication, down to those fine details that are necessary to make a book successful – which I hope this book will be.

Shlomo Stern

1

Silent myocardial ischemia: the early years

Peter F Cohn

In the beginning there was doubt that a condition such as 'silent' myocardial ischemia could exist. This was because the concept of angina as being synonymous with myocardial ischemia was very much part of the structure of established medicine. Although the realization that not all coronary artery disease must be symptomatic is not a new one, it has not always received the attention it deserved. It is safe to say that it was not until patients with coronary artery disease were actually observed to be free of pain during episodes of transient myocardial ischemia on exercise tests and during ambulatory electrocardiographic monitoring that interest in the subject increased.

The term 'angina pectoris' was used by Heberden in the 1770s,[1] but only at the beginning of this century did the cause-and-effect relationship between ischemia and pain become clearer, mainly because of the pioneering work of Herrick.[2] This doctrine became then so rigid that for generations physicians have been taught that myocardial ischemia and angina pectoris are synonymous, and, if chest pain was not present, myocardial ischemia was not suspected. Interestingly, Herrick, in his original and now classic description of acute coronary occlusion and myocardial infarction, stated that in two of six of his patients pain was not experienced during the acute event. Despite this, the concepts of painless infarctions and painless ischemia remained dubious. When Master in the late 1920s introduced his two-step effort test aimed at the provocation of transient myocardial ischemia,[3] the presence of pain during the

period of ST depression was not a prerequisite for diagnosing an ischemic response to the test. Wood and associates[4] pointed out that even in a 'positive' stress test, with electrocardiographic changes during the exercise, pain is frequently absent. Kemp and Ellestad[5] also noted anecdotally in 1968 that during exercise testing ischemia could be provoked without pain.

Because of the pioneering work of Holter it became possible to obtain ambulatory ECG recordings of active subjects during daily life.[6] It was soon shown that during everyday activities episodes of ST depression without pain could occur.[7] The ischemic nature of these ST depression episodes was proved subsequently by several sophisticated methods used as adjuncts to electrocardiography. Thus, it is perhaps best to think of the early years of active research (the 1970s and the first part of the 1980s) in terms of either exercise testing or ambulatory monitoring. In the exercise testing field the author and colleagues helped popularize the concept of silent ischemia in clinical studies, editorial reviews, and books, while three distinct groups did the same with ambulatory electrocardiology: Stern and Tzivoni in Israel, Pepine and colleagues in Florida, USA, and Maseri, Selwyn and Deanfield in the United Kingdom.

EXERCISE TESTING

The present author's interest in asymptomatic coronary artery disease began in the early 1970s and initially involved ECG responses during exercise testing. His first study was reported at

Table 1.1 Types of cases in which silent myocardial ischemia may be found.
1) In persons who are totally asymptomatic
2) In persons who are asymptomatic following a myocardial infarction, but still demonstrate active ischemia
3) In persons with angina who are asymptomatic with some episodes of myocardial ischemia, but not others
Source: Cohn.[9]

the American Heart Association meetings in 1975[8] and subsequently published as a full paper in 1978.[9] This study from the Peter Bent Brigham Hospital evaluated the exercise responses of 122 consecutive patients studied between 1972 and 1974 with chest pain syndromes, angiographically documented coronary artery disease, and an abnormal response to exercise testing. Of the 122 patients, 44 had neither angina nor commonly recognized anginal equivalents during the test, and 32 had no symptoms at all. Extent of coronary artery disease was similar in patients with and without anginal complaints, as were other features. Shortly afterwards, the author published a review calling attention to the phenomenon of silent ischemia and noting its presence in about one-third of all diagnostic tests that were 'positive' for ischemia: exercise ECGs, radionuclide stress tests, metabolic determinations, etc. (Table 1.1).[10] Speculation about the reason for the lack of pain increased but has been difficult to prove despite intense investigation. The early pain threshold works of Droste and Roskamm[11] were particularly important in this regard. They indicated that although patients with silent ischemia have on average a reduced general pain perception, a generalized reduction in sensitivity to pain does not explain all cases of silent ischemia. Other noteworthy studies involved estimations of the amount of myocardium at jeopardy in painless compared with painful ischemia.[12–14]

During these early years, some investigators studied thallium-201 myocardial imaging in asymptomatic individuals while others[15,16] evaluated enhanced ST-segment criteria (such as depth of depression and persistence into recovery time) in asymptomatic subjects[17] to increase the diagnostic accuracy of the exercise electrocardiogram. Survey programs using the Framingham risk profile index and abnormal exercise tests were adopted by the United States Army with about 2.5% of individuals 'failing' the screening procedures,[18] a statistic similar to that reported in the asymptomatic population screened by the Oslo Ischemia Study and initially reported in 1976.[19] The Oslo Ischemia Study merits further elaboration. This unique enterprise consisted of a base population of approximately 2000 presumably healthy males aged 40–59 years employed in five companies in Oslo, Norway. Initial examination included history and physical as well as baseline laboratory tests (including a resting ECG) and a stress test utilizing a bicycle ergometer. Of the 2014 men screened, 115 fulfilled one or more criteria suggestive of coronary artery disease. Six of the 115 refused consent for coronary angiography and four others were excluded later. The angiographically studied population thus totaled 105, of whom 69 were found to have at least 50% stenosis in one coronary artery and 50 of these (15 with three-vessel disease, 18 with two-vessel disease and 17 with one-vessel disease), or 2.5% of the total of 2014 men, were completely asymptomatic. This figure is similar to that reported in the United States Army study cited earlier, as well as a United States Air Force Study[20] of 1390 men in which 34 (or about 2.5%) had at least over 50% stenosis in one major coronary artery. The United States Air Force study had several subsequent publications that provided other important confirmatory data.

AMBULATORY MONITORING

The other main line of research – ambulatory monitoring – has had a more controversial history, mainly because of questions concerning the reliability of the electrical signal, especially in amplitude-modulated systems. The technical considerations notwithstanding (and with contemporary equipment they are no longer considered relevant) it is important to note that Stern and Tzivoni[7] were the first to demonstrate ST-segment abnormalities on Holter monitoring in a series of studies reported in the early 1970s. In a typical study, 37 of 80 patients with chest pain syndromes had abnormal ST-segment recordings and developed overt coronary artery disease during the course of the one-year follow-up. In another study, they correlated the results of Holter monitoring with coronary arteriography and found that ambulatory ECGs identified nearly 80% of patients with angiographically documented coronary artery disease.[21]

In the late 1970s and early 1980s, other groups attempted similar correlations using ambulatory ECGs but the reliability of the electrocardiographic changes cited earlier clouded the issue. Two studies helped resolve the matter. Schang and Pepine[22] studied 20 patients with angiographically confirmed coronary artery disease and positive exercise tests, each monitored for several 10-hour periods over the course of 16 months. In the total of 2826 hours of technically adequate records, 411 episodes of transient ST-segment abnormalities were documented. Of the 411 episodes, 308 (or 75%) were asymptomatic. By markedly reducing their occurrence with the frequent, prophylactic use of a nitrate preparation Schang and Pepine indirectly 'proved' that the silent ST-segment episodes were truly ischemic. Deanfield and co-workers[23] succeeded in refuting much of the skepticism concerning the occurrence and significance of symptomatic versus asymptomatic episodes. In patients with stable angina and positive exercise tests, ambulatory ST-segment monitoring was used to record episodes of transient ischemia during daily life. All patients had four consecutive days of monitoring, and in many patients long-term variability was evaluated by repeated 48-hour monitoring and exercise testing over an 18-month period. Only 17–37% of the episodes of horizontal or downsloping ST-segment depression were

accompanied by angina – a figure similar to that of Schang and Pepine in their study published six years earlier. Physiologic confirmation of the ST-segment change was an especially important part of their study. That ischemia could occur without angina was validated by positron emission tomography, which documented that silent episodes of ST-segment depression were associated with severe regional defects in myocardial perfusion. Heart rate increase was not common, suggesting that transient increases in coronary vasomotor tone were a major contributor to myocardial ischemia – with or without symptoms – during daily activities. (More recent work has moderated this view.)

It became apparent that if the subject of silent myocardial ischemia were to be investigated fully, a classification system for asymptomatic coronary artery disease was necessary. Accordingly, in 1981, the author proposed that silent myocardial ischemia be thought of as occurring in three types of patients with coronary artery disease (Table 1.2).[24] The first group consisted of persons who were totally asymptomatic and the second group of persons who were asymptomatic after an infarction. In addition, silent myocardial ischemia can be seen in patients with angina who also have asymptomatic episodes. The key to this classification is in documentation of active ischemia; persons who have asymptomatic coronary artery disease but are not experiencing active ischemia are purposely not involved in this classification. Thus, someone with an infarction, a totally occluded vessel and no ongoing ischemia by objective criteria would be excluded.

Finally, the five major questions that were posed in the 1981 review are still pertinent today. They are:

1) What is the pathophysiologic basis of silent myocardial ischemia?
2) What is the prevalence of the different types of silent myocardial ischemia, and of silent myocardial infarction?
3) What are the most reliable noninvasive methods of detecting the syndrome of silent myocardial ischemia, and what are the

Table 1.2   Myocardial ischemia without anginal symptoms.

| Abnormality suggestive of myocardial ischemia | Total group (n) | Patients with CAD manifesting abnormality | |
| | | Group with angina[a] | |
		No.	%
Abnormal left ventricular wall motion	87	33	39
Pacing contrast ventriculogram	8	3	38
Pacing contrast ventriculogram	8	6	75
Exercise radionuclide ventriculogram	63	18	29
Exercise radionuclide ventriculogram	8	6	75
Abnormal lactate metabolism	36	9	25
Pacing study	14	1	7
Pacing study	22	8	36
Abnormal myocardial perfusion scintigrams	64	26	40
Thallium-201 study	35	20	57
Rubidium-81 study	29	6	19
Electrocardiographic stress test	568	186	32
Treadmill test	135	23	17
Treadmill test	122	32	26
Bicycle and two-step test	59	15	26
Treadmill test	146	68	45
Treadmill test	102	48	47
Total	755	254	34

[a]Although not symptomatic during this test, almost all patients in these studies had a history of angina or prior myocardial infarction.
CAD: coronary artery disease.
Source: Cohn.[9]

indications for cardiac catheterization in asymptomatic persons?

4) What is the prognosis of patients with silent myocardial ischemia and/or silent myocardial infarction?

5) How should silent myocardial ischemia be treated, if at all? Perhaps most importantly: does treatment affect prognosis?

The first attempt at answering these questions in a systematic way was in a seminar that appeared in 1983 in the *Journal of the American College of Cardiology*.[25] This was followed by the first international symposium on silent myocardial ischemia held in Geneva, Switzerland, in 1984, under the auspices of the European Society of Cardiology, which in a way concluded the first decade of 'silent ischemia'. Numerous other important national and international symposia have been held since then but the exciting atmosphere of the early years was truly unique – as all involved will attest to.

REFERENCES

1. Heberden W. Some accounts of a disorder of the breast. *Med Trans Coll Physicians (Lond)* 1772; **2**: 59–62.
2. Herrick JB. Clinical features of sudden obstruction of the coronary arteries. *JAMA* 1992; **59**: 2015–17.
3. Master AM. The Master two-step test. *Am Heart J* 1968; **75**: 810–37.
4. Wood P, McGregor M, Magidson O, Whittaker W. The effort test in angina pectoris. *Br Heart J* 1950; **12**: 363–71.
5. Kemp GL, Ellestad MH. The incidence of 'silent' coronary heart disease. *Calif Med* 1968; **109**: 303–5.
6. Holter NJ. New method for heart studies. Continuous electrocardiography of active subjects over long periods is now practical. *Science* 1961; **134**: 1214–20.
7. Stern S, Tzivoni D. Early detection of silent ischemic heart disease by 24-hour electrocardiographic monitoring of active subjects. *Br Heart J* 1974; **36**: 481–8.
8. Lindsey HE Jr, Cohn PF. 'Silent' ischemia during and after exercise testing in patients with coronary artery disease. *Circulation* 1975; **52 (suppl 2)**: 47.
9. Lindsey HE Jr, Cohn PF. 'Silent' myocardial ischemia during and after exercise in patients with coronary artery disease. *Am Heart J* 1978; **95**: 441–7.
10. Cohn PF. Silent myocardial ischemia in patients with a defective angina warning system. *Am J Cardiol* 1980; **45**: 697–702.
11. Droste C, Roskamm H. Experimental pain measurement in patients with asymptomatic myocardial ischemia. *J Am Coll Cardiol* 1983; **1**: 340–5.
12. Chierchia S, Lazzari M, Freedman B, Brunelli C, Maseri A. Impairment of myocardial perfusion and function during painless myocardial ischemia. *J Am Coll Cardiol* 1983; **1**: 923–30.
13. Cohn PF, Brown EJ, Wynne J, Holman BL, Atkins HL. Global and regional left ventricular ejection fraction abnormalities during exercise in patients with silent myocardial ischemia. *J Am Coll Cardiol* 1983; **1**: 931–3.
14. Iskandriam AS, Hakki A-H. Left ventricular function in patients with coronary heart disease in the presence or absence of angina pectoris during exercise radionuclide ventriculography. *Am J Cardiol* 1984; **53**: 1239–43.
15. Guiney TE, Pohost GM, McKusick KA, Beller GA. Differentiation of false- from true-positive ECG responses to exercise stress by thallium 201 perfusion imaging. *Chest* 1981; **80**: 4–10.
16. Caralis DG, Bailey I, Kennedy HL, Pitt B. Thallium-201 myocardial imaging in evaluation of asymptomatic individuals with ischemic ST segment depression on exercise electrocardiogram. *Br Heart J* 1979; **42**: 562–7.
17. Lozner EC, Morganroth J. New criteria to enhance the predictability of coronary artery disease by exercise testing in asymptomatic subjects. *Circulation* 1977; **56**: 799–802.
18. Zoltick JM Maj, McAllister HA Col, Bedynek JL Col Jr. The United States Army Cardiovascular Screening Program. *J Cardiac Rehabil* 1984; **4**: 530–5.
19. Erikssen J, Enge I, Forfang K, Storstein O. False positive diagnostic tests and coronary angiographic findings in 105 presumably healthy males. *Circulation* 1976; **54**: 371–6.
20. Hickman JR Jr, Uhl GS, Cook RL, Engel PJ, Hopkirk A. A natural history study of asymptomatic coronary disease. *Am J Cardiol* 1980; **45**: 422 (abst).
21. Stern S, Tzivoni D. Diagnostic accuracy of ambulatory ECG monitoring in ischemic heart disease. *Circulation* 1975; **52**: 1045–9.
22. Schang SJ, Pepine CJ. Transient asymptomatic ST-segment depression during daily activity. *Am J Cardiol* 1977; **39**: 396–402.
23. Deanfield JE, Maseri A, Selwyn AP et al. Myocardial ischemia during daily life in patients with stable angina: its relation to symptoms and heart rate changes. *Lancet* 1983; **1**: 753–8.
24. Cohn PF. Asymptomatic coronary disease: pathophysiology, diagnosis, management. *Mod Conc Cardiovasc Dis* 1981; **50**: 55–60.
25. Cohn PF. Introduction to the seminar on asymptomatic coronary artery disease. *J Am Coll Cardiol* 1983; **1**: 922–3.

2

Exercise testing in silent ischemia

Myrvin H Ellestad

INTRODUCTION

In preparing a chapter on exercise testing in silent ischemia, several questions arise. What type of silent ischemia are we considering? Controversy has raged, and still continues, as to the appropriateness of exercise tests for screening.[1] The data establish that from 8 to 10% of men over 40 years of age have significant coronary artery disease (CAD), and that most are asymptomatic.[2,3] If one restricts the use of exercise testing of those with risk factors, the prevalence of CAD will be a good deal greater. It is of interest that the paper by Froelicher et al.,[4] describing the usefulness of exercise testing in asymptomatic Air Force personnel, published in 1973, reports a 60% sensitivity and a 92% specificity, and was considered to be an excellent case-finding methodology; but by 1983, when working with the Veteran's Administration, Uhl and Froelicher report that exercise testing is not indicated in asymptomatic men.[5] It seems that screening means different things depending on what population of silent ischemia is under consideration. It is now recognized that silent ischemia can be lethal[6] and approximately 400 000 people die unexpectedly each year in the USA. Many of these undoubtedly had silent ischemia.

When the present author first became involved in exercise testing in 1962, it was thought that a careful history was a reliable way to diagnose coronary disease. If a patient failed to have a typical pain pattern, it was

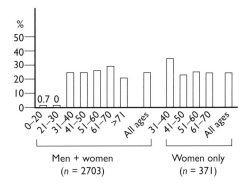

Figure 2.1 Incidence of anginal pain. The percentage of patients with ST-segment depression who had anginal pain during exercise testing stratified according to sex and age. Note that young women, a cohort who are unlikely to have CAD, have more pain than any other group. (Reproduced with permission from Kemp and Ellestad.[8])

believed that one could be quite certain that he did not have significant ischemia. Surprisingly, it was found that more than half of patients with ST depression on the treadmill failed to have angina during the test (Fig. 2.1).[7] Over time, as more and more angiograms were carried out, it became evident that even those with significant coronary narrowing were often completely free of angina, and others who had angina at one time or another might go to a high level of exercise and have ST changes but without any pain at the time of the test.[8]

MECHANISM

A few comments are in order to understand the application of exercise testing in this cohort. Although it has been common knowledge for many years that ischemic muscle causes pain, whether it be skeletal or cardiac, the exact mechanism is still only partly understood. There is a paradox that patients who are able to exercise to high workloads are less likely to have chest pain and are usually believed to have a reduced probability of ischemia, even though more patients with severe three-vessel disease have silent ischemia than those with one- or two-vessel disease.[9,10] The data suggest that a short period of ischemia of 3 minutes or less during Holter recording is less likely to be associated with pain, but the time from the onset of ischemia to the onset of pain[10] has not been examined in exercise testing to the author's knowledge. Failure to increase the left ventricular end-diastolic pressure above 7 mm has also been associated with reduced incidence of pain,[6] suggesting that silent ischemia equates with less severe ischemia. It has long been recognized that there are many patients who never have angina even with the most severe ischemia, including a myocardial infarction.[12] Alterations in pain perception have been detected in some of these patients;[12] however, the failure of Naloxone to initiate chest pain during exercise-induced ST depression suggests that endorphins do not have much influence.[13]

Pain is more common during percutaneous transluminal coronary angioplasty (PTCA), which produces ST elevation, than exercise-induced ischemia. When the artery is occluded by a balloon, ischemia of a greater amount of myocardium is more likely, therefore inducing pain, than when less muscle is involved, as might be postulated in exercise angina where the subendocardium is the most ischemic tissue. This conflicts with the previous reports just cited. From the contradictions described, it seems evident that the mechanism is still poorly understood.

PREVALENCE OF ASYMPTOMATIC ISCHEMIA IN THE EXERCISE LABORATORY

Referral pattern is one of the factors that will dictate how often ischemia occurs during exercise testing in the laboratory.[11] During a visit to Hammersmith Hospital in London, years ago, it appeared to the author that almost all the patients had angina pectoris and more than half had pain during the exercise test. In the early years (1965–70) exercise testing was used in many cases to screen asymptomatic patients who had several risk factors.[14] This resulted in the reporting of a low prevalence of pain in patients with ST depression. On the other hand, follow-up data of asymptomatic patients in 1975 were among the first to demonstrate the clinical importance and predictive implications of ST depression, which has been confirmed by many subsequent studies.[7,15]

MANAGEMENT DURING THE EXERCISE TEST

The indications and contraindications are very similar in silent ischemia to those in any other exercise test. Patients who have resting ST depression in the absence of LVH, even though asymptomatic, must be watched very closely. If their ST depression increases significantly—especially at low workloads—they are at risk of global ischemia and may have left main disease. Most of the catastrophies in the exercise laboratory occur in this subset.

Many laboratories use some predetermined magnitude of ST depression as an indication to terminate. If this is done, exercise time, an important prognostic predictor,[16] can be compromised. With some important exceptions, the magnitude of ST depression need not dictate the degree of ischemia in patients without exercise-induced pain. Recent reports have documented that, despite popular belief to the contrary, the magnitude of exercise-induced ST depression does not correlate with the number of diseased coronary vessels nor the area of ischemia on the thallium centigram (Fig. 2.2).[17,18] The author has found, for example,

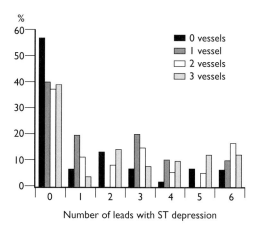

Figure 2.2 Magnitude of ST depression. The mean magnitude of ST depression is shown categorized according to the number of coronary arteries over 70% obstructed. (Reproduced with permission from Ellestad et al.[19])

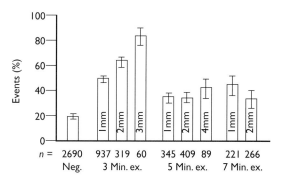

Figure 2.3 Effect of time onset of ST depression in prognosis. The time of onset of ST depression, subgrouped by magnitude of ST deviation is depicted according to mean number of cardiac events in a 6-year follow-up. (Reproduced with permission from Ellestad[36])

that those with LVH may have more profound ST depression with lesser amounts of ischemia, as do those with previous myocardial infarction or reduced R-waves.[19]

One millimeter of ST depression has been accepted as the threshold of significant ischemia for many years. It is obvious that there is probably no difference between 0.9 and 1.1 mm of ST depression physiologically, but it has been generally accepted that the greater the ST depression, the more reliable the diagnosis of ischemia. Using any cut-off, it must be recognized that the more specific the finding, that is, the greater the ST depression, the more sensitivity will be reduced. The question must be then, is more ST depression required in order to be diagnostic for ischemia in patients with silent ischemia than those with angina? The answer to this question will be forthcoming.

DATA FROM MEMORIAL HEART INSTITUTE

Exercise files were compared where an angiogram had been carried out within 90 days and there had been no intervention to invali-

date the comparison. An obstruction of 70% in at least one coronary artery was required in order to call it an abnormal angiogram.

In order to explore the use of exercise testing in silent ischemia the data were analyzed in two ways. First, the sensitivity, specificity and predictive value of a number of variables were examined and categorized according to whether a patient had a reported history of angina or not when they had their exercise test. A similar analysis was then performed but the patients were divided according to whether they had chest pain during the exercise test.

TIME OF ONSET OF ST DEPRESSION

It has long been recognized that ST-segment depression at low workloads is associated with a poor prognosis in patients with coronary disease. Figure 2.3 illustrates the follow-up data, without separating patients as to whether or not they have pain.

When the coronary anatomy is used to stratify these patients, it can be seen from Table 1 that ST depression occurring early has a higher

Table 2.1 Time of onset of ST depression.

	Sensitivity	Specificity	PPV
No-exercise angina			
≤ 3 minutes	0.36	0.73	0.73
> 3 and < 5 minutes	0.24	0.76	0.66
> 5 minutes	0.40	0.512	0.62
Exercise angina			
≤ 3 minutes	0.34	0.77	0.83
> 3 and < 5 minutes	0.32	0.92	0.93
> 5 minutes	0.34	0.31	0.62

Most studies on silent ischemia have concentrated on patients who fail to have angina during testing. Although it is well known that even though most patients sent for exercise testing are referred because of a history of pain, only a few actually have pain during the test. Table 2.2 illustrates that when comparing patients according to whether or not they have a history of angina, the sensitivity and specificity of most of the markers of ischemia are quite similar. On the other hand, the positive predictive value, considered by some to be the most acceptable measure of utility or reliability of exercise testing, is consistently higher in those with a history of angina. This is particularly true when testing females, where we find a very low positive predictive value in those who do not give a history of angina as compared with those who do. The high incidence of false-positive exercise tests in women has been well documented.[20,21]

The specificity of conventional ST depression in the author's database is below that usually reported by others. Be that as it may, the PPV is significantly lower in silent ischemia than in those with a history of angina. The high specificity seen in those with a short exercise time is noteworthy.

The high specificity when ST depression is combined with either ST elevation in AVR, or with R-wave increase in V_5, illustrates the importance of two separate markers to increase reliability. Also, the high specificity of an increase in T-waves in V_2, and ST elevation in the anterior precordial leads, should not be overlooked.

The magnitude of ST depression is compared in those with a history of angina versus those without. It is found that the specificity is about the same in both groups and increases with the magnitude of ST depression, as might be suspected (Table 2.3). On the other hand, the positive predictive value is higher with each increase in ST depression in those with an anginal history. The sensitivity is also considerably higher in patients with a history of chest pain. These data then suggest that exercise-induced ST depression is somewhat more

specificity and positive predictive value, particularly in patients with exercise angina, and can help to identify ischemia. Even when the patient is not experiencing angina this trend persists but is not nearly so significant.

HISTORY OF ANGINA VERSUS NO ANGINA

This section presents data on two groups of markers that have been used in the author's laboratory. First, the conventional markers that have been recognized for years and which are the ones most physicians think of when examining exercise tests. The second group, unconventional markers, have all been found to have merit but to the author's knowledge are not in common usage. The unconventional markers are often very helpful and readers may be assured that using them will increase their ability to identify patients with myocardial ischemia. If one averages the positive predictive value of the unconventional markers, it comes to 0.69, just slightly better than the 0.67 for the conventional ones.

Table 2.2 Markers for ischemia according to history of angina compared with no history.

	No history of angina			History of angina		
	Sensitivity	Specificity	PPV	Sensitivity	Specificity	PPV
Conventional markers						
1) ST ↓ >1 mm (any lead)	0.64	0.51	0.57	0.69	0.51	0.70
2) ST ↓ >1 mm V$_5$	0.44	0.77	0.66	0.50	0.74	0.77
3) Downslope in recovery	0.64	0.51	0.57	0.69	0.50	0.70
4) Exercise time						
<3 min	0.07	0.95	0.60	0.76	0.93	0.64
>5 min	0.79	0.19	0.50	0.75	0.19	0.60
5) ST in males	0.66	0.51	0.67	0.69	0.55	0.75
6) ST in females	0.57	0.50	0.36	0.71	0.45	0.60
Unconventional markers						
1) ST/R >0.1 mm	0.51	0.66	0.60	0.55	0.73	0.77
2) ST ↓ >1 + ST ↑ AVR	0.13	0.95	0.75	0.12	0.99	0.93
3) Δ HR <50	0.33	0.78	0.60	0.26	0.73	0.61
4) Δ T ↑ >2.5 mm V$_2$	0.18	0.84	0.53	0.23	0.81	0.66
5) Δ R >2 mm V$_5$	0.36	0.64	0.51	0.33	0.60	0.57
6) Δ R and ST ↓	0.28	0.78	0.56	0.26	0.84	0.72
7) ST ↑ >2 mm V$_2$ or V$_3$	0.15	0.91	0.63	0.07	0.92	0.57

Table 2.3 Exercise angina: magnitude of ST depression.

ST depression (mm)	Sensitivity		Specificity		PPV	
Angina	No	Yes	No	Yes	No	Yes
1.0–1.4	0.21	0.19	0.78	0.71	0.53	0.54
1.5–2.0	0.22	0.22	0.85	0.87	0.62	0.75
>2.0	0.33	0.43	0.82	0.79	0.68	0.79

reliable as a predictor in patients with a history of chest pain. In the population reported here, where all patients have had an angiogram, this effect is probably minimized. When examining a large population for screening, a history of chest pain combined with ST depression is obviously more reliable than ST depression without symptoms.[22]

Table 2.4 Markers for ischemia stratified according to angina during the test compared with no angina.

Markers	No angina			Angina		
	Sensitivity	Specificity	PPV	Sensitivity	Specificity	PPV
Conventional markers						
1) ST ↓ >1 mm (any lead)	0.66	0.51	0.60	0.70	0.47	0.70
2) ST ↓ >1 mm V$_5$	0.43	0.77	0.68	0.58	0.71	0.78
3) Downslope in recovery	0.66	0.51	0.60	0.70	0.47	0.70
4) Exercise time						
<3 min	0.70	0.96	0.65	0.07	0.90	0.56
>5 min	0.77	0.18	0.51	0.78	0.21	0.64
Average			0.60			0.67
Unconventional markers						
1) ST/R >0.1 mm	0.53	0.67	0.65	0.52	0.73	0.78
2) ST ↓ >1 + ST ↑ AVR	0.13	0.96	0.80	0.12	0.94	0.89
3) Δ HR <50	0.30	0.78	0.61	0.26	0.66	0.58
4) Δ T ↑ >2.5 mm V$_2$	0.19	0.84	0.57	0.23	0.79	0.67
5) Δ R >2 mm in V$_5$	0.36	0.63	0.52	0.30	0.60	0.58
6) Δ R and ST ↓	0.27	0.79	0.59	0.35	0.84	0.70
7) ST ↑ >2 mm V$_2$ or V$_3$	0.11	0.92	0.59	0.11	0.90	0.67
Average			0.61			0.69

PATIENTS WHO HAVE PAIN DURING THE TEST VERSUS THOSE WHO ARE SILENT

Stratification according to pain during the test has been used by the majority of those who have studied silent ischemia. Many patients who have a history of angina will be classified as having silent ischemia when this criterion is utilized. Table 2.4 illustrates the previously reported markers in this way. Although the specificity of the conventional markers is slightly higher in patients without pain, the sensitivity and the positive predictive value is better in patients with angina, although the difference is usually not significant, except for the unconventional markers where the average positive predictive value in patients with silent ischemia is 0.61, as compared to 0.69 in those with pain during the test.

It will be noticed that the average sensitivity of the unconventional markers is far below that of the conventional ones, but the specificity is a good deal better. Therefore, many patients with ischemia will not have the findings categorized as unconventional, but when they occur one can be quite confident that they are reliable and that the false-positives will be uncommon. One should learn to look for these changes in order to understand better the patient's pathology.

Table 2.5 Markers for ischemia stratified as to history of angina or angina during exercise test.

Markers	PPV		Specificity	
Conventional markers	No ex. angina	No hx angina	No ex. angina	No hx. angina
1) ST ↓ >1 mm (any lead)	0.60	0.57	0.52	0.57
2) ST ↓ >1 mm in V_5	0.68	0.67	0.68	0.66
3) Downslope ST in recovery	0.60	0.57	0.51	0.60
4) Exercise time				
<3 min	0.65	0.60	0.65	0.95
>5 min	0.51	0.50	0.18	0.18
Unconventional markers	No ex. angina	No hx angina	No ex. angina	No hx. angina
1) ST/R	0.65	0.60	0.65	0.66
2) ST ↓ >1 + ST ↑ in AVR	0.80	0.75	0.96	0.95
3) Δ HR <50	0.61	0.53	0.78	0.78
4) Δ T ↑ >2.5 mm V_2	0.57	0.55	0.84	0.84
5) Δ R V_5 >2 mm	0.52	0.51	0.63	0.64
6) Δ R >2 mm and ST ↓ >1 mm	0.59	0.50	0.79	0.78
7) ST ↑ >2 mm V_2 or V_3	0.59	0.65	0.91	0.90

When conventional ST depression is combined with other findings, such as ST elevation in AVR, a change that may well be reciprocal, the specificity increases from 51% to 96%. Combining ST depression with an increase in R-amplitude has a specificity of 79%, again considerably better than that of ST depression alone.

The comparison of data using history of angina, or the absence of an anginal history versus absence of pain during the exercise test, reveals that these groups are surprisingly similar. Table 2.5 compares the positive predictive value and the specificity of the two groups for the various markers. It would appear that regardless of which criteria one uses to classify silent ischemia, the exercise test findings are almost equivalent.

SILENT ISCHEMIA AFTER AN ACUTE MYOCARDIAL INFARCTION

Exercise testing prior to discharge after an acute myocardial infarction (MI) used to be a common practice.[23] There was evidence that those who had no ischemia would do relatively well compared with those who had ST depression.[23] In many centers, exercise-induced ST depression was considered an indication to proceed with angiography after acute MI, with the expectation that revascularization might be indicated.[24] This is partly because patients with so-called non-Q infarcts, which include many with posterior wall necrosis due to circumflex occlusion, made up a significant portion of this cohort. In these patients, a coexisting lesion in either the right coronary or the left anterior descending artery (LAD) was often present and, if it could be identified, would often lead to coronary revascularization surgery. Since widespread use of thrombolytic agents has occurred, there are no current data to support this practice.

In the author's institution, 65% of those with a diagnosis of acute MI have an angiogram prior to discharge and 26% are treated primarily with angioplasty during an acute event. Thus, in these patients, the coronary anatomy is known and therefore only those patients with distal lesions or obstructions considered to be of marginal significance are referred for post-MI testing. In TIMI-II (Thrombolysis in Myocardial Infarction), ST depression found on testing was not predictive of 1-year cardiac events, but this was probably because all the high-risk patients were preselected after angiography for revascularization prior to their exercise test.[25]

The best recent data in post-MI exercise testing are from Il Gruppo Italiano per lo Studio della Supravvivenza nell'Infarto Miocardioco (GISSI-II). In this study, 6296 patients were tested an average of 28 days after therapy.[26] They found that asymptomatic ST-segment depression was not predictive of 6-month mortality. It may be that with a longer follow-up these changes may still be useful.

This does not mean that exercise testing after an infarction was not useful, because those with a very low work capacity had a higher mortality, which was also the case in TIMI-II. Thus, it appears evident that functional testing after an infarction is often very useful in stratifying patients even though the ST-segment itself may not always be as predictive as previously reported.

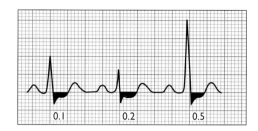

Figure 2.4 Lead strength. The ST depression that is significant is related to the R-wave amplitude, where a ratio of 0.1 was found to be the most useful cut-off. (Reproduced with permission from Ellestad et al.[19])

DISCUSSION OF UNCONVENTIONAL MARKERS

ST/R or lead strength

It has been recognized that false-negative exercise tests using ST depression are very common in patients with low voltage. Indeed, Hakki et al.[27] reported that when the lateral precordial R-waves were less than 10 mm the sensitivity was only 11%. It has also been recognized that patients with left ventricular hypertrophy and very tall R-waves are more likely to have false-positive exercise tests. Accordingly, the author studied the benefit of correcting the ST depression for R-wave amplitude and found that a ratio of 0.1 was a good cut-off. In patients with an R-wave of 5 mm and ST depression of 0.5 mm, the ratio was equivalent to 1 mm of ST depression in a patient with a 10 mm R-wave (see Fig. 2.4).[19] Using this correction, it was possible to increase the sensitivity in patients with R-waves less than 10 mm from 31% to 82%. It also corrected the specificity in patients with tall R-waves but, as might be expected, reduced the sensitivity somewhat.

Delta heart rate less than 50

Many years ago it was reported that chronotropic incompetence, a failure of the heart rate to increase normally during exercise, identified a cohort of patients who had a higher mortality.[14] Recently, Sandvik et al.[28] and Lauer et al.[16] have confirmed this by correlating the delta heart rate (difference between resting and maximum exercise) with mortality in normal populations. For the purposes of this study a maximum heart rate change of less than 50 beats per minute was selected. A patient with a resting rate of 70 beats per minute and a change of heart rate less than 50 would not be able to generate a heart rate of over 120 with exercise. This finding has a low sensitivity, but a specificity of almost 80%. The author believes the use of some measure of chronotropic incompetence will be very useful in evaluating a patient with silent ischemia.

R-wave increase with exercise

The R-wave in the lateral precordial leads usually decreases with exercise in normal subjects. It was first reported that an increase in R-wave amplitude with exercise was a marker of ischemia in 1978.[28] Subsequently, several papers have either supported or refuted the original data.[29–31] This measurement has been found to have a relatively low sensitivity, but if an increase of 2 mm is used in association with a good exercise tolerance, the specificity is fairly good (see Table 2.4).

Increase in T-amplitude in V_2 with exercise

This was first reported in 1995 and, like many of the unconventional markers, has a low sensitivity.[32] A high specificity (over 80%), however, makes it very useful when it does occur (Fig. 2.5).

Combinations: ST depression and ST elevation in AVR

ST elevation in AVR has been reported to be useful when exercise-testing patients who have had a previous MI.[33] The author has found that when combined with ST depression in other leads, the specificity is over 95%. Again, the combination has only a sensitivity of about 13%. When combining ST depression with R-

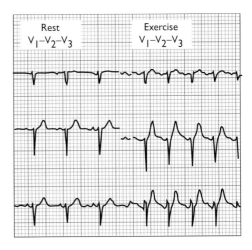

Figure 2.5 Amplitude of T-V_2. The difference between the T-wave amplitude from rest to maximum exercise of >2.5 has been found to be specific for LAD disease. (Reproduced with permission from Lee et al.[33])

wave increase, the sensitivity is also low but the specificity is 97%. Other combinations will also increase specificity.

ST elevation

This event, when it occurs during exercise in patients without a previous myocardial infarction, is not only very specific for ischemia but can localize the culprit artery.[34] ST elevation in V_2 or V_3 identifies a high-grade LAD lesion in over 90% of cases. If it occurs in lead 3 and AVF, it will identify ischemia in the inferior wall due to the right coronary or the circumflex artery.[35]

In order to answer the question, 'Does it take more ST depression in the absence of chest pain to identify ischemia?', we must return to Table .3 which compares sensitivity, specificity and positive predictive value in those who have pain during exercise and those who do not.

If more ST depression were required to identify ischemia in patients without pain, the sensitivity of a 2 mm ST depression might be expected to be similar to that of a 1 mm depression in someone who had angina. Table .3 demonstrates that this is not the case. Indeed, the sensitivities and specificities of the various degrees of ST depression are quite similar. This is not surprising, as it has been demonstrated that there is a poor correlation between the magnitude of ST depression and the magnitude of ischemia, judged by either the thallium scintigram or the number of narrowed coronary arteries.[16]

CONCLUSION

In summary, then, although the diagnosis of silent ischemia is predicated on finding ST depression during exercise testing, the reliability of this response is somewhat reduced when compared with those with symptomatic ischemia. The use of unconventional markers, however, is very important and will improve the diagnostic power when evaluating this class of patients. Because most patients who are diagnosed as having silent ischemia are identified by the presence of ST-segment depression, it is important to remember that these electrocardiographic changes may possibly be the penultimate event in the ischemic cascade, with anginal pain being the last event in the process.[36,37]

REFERENCES

1. Redwood DR, Borer JS, Epstein SE. Whither the ST-segment during exercise. *Circulation* 1976; **54**: 703–6.
2. Allen WH et al. Five-year follow-up of maximal treadmill stress test in asymptomatic men and women. *Circulation* 1980; **62**: 522–7.
3. Erikssen J et al. False positive diagnostic tests and coronary angiographic findings in 105 presumably healthy males. *Circulation* 1976; **54**: 371–6.
4. Froelicher VF Jr, Thomas MM, Pillow C, Lancaster MC. Epidemiologic study of asymptomatic men screened by maximal treadmill testing for latent coronary artery disease. *Am J Cardiol* 1974; **34**: 768–76.
5. Uhl GS, Froelicher V. Screening for asymptomatic coronary artery disease. *Am Coll Cardiol* 1983; **3**: 946–55.
6. Sharma B et al. Demonstration of exercise-induced painless ischemia in survivors of out-of-hospital ventricular fibrillation. *Am J Cardiol* 1987; **59**: 740–5.
7. Kemp GL, Ellestad MH. Incidence of 'silent' coronary disease. *Calif Med* 1968; **109**: 363–7.
8. Weiner DA, Ryan TJ, McCabe CH et al. Value of exercise testing in determining the risk classification and the response to coronary artery bypass grafting in three-vessel coronary artery disease: a report from the Coronary Artery Surgery Study (CASS) registry. *Am J Cardiol* 1987; **60**: 262–6.
9. Falcone C, DeServi S, Poma E et al. Clinical significance of exercise-induced silent myocardial ischemia in patients with coronary artery disease. *J Am Coll Cardiol* 1987; **9**: 295–9.
10. Lindsey HE, Cohn PF. 'Silent' myocardial ischemia during and after exercise testing in patients with coronary artery disease. *Am Heart J* 1978; **95**: 441–7.
11. Kannel WB, Abbott RD. Incidence and prognosis of unrecognized myocardial infarction. An update on the Framingham study. *N Engl J Med* 1984; **311**: 1144–7.
12. Droste C, Roskamm H. Experimental pain measurement in patients with asymptomatic myocardial ischemia. *J Am Coll Cardiol* 1983; **1**: 940–5.
13. Ellestad MH, Kuan P. Naloxone and asymptomatic ischemia: failure to induce angina during exercise testing. *Am J Cardiol* 1984; **54**: 982–4.
14. Ellestad MH, Wan MKC. Predictive implications of stress testing: follow-up of 1700 subjects after maximum treadmill stress testing. *Circulation* 1975; **51**: 363–9.
15. Callaham PR, Froelicher VF, Klein J, Risch M, Dubach P, Friis R. Exercise-induced silent ischemia: age, diabetes mellitus, previous myocardial infarction and prognosis. *J Am Coll Cardiol* 1989; **14**: 1175–80.
16. Lauer MS, Okin PM, Larson MG, Evans JC, Levy D. Impaired heart rate response to graded exercise: prognostic implications of chronotropic incompetence in the Framingham Heart Study. *Circulation* 1996; **93**: 1520–6.

17. Husted R, Crump R, Mishkin F, Stavitsky Y, Ellestad MH. The failure of multilead ST depression to predict severity of ischemia. *Am J Noninvas Cardiol* 1994; **8**: 386–90.
18. Bogaty P et al. Does more ST-segment depression on the 12 lead ECG signify more severe ischemic heart disease? *Circulation* 1993; **88**: 1–22.
19. Ellestad MH, Crump R, Surber M. The significance of lead strength on ST changes during treadmill stress tests. *J Electrocardiogr* 1993; **25** (suppl): 31–4.
20. Amsterdam EA et al. Exercise stress testing in patients with angiographically normal coronary arteries: similar frequency of false positive ischemic responses in males and females. *Am J Cardiol* 1978; **41**: 378.
21. Weiner DA et al. Correlations among history of angina, ST-segment response and prevalence of coronary artery disease in the Coronary Artery Surgery Study (CASS). *N Engl J Med* 1979; **301**: 230–9.
22. Cole JP, Ellestad MH. Significance of chest pain during treadmill exercise: correlation with coronary events. *Am J Cardiol* 1978; **41**: 277–81.
23. Ericsson M et al. Arrhythmias and symptoms during treadmill testing three weeks after myocardial infarction in 100 patients. *Br Heart J* 1973; **35**: 787–90.
24. Taylor GJ et al. Predictors of clinical course, coronary anatomy and left ventricular function after recovery from acute myocardial infarction. *Circulation* 1980; **62**: 960–70.
25. Chaitman BR, McMahon RP, Terrin M et al. Impact of treatment strategy on predischarge exercise test in the Thrombolysis in Myocardial Infarction (TIMI) II trial. *Am J Cardiol* 1993; **71**: 131–8.
26. Chaitman BR. What has happened to risk stratification with noninvasive testing? *ACC Curr J Rev* 1996; **5**(5): Sept/Oct.
27. Hakki AH, Iskandrian SD, Kutalek et al. R-wave amplitude: a new determinant of failure of patients with coronary heart disease to manifest ST-segment depression during exercise. *J Am Coll Cardiol* 1984; **3**: 1155–60.
28. Sandvik L, Erikssen J, Ellestad M et al. Heart rate increase and maximal heart rate during exercise as predictors of cardiovascular mortality: 16-year follow-up study of 1960 healthy men. *Coron Artery Dis* 1995; **6**: 667–8.
29. Bonoris PE, Greenberg PS, Chxistism GW, Castellanett MJ, Ellestad MH. Evaluation of R-wave changes vs. ST-segment depression in stress testing. *Circulation* 1978; **57**: 904–10.
30. Berman JL, Wynne K, Cohn P. Multiple lead treadmill exercise tests. *Circulation* 1980; **61**: 53.
31. Degre S et al. Analysis of exercise-induced R-wave changes in detection of coronary artery disease in patients with typical or atypical chest pain under digitalis treatment. *Cardiology* 1981; **68** (suppl 2): 178–85.
32. Fox K et al. Inability of exercise-induced R-wave changes to predict coronary artery disease. *Am J Cardiol* 1982; **49**: 674–9.
33. Lee JH, Crump R, Ellestad MH. Significance of precordial T-wave increase during treadmill testing. *Am J Cardiol* 1995; **76**: 1297–9.
34. Nakamori H, Iwasaka T, Shimada T et al. Clinical significance of ST-segment elevation in lead AVR in anterior myocardial infarction. *Cardiol* 1995; **86**: 147–51.
35. Calahine RA, Raezner AE, Ischimori T. The clinical significance of exercise-induced ST-segment elevation. *Circulation* 1976; **54**: 209–13.
36. Ellestad MH. *Stress Testing Principles and Practice*, 4th edn (Philadelphia, PA: FA Davis, 1995).
37. Grossman W. Why is left ventricular diastolic pressure increased during angina pectoris? *J Am Coll Cardiol* 1985; **5**: 607–8.

3

Prognostic significance of exercise testing: the CASS study

Donald A Weiner

The clinical indications for exercise testing to assess patients with ischemic heart disease have evolved in the past decade. New information has been obtained from correlative studies between electrocardiographic, angiographic, and outcome parameters in large-database studies. Whereas at one time the exercise test was used almost exclusively as a diagnostic method to assess patients with chest pain syndromes, it is now predominantly used to evaluate the prognostic outcome in patients with ischemic heart disease and to identify patients who might benefit from revascularization procedures.[1–7]

This review will attempt to place the exercise electrocardiogram in perspective as a tool to assess the prognosis of patients with ischemic heart disease. Prior studies will be reviewed using data from the Coronary Artery Surgery Study (CASS) registry in which a large group of patients with exercise testing and complete cardiac catheterization analyses were followed prospectively for over 10 years.

THE CASS TRIAL

Study population

The design, study protocol, procedures for randomization, quality control measures and baseline characteristics of the patients participating in CASS have been published previously.[8] The CASS registry comprises 24 959 consecutive patients who underwent coronary arteriography at 14 cooperating clinical sites between 1974 and 1979. From this registry, 780 consenting patients with at least a 70% diameter stenosis of one or more operable vessels were randomly assigned to receive medical or surgical treatment at 11 participating sites. Clinical criteria for entry into the randomized trial included age ≤ 65 years and either angina or Canadian Cardiovascular Society Class I or II or no symptoms with a well documented myocardial infarction more than 3 weeks before enrollment.

Study protocol

The following information was collected prospectively on each patient and recorded on standardized forms: a clinical profile, data from physical examination and laboratory studies, exercise test results, chest X-ray findings, precise angiographic characterization of the coronary arteries and left ventricle, electrocardiographic findings, and information on surgical procedures (if applicable). All patients were followed up at yearly intervals for a minimum of 10 years to ascertain health status. Overall, the follow-up was 99% complete.

Selective coronary arteriograms were obtained in multiple projections with either the brachial or femoral artery technique. Clinically important coronary artery disease was defined as 70% or greater narrowing of the diameter in either the left anterior descending, left circumflex or right coronary artery or their major branches or 50% or greater stenosis of the left main segment. Left ventriculography was performed using a single plane adaptation of the area-length method, and the ejection fraction was determined from the right anterior oblique projection. In addition, a left ventricular contraction score (ranges 5 to 30) was calculated on the basis of a subjective grading of the left ventricular angiogram as described previously.[8]

Although a graded treadmill exercise test using the Bruce protocol[9] was a study requirement, its absence did not constitute a reason for exclusion from randomization. The exercise test was analyzed for the presence of ≥1 mm of horizontal or downward ST-segment depression measured 0.08 seconds after the J point of the electrocardiogram and for the occurrence of angina chest pain either during exercise or during recovery.

The prognostic exercise test studies were based on an analysis of 5303 registry patients with no previous coronary bypass surgery who underwent graded treadmill exercise testing between 1974 and 1979 at one of the participating institutions within 1 month of catheterization.

The noninvasive and invasive data analyzed consisted of 18 clinical or historic variables, eight variables obtained from the exercise test and five obtained from cardiac catheterization as delineated in Table 3.1 and described previously in detail.[8] The variables were selected because they were thought to be related to survival on the basis of clinical judgment or previous publications.

The advantages of the CASS registry population included: (1) a large number of patients who had standard exercise testing using a common protocol; (2) precise angiographic characterization of the coronary arteries and left ventricle with quality control; and (3) excellent follow-up.

CLINICAL FACTORS

Evaluation of data from the CASS registry patients who underwent medical therapy and

---

Table 3.1 Baseline variables analyzed.

Clinical
  Gender
  Age
  Chest pain
    Description (definite angina, probable angina, nonischemic chest pain, none)
    Severity (I to V)
  Congestive heart failure
    History
    Functional impairment (none, mild, moderate, severe)
    Rales by examination
    Cardiac enlargement
    Score (0 to 4)[a]
  Family history of coronary disease
  History of hypertension
  Previous myocardial infarction
  Risk factor index
  Previous cardiac arrest
  Drug therapy
    Digitalis
    Diuretics
    Beta-adrenergic blockade
  No. of associated illnesses (0 to 5)[b]
Exercise test
  Limiting symptom
  Angina
  Ventricular arrhythmias
  Peak heart rate
  Peak systolic blood pressure
  Baseline ST-segment on rest electrocardiogram
  ST-segment response
  Final exercise stage
Catheterization
  No. of stenotic coronary vessels ≥ 70%
  Left ventricular score (5 to 30)[c]
  Left ventricular ejection fraction
  Left main coronary disease ≥ 50% luminal stenosis
  Left ventricular end-diastolic pressure

[a]One point was assigned for each of the following factors: history of heart failure, use of digitalis, use of diuretics and presence of pulmonary rales or an S_3 gallop on auscultation.
[b]One point was assigned for each of the following factors: diabetes mellitus, hypertension, cerebrovascular disease, peripheral vascular disease and chronic pulmonary disease.
[c]A wall motion score for each of five different segments of the left ventricular silhouette was calculated as follow: 1 = normal; 2 = mild hypokinesia; 3 = moderate hypokinesia; 4 = akinesia; 5 = dyskinesia; 6 = aneurysm.

were observed prospectively revealed that the presence of cardiac enlargement, prior myocardial infarction, and the congestive heart failure score were the three clinical factors that best predicted subsequent cardiac mortality.[1] Patients with no or minimal heart failure had a 4-year survival of 90%, whereas those with moderate or severe heart failure had survival rates of 62% and 18%, respectively. These results confirmed the findings of another large databank study, the Seattle Heart Watch study,[10] which identified several clinical variables relating to the functional state of the left ventricle to be the most important predictors of survival. These parameters included the presence of cardiac enlargement, the use of diuretics, S_3 gallop, and congestive heart failure.

EXERCISE TEST PARAMETERS

Evaluation of the CASS registry patients who underwent exercise testing and who were prospectively followed on medical therapy revealed that the best predictors of cardiac mortality on the exercise test were the exercise capacity and the amount of ischemic ST depression.[1] The subset of patients who had at least 1 mm of ST-segment depression and could only achieve Stage I or less on the Bruce protocol had an annual mortality in excess of 5%. This higher-risk subgroup contrasted with a lower-risk one consisting of patients who did not have ischemic ST-segment depression and who could exercise into Stage III or more. The annual mortality in this lower-risk subset was less than 1%. Thus risk stratification created subsets of patients with a five-fold difference in annual mortality rates (Table 3.2).

Among the patients with three-vessel coronary artery disease (CAD), those with limited exercise tolerance had a much worse survival rate (average annual mortality of 12% for those patients unable to complete Stage I versus annual mortality of 0% for those able to achieve Stage V).[1] Thus, patients with moderate or significant ischemia and poor exercise tolerance, especially in the presence of three-vessel CAD, constitute a high-risk group.

Table 3.2 Exercise test risk classification.

Variable	Risk		
	Low	Intermediate	High
ST-segment depression (mm)	None	1–2	
Final exercise stage (Bruce protocol)	≥ 3	≥ 2	≤ 1
Peak heart rate (beats/min)	≥ 160	≥ 130	< 130
Peak systolic blood pressure (mmHg)	≥ 160	130–160	< 130

CORONARY BYPASS SURGERY

To determine whether exercise testing could identify patients whose survival might be prolonged by coronary bypass surgery, the results of bypass surgery were compared with those of medical therapy alone in the 5303 CASS registry patients who underwent exercise testing.[7] The results revealed that among patients with early positive exercise test results, survival at 7 years was 82% after surgical therapy and 72% after medical therapy. By contrast, survival was not different between surgical and medical therapy among patients without ischemic ST depression who could exercise into Stage III or greater (Fig. 3.1). The greatest difference in survival was found in patients with severe CAD. Among the 398 patients with three-vessel CAD and with an early positive exercise test result, 7-year survival was 58% for the medical group and 81% for the surgical group (Fig. 3.2).[7] Thus, results from the CASS exercise test analysis suggest that the prognosis of patients with

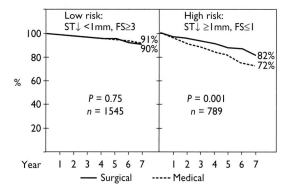

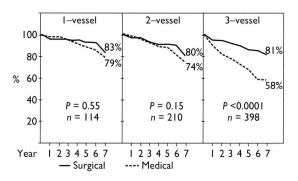

Figure 3.1 Cumulative survival rates for medical and surgical patients according to exercise risk classification. A lower-risk subgroup comprised patients with less than 1 mm ST-segment depression and a final exercise level of Stage III or higher, whereas a higher-risk subgroup consisted of patients with 1 mm or greater ST-segment depression and a final exercise level of Stage I or less. (Adapted from Weiner et al.[7])

Figure 3.2 Cumulative survival rates for medical and surgical patients with the higher-risk exercise classification and single-, double-, or triple-vessel coronary disease. (Adapted from Weiner et al.[7])

CAD can be based not only on the anatomic finding of CAD but also on the physiologic assessment of the disease utilizing results of an exercise test.

SILENT ISCHEMIA

To assess the significance of ischemic ST-segment depression without chest pain (Group 1), the long-term survival of patients with these exercise test characteristics was compared with three other groups of CAD patients: those with angina but no ischemic ST depression (Group 2); those with both ischemic ST depression and angina (Group 3); and those with neither ischemic ST depression nor angina (Group 4).[11] All the 1351 patients in this analysis had documented CAD. The cumulative seven-year survival rates (Fig. 3.3) were similar for patients in Groups 1 (76%), 2 (77%), and 3 (78%), but were significantly better for patients in Group 4 (88%).[11] Among patients with silent myocardial

ischemia during exercise testing (Group 1), the seven-year survival among patients with one-, two-, and three-vessel CAD was 88%, 73%, and 57%, respectively (Fig. 3.4).

Analysis of the combination of the two catheterization variables, extent of CAD and left ventricular function, yielded a continuum of risk among patients with silent ischemia. Patients with one-vessel CAD and preserved left ventricular function had a 90% probability of being free of an acute myocardial infarction or sudden death at 7 years.[12] By contrast, only 37% of Group 1 patients with three-vessel CAD and impaired left ventricular function remained free of these end-points at 7 years.

A nonrandomized comparison was performed among the 424 patients with silent ischemia who received medical therapy and the 268 patients with silent ischemia who underwent coronary artery bypass graft surgery.[13] A multivariate stepwise discriminate function analysis revealed that the most important independent predictors of survival were

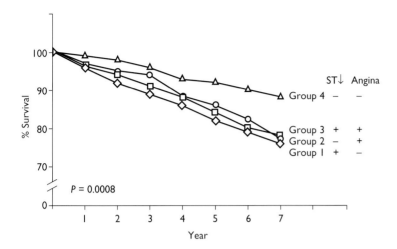

Figure 3.3 Cumulative 7-year survival curves for four groups of patients with coronary disease, three with some combination of ST-segment depression and angina and the fourth with no ST-segment depression or angina. Patients without ischemia (Group 4) had substantially better 7-year survival.

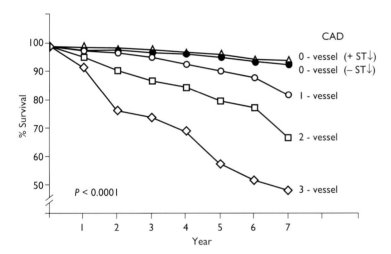

Figure 3.4 Seven-year survival rates for patients with silent ischemia based on the severity of CAD.

the severity of CAD, the left ventricular function, and coronary artery bypass graft surgery.

By stratifying the patients into subsets based upon the severity of CAD and the left ventricular function, the present author attempted to determine in which subset of patients with silent ischemia coronary artery bypass graft surgery would make the greatest impact on survival. Among patients with one- and two-vessel CAD, medical therapy resulted in 7-year survival rates of 88% and 81%, respectively. Survival rates after surgery were similar: 91%

and 84%, respectively.[13] By contrast, among patients with three-vessel CAD, the surgical group had a substantially improved survival rate compared with the medical group (85% versus 58%, respectively, $P < 0.001$). This significant difference between the medical and surgical results among patients with silent ischemia and three-vessel CAD was even more marked if the patients had impaired left ventricular function. In this subset of patients, surgery resulted in an 83% survival compared with a 37% survival for the medically treated patients.[14]

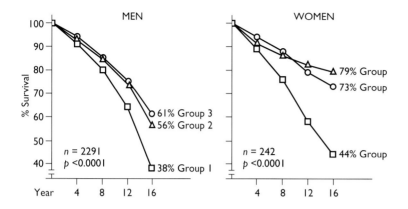

Figure 3.5 Cumulative survival for men and women based on the results of exercise testing. Group 1 (high risk): ≥ 1 mm ST depression, final stage ≤ 1; Group 2 (intermediate risk): ≥ 1 mm ST depression, final stage > 1 or no ST depression, final stage < 2; Group 3 (low risk): no ST depression, final stage ≥ 3.

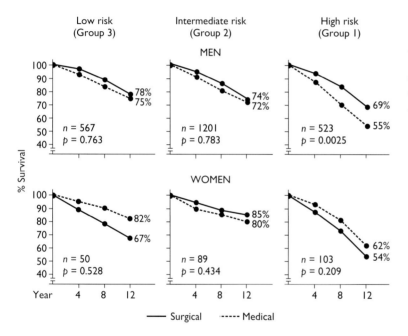

Figure 3.6 Cumulative survival rates for medically (dashed line) and surgically (solid line) treated men and women according to exercise test risk classification. Coronary artery bypass surgery was associated with improved survival in Group 1 men.

EXERCISE TESTING IN WOMEN

The long-term prognostic value of exercise testing was analyzed in 3086 men and 747 women from the CASS registry.[15] The exercise test was classified as high, intermediate, and low risk based on the degree of ST-segment depression and the final exercise stage achieved. Among men, 16-year survival varied from 74% with a low-risk exercise test to 48% with a high-risk test; similarly, among women, corresponding 16-year survival rates ranged from 91% to 58% (Fig. 3.5). Thus the exercise test was useful in assessing the long-term survival for both men and women. The men and women in the three exercise test group classifications who were treated medically were then compared with those who underwent coronary artery bypass surgery (Fig. 3.6). Among men with a high-risk exercise test classification, surgery was associated with a survival advantage at 68% when compared

Table 3.3 Exercise test parameters associated with poor prognosis and/or increased severity of coronary artery disease.

1) Duration of symptom-limiting exercise:
   a) Failure to complete Stage I of Bruce protocol or equivalent workload (i.e. < 5 METs)
2) Exercise heart rate at onset of limiting symptoms:
   a) Failure to attain HR ≥ 120/min (without medication)
3) Time of onset, magnitude, morphology, and postexercise duration of abnormal horizontal or downsloping ST-segment depression:
   a) Onset at HR < 120/min or ≤ 6.5 METs
   b) Magnitude ≥ 2.0 mm
   c) Postexercise duration ≥ 6 min
   d) Depression in multiple leads
   e) Downsloping configuration
4) Systolic BP response during or following progressive exercise:
   a) Sustained decrease of > 10 mmHg or flat BP response (≤ 130 mmHg) during progressive exercise
5) Other potentially important determinants:
   a) Exercise-induced ST-segment elevation in leads other than AVR
   b) Angina pectoris during exercise
   c) Exercise-induced ventricular tachycardia
   d) ST/HR slope ≥ 26 μV/beats/min

METs: metabolic equivalents; HR: heart rate; BP: blood pressure.

with medical therapy at 57%. The difference was especially true for men with three-vessel CAD. By contrast, among women, there was no subgroup based on exercise test results in which coronary bypass surgery was associated with increased survival. These results occurred even among women with three-vessel CAD.

SUMMARY AND CONCLUSIONS

The use of exercise testing to assess the prognosis of patients with CAD has been designated as a Class I (that is, justified) indication for exercise testing according to a joint report from the American Heart Association and the American College of Cardiology Task Force.[16]

The initial evaluation of the patient with angina should involve a comprehensive history and a careful physical examination to detect signs of congestive heart failure, since the latter finding is one of the best predictors of prognosis.[17] If the patient is severely limited by anginal symptoms despite adequate medical therapy, a coronary angiogram should be performed to determine whether coronary artery bypass graft surgery or coronary angioplasty is indicated. An exercise test might be helpful to assess the degree of ST-segment depression, to quantify the exercise limitation, and to serve as a baseline evaluation for comparison to an exercise test performed after a revascularization procedure.

For patients with milder symptoms of angina pectoris, or for those who are asymptomatic following an acute myocardial infarction, an exercise test is useful to stratify the risk of the patient for future coronary events. The use of multivariate analysis of multiple exercise test variables becomes important when using the exercise test to evaluate the prognosis of patients with known CAD.[18] Patients who demonstrate marked exercise test abnormalities (Table 3.3), such as substantial ST-segment depression at an early workload, would have a much higher mortality risk. Once identified, such patients would be candidates for cardiac catheterization procedures and would likely benefit from coronary revascularization procedures if severe coronary anatomic disease were present.[19]

Among patients in a lower-risk exercise category, characterized by a good exercise capacity and lack of ischemic ST depression, the prognosis is very good, especially if left ventricular function is normal. Medical therapy would be indicated to abolish the symptoms of angina.

Unless these patients become severely symptomatic they do not require cardiac catheterization in most situations.[20]

Finally, for the mildly symptomatic patient who has a borderline abnormal or equivocal exercise test result, risk stratification using exercise imaging studies would be indicated. If these tests demonstrated substantial abnormalities, cardiac catheterization would be indicated.

REFERENCES

1. Weiner DA, Ryan TJ, McCabe CH et al. Prognostic importance of a clinical profile and exercise test in medically treated patients with coronary artery disease. *J Am Coll Cardiol* 1984; **3**: 772–9.
2. Morrow K, Morris CK, Froelicher VF et al. Prediction of cardiovascular death in men undergoing noninvasive evaluation for coronary artery disease. *Ann Intern Med* 1993; **118**: 689–95.
3. McNeer JF, Margolis JR, Lee KL et al. The role of the exercise test in the evaluation of patients for ischemic heart disease. *Circulation* 1979; **57**: 64–70.
4. Bruce RA, DeRouen TA, Hammermeister KE. Noninvasive screening for enhanced 4-year survival after aortocoronary bypass surgery. *Circulation* 1979; **60**: 638–46.
5. Mark DB, Hlatky MA, Harrell FE Jr et al. Exercise treadmill score for predicting prognosis in coronary artery disease. *Ann Intern Med* 1987; **106**: 793–800.
6. Peduzzi P, Hultgren H, Thomsen J et al. Prognostic value of baseline exercise tests. *Prog Cardiovasc Dis* 1986; **28**: 285–92.
7. Weiner DA, Ryan TJ, McCabe CH et al. The role of exercise testing in identifying patients with improved survival after coronary artery bypass surgery. *J Am Coll Cardiol* 1986; **8**: 741–8.
8. Principal Investigators of CASS and their Associates. National Heart, Lung and Blood Institute Coronary Artery Surgery Study. *Circulation* 1981; **63** (suppl I): 1-81.
9. Bruce RA, Hornsten TR. Exercise stress testing in evaluation of patients with ischemic heart disease. *Prog Cardiovasc Dis* 1979; **11**: 371–90.
10. Hammermeister KE, DeRouen TA, Dodge HT. Variables predictive of survival in patients with coronary disease—selection by univariate and multivariate analyses from the clinical, electrocardiographic, exercise, arteriographic, and quantitative angiographic evaluation. *Circulation* 1979; **59**: 421–30.
11. Weiner DA, Ryan TJ, McCabe CH et al. Significance of silent myocardial ischemia during exercise testing in patients with coronary artery disease. *Am J Cardiol* 1987; **59**: 725–9.
12. Weiner DA, Ryan TJ, McCabe CH et al. Risk of developing an acute myocardial infarction or sudden coronary death in patients with exercise-induced silent myocardial ischemia: a report from the Coronary Artery Surgery Study (CASS) registry. *Am J Cardiol* 1988; **62**: 1155–8.
13. Weiner DA, Ryan TJ, McCabe CH et al. Comparison of coronary artery bypass surgery and medical therapy in patients with exercise-induced silent myocardial ischemia: a report from the Coronary Artery Surgery Study (CASS) registry. *J Am Coll Cardiol* 1988; **12**: 595–9.
14. Weiner DA, Ryan TJ, McCabe CH et al. The role of exercise-induced silent myocardial ischemia in patients with abnormal left ventricular function. A report from the Coronary Artery Surgery Study (CASS) registry. *Am Heart J* 1989; **118**: 649–54.
15. Weiner DA, Ryan TJ, Parsons L et al. Long-term prognostic value of exercise testing in men and women from the Coronary Artery Surgery Study (CASS) registry. *Am J Cardiol* 1995; **75**: 865–70.
16. Subcommittee on Exercise Testing. Guidelines for exercise testing. A report of the American College of Cardiology/American Heart Association Task Force of Assessment of Cardiovascular Procedures. *Circulation* 1986; **74**: 653A–67A.
17. Weiner DA. Risk stratification in angina pectoris. In: Abrams J, ed. *Angina Pectoris: Mechanisms, Diagnosis, and Therapy.* (Philadelphia, PA: WB Saunders, 1991) 39–47.
18. Chaitman BR. The changing role of the exercise electrocardiogram as a diagnostic and prognostic test for chronic ischemic heart disease. *J Am Coll Cardiol* 1986; **8**: 1195–210.
19. Kirklin JW, Akins CW, Blackstone EH et al.

ACC/AHA guidelines and indications for coronary artery bypass graft surgery. A report of the American College of Cardiology/American Heart Association task force on assessment of diagnostic and therapeutic cardiovascular proce- dures (subcommittee on coronary artery bypass graft surgery). *Circulation* 1991; **83**: 1125–41.

20. Weiner DA, Kannel WB. A comparison of surgi- cal and medical therapy for coronary artery disease. *Cardiovasc Rev Rep* 1987; **8**: 43–6.

4

Observations of silent myocardial ischemia by nuclear cardiology techniques

Dennis A Calnon and George A Beller

The field of nuclear cardiology is uniquely suited for the evaluation of silent myocardial ischemia. Nuclear studies have provided insight into the pathophysiology, prevalence, and prognostic importance of silent ischemia in a wide spectrum of clinical settings, from totally asymptomatic subjects to those with severe multivessel coronary artery disease and ischemic left ventricular dysfunction. Nearly all the measurable manifestations of myocardial ischemia (myocardial blood flow heterogeneity, regional and global systolic dysfunction, and abnormalities in myocardial metabolism) can be accurately quantitated by nuclear techniques.[1]

Because abnormalities in regional myocardial perfusion occur early in the cascade of myocardial ischemia, radionuclide perfusion studies are inherently more sensitive than other techniques in detecting silent ischemia. However, it is important to make the distinction between myocardial flow heterogeneity and myocardial ischemia. Myocardial ischemia implies an imbalance in myocardial oxygen supply and demand. Radionuclide measures of regional perfusion by single-photon perfusion scintigraphy are made relative to normally perfused reference regions. If myocardial blood flow reserve is globally impaired due to diffuse multivessel coronary artery disease, it is feasible that diffuse myocardial ischemia could occur under conditions of increased myocardial oxygen demand despite little or no regional heterogeneity in blood flow. Alternatively,

under conditions of vasodilator stress with adenosine or dipyridamole in patients with flow-limiting coronary stenoses,[2] myocardial oxygen demand increases only modestly, and myocardial blood flow heterogeneity can occur in the absence of myocardial ischemia. Similarly, at low levels of exercise in patients with coronary artery disease (CAD), regional abnormalities in radionuclide uptake may be detectable in the absence of other objective evidence of myocardial ischemia. Heller et al.[3] studied a group of patients with CAD who developed ST depression and thallium-201 (Tl-201) defects on maximal exercise. Most patients (84%) had angina as well. At low-level exercise in these same patients (to 70% of the heart rate achieved on maximal exercise), angina occurred in only 26%, ST depression in only 47%, but Tl-201 defects were seen in 89% of patients. Whether or not this symptomatically and electrocardiographically silent flow heterogeneity represented true myocardial ischemia at the tissue level, this study clearly demonstrates the greater sensitivity of perfusion imaging for detecting flow-limiting coronary stenoses and the potential to develop myocardial ischemia.

Similarly, left ventricular systolic dysfunction occurs early in the ischemic cascade. In 25 patients with treadmill-exercise-induced ST depression and documented CAD, Upton et al.[4] measured regional and global left ventricular function during upright bicycle exercise. At low-level exercise, end-systolic left ventricular volume increased in 19 patients (76%), and regional wall motion abnormalities developed in 14 patients (56%), in the absence of angina or ST-segment depression. Kayden et al.[5] demonstrated ischemic systolic dysfunction during balloon angioplasty of the left anterior coronary artery. Using an ambulatory ventricular function monitoring device (VEST), a $\geq 10\%$ reduction in left ventricular ejection fraction (LVEF) was observed in 94% of balloon inflations, while ST depression and angina occurred in only 39% and 56% of inflations, respectively. The decrease in LVEF was apparent within 15 seconds of balloon inflation, while ST depression and angina (when present) were seen 18 ± 7 seconds and 41 ± 8 seconds after inflation, respectively. However, like myocardial flow heterogeneity, stress-induced systolic dysfunction does not always imply true myocardial ischemia.[6] Global (and to a lesser extent regional) left ventricular systolic function is affected by changes in heart rate, preload, and afterload. For example, a stress-induced increase in systemic blood pressure may induce a measurable decrease (or suboptimal increase) in the left ventricular ejection fraction in the absence of myocardial ischemia. Similarly, akinetic myocardial regions in areas of prior myocardial infarction may become dyskinetic during exercise or dobutamine stress due to increases in left ventricular systolic pressure in the absence of regional myocardial ischemia.

Despite these potential limitations, myocardial perfusion imaging (and radionuclide angiography) remain the most reliable noninvasive indicators of inducible myocardial ischemia, silent or symptomatic.

PATHOPHYSIOLOGY OF SILENT MYOCARDIAL ISCHEMIA: INSIGHTS FROM NUCLEAR STUDIES

Why is myocardial ischemia totally silent in some patients, and silent in the majority of episodes in patients who also experience angina? Are there fundamental differences in the pathophysiologic mechanisms of silent and symptomatic ischemia? Is silent ischemia less severe than symptomatic ischemia and, if so, does it carry a more favorable prognosis? Nuclear cardiology techniques have provided much of the insight into these fundamental questions.

Why is silent ischemia silent?

One proposed mechanism for the absence of angina in silent myocardial ischemia is the presence of a global or regional abnormality in left ventricular sympathetic afferent innervation. Such an abnormality might occur as part of a diffuse metabolic autonomic neuropathy in diabetes mellitus, following surgical denervation during coronary artery bypass grafting (CABG) or cardiac transplantation, or following ischemic regional nerve injury by myocardial infarction (MI). Iodine-123 (I-123) metaiodobenzylguanidine (MIBG) is a norepinephrine analog which is taken up by sympathetic efferent nerve terminals, and which allows for a noninvasive and quantitative assessment of cardiac autonomic function.[7-9]

In diabetic patients with autonomic dysfunction, Langer et al.[7] demonstrated more MIBG mismatch (decreased MIBG uptake in the presence of preserved perfusion) than in diabetic patients without autonomic dysfunction ($P = 0.0001$). Abnormalities in MIBG uptake correlated with the presence of silent ischemia as well ($P = 0.001$). However, few studies have shown a significantly higher prevalence of silent ischemia among diabetic patients.

Shimonagata et al.[8] compared the uptake of MIBG and Tl-201 early and late (3 months) after MI. In those patients with silent ischemia early after MI, resting regional uptake of MIBG was reduced proportionally more than the uptake of Tl-201 during exercise as defined by quantitative defect scores ($P < 0.01$). At repeat testing 3 months later, this pattern was reversed, with relatively smaller MIBG than Tl-201 defect scores ($P < 0.05$), and correlated with the development of exertional angina in five of the seven

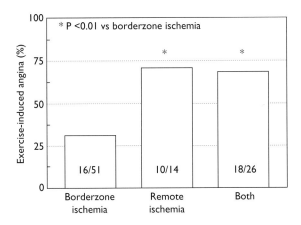

Figure 4.1 Comparison of frequency of angina during exercise testing among patients with ischemia confined to the zone of prior infarction (borderzone ischemia), ischemia remote from the zone of prior infarction (remote ischemia), and ischemia in both distributions (both). Ischemia confined to the zone of prior infarction was significantly more likely to be symptomatically silent. (Adapted from Kurata et al.[10])

previously asymptomatic patients. These results suggest that there was a reversible regional injury to the sympathetic innervation of the infarct zone, presumably reflecting residual ischemic but viable myocardium in the 'borderzone'. The results of Kurata et al.[10] support this contention. In patients with Tl-201 evidence of myocardial ischemia following myocardial infarction, angina was more likely to be present when the ischemia occurred in myocardium remote from the infarction than when it occurred in the infarction 'borderzone' (Fig. 4.1).

Ribeiro et al.[11] examined the effects of CABG surgery on myocardial ischemia as evidenced by exertional angina and perfusion defects on rubidium-82 (Rb-82) positron emission tomography (PET) imaging. While normalization of myocardial perfusion after CABG could explain the relief of angina in 10 of 15 patients, one patient had relief of angina on the basis of silent MI (in a previously viable but ischemic region),

and others had persistent evidence of ischemia (by Rb-82 PET and ambulatory ST depression) with no accompanying angina (silent ischemia). Williams et al.[12] also noted a higher incidence of ischemia (by exercise Tl-201 imaging) in patients with a history of CABG than in those without prior CABG (80% versus 33%, respectively; $P = 0.01$). Thus, there is evidence that abnormalities in cardiac innervation may play a role in silent myocardial ischemia, although these abnormalities do not explain all (or even most) of the silent myocardial ischemia observed clinically.

Pathophysiologic differences between silent and symptomatic ischemia

Myocardial ischemia (silent or symptomatic) can be caused by an increase in myocardial oxygen demand accompanied by an inadequate increase in myocardial oxygen delivery, a primary reduction in myocardial blood flow, or a combination of these mechanisms. Reductions in blood flow might be due to transient coronary vasoconstriction, platelet aggregation, and, in more extreme cases, atherosclerotic plaque rupture and thrombus formation. Deanfield et al.[13] demonstrated a reduction in regional myocardial blood flow by Rb-82 PET during mental stress in 12 of 16 patients with CAD and exercise-induced ST depression. Although most (94%) of these patients had angina during treadmill exercise, only 33% had angina during this mental-stress-induced hypoperfusion. Although the systolic blood pressure response to mental stress was similar to that during exercise, the heart rate response was significantly less (87 ± 12 versus 108 ± 10 beats/min; $P < 0.01$), implying a pathologic role for a reduction in myocardial blood flow during mental stress. Rozanski et al.[14] documented myocardial ischemia by radionuclide angiography (RNA) during mental stress, the majority of which was silent (83%). They also noted a smaller increase in heart rate during mental stress than during exercise ($P < 0.05$), although the systolic blood pressure response was comparable, and the diastolic blood pressure response was even greater with mental stress ($P < 0.05$ versus exercise). These observations, confirmed in similar studies,[15,16] suggest that the increases in blood pressure induced by mental stress (and increases in myocardial oxygen demand) may play a role in the pathophysiology of mental-stress-induced myocardial ischemia. Despite the development of new regional wall motion abnormalities (by RNA) during mental stress in 34% of patients,[16] not one patient developed ST depression. Williams et al.[12] noted that leg cycling was also less likely than treadmill exercise to produce both angina ($P = 0.008$) and ST depression ($P = 0.003$). In similarity to mental stress, leg cycling produced relatively lower peak heart rates (136 ± 18 versus 152 ± 22 beats/min; $P < 0.001$), but higher systolic blood pressure (193 ± 29 versus 183 ± 29 mmHg; $P < 0.01$) compared with treadmill exercise. Thus, it appears that the expression of angina during myocardial ischemia may be dependent on the relative increases in heart rate versus blood pressure. Alternatively, some of the observed reductions in left ventricular systolic function during mental stress and leg cycling may represent hemodynamic (nonischemic) responses to the acute elevation in blood pressure.

Global left ventricular systolic function can now be monitored in the ambulatory setting with the VEST device.[5,6,17] The VEST is a portable, nonimaging gamma detector capable of ECG-gated analysis of LVEF and relative end-diastolic and end-systolic volumes. Burg et al.[18] have used this device to identify personality traits which predicted the development of LV dysfunction during mental stress. The use of this device (together with continuous electrocardiographic and blood pressure monitoring) should provide additional insight into the silent ischemia that occurs during activities of daily living, as abnormalities in LV systolic function are more sensitive and specific indicators of myocardial ischemia than are ST-segment changes on conventional ambulatory electrocardiographic monitoring.[5]

Is silent ischemia less severe than symptomatic ischemia, and does it imply a more favorable prognosis?

Perhaps no other aspect of silent myocardial ischemia has been as extensively studied as this fundamental question, with at least 18 studies[10,12,19–34] involving nuclear cardiology techniques alone (Tables 4.1 and 4.2). Despite this wealth of clinical experience, the issue remains unsettled because the available data are conflicting. The conflicting results are understandable given the many important differences in study design.

Effects of patient selection criteria
Twelve studies reached the conclusion that the severity and prognosis of silent ischemia are similar to that of symptomatic ischemia (Table 4.1), while six studies concluded that silent ischemia is less severe and less important than symptomatic ischemia (Table 4.2).

The studies in Table 4.1 tended to require objective evidence of inducible myocardial ischemia by Tl-201 perfusion imaging, RNA, or both. In addition, in seven of these twelve studies, over 30% of patients had a history of recent or remote MI. Furthermore, patients with a history of CABG were excluded from only two of these studies.[19,20] The result of selecting a higher-risk, homogeneous group of patients with objective evidence of inducible myocardial ischemia, prior MI, and prior CABG surgery is that those patients without exercise-induced angina are likely to represent 'true silent ischemia', and to be similar in other aspects to those with symptomatic ischemia.

In contrast, the studies in Table 4.2 tended to select a more heterogeneous and lower-risk patient population. Only one of the six studies[21] required objective evidence of inducible myocardial ischemia on perfusion scintigraphy, while two required only an abnormal ECG response to exercise,[22,23] and the remaining three studies did not require any evidence of inducible myocardial ischemia on entry.[10,24,25] In addition, half of these studies excluded patients with recent MI (< 6 months), and four of the six

Table 4.1   Studies suggesting that the severity of ischemia and/or prognosis are similar in silent and symptomatic ischemia.

Author	Patients	Selection criteria	With silent ischemia (%)	Exercise variables (silent ischemia)	End-points
Gasperetti et al.[31]	103	+ Exercise TI-201[a]	57	Similar	TI-201 ischemia, coronary anatomy
Mahmarian et al.[19]	219	+ Cath[a,b]	83	Higher HR, RPP	TI-201 ischemia, coronary anatomy
Hecht et al.[30]	112	+ Exercise TI-201, + Cath[a]	75	Similar	TI-201 ischemia, coronary anatomy
Heller et al.[26]	234	+ Exercise TI-201[a]	45	Higher HR, SBP, duration	Death, MI, USAP, revasc. (> 3 months)
Breitenbücher et al.[27]	140	+ Exercise RNA[a]	60	Similar	Death, MI, unstable angina
Reisman et al.[32]	96	+ Exercise TI-201	50	Higher HR, duration	TI-201 ischemia, coronary anatomy
Bandu et al.[29]	136	+ Exercise TI-201	68	Higher HR, duration	TI-201 ischemia, coronary anatomy
Williams et al.[12]	38	+ TI-201, + RNA, + Cath[a]	71	Similar	TI-201 ischemia, exercise RNA
Assey et al.[34]	55	+ Exercise TI-201, + Cath	49	Higher RPP, duration	Death, MI, unstable angina[c]
Cohn et al.[33]	40	+ Exercise ECG[a]	40	Not reported	Exercise RNA, coronary anatomy
Bech et al.[28]	28	+ Exercise TI-201	N/A	Similar	Exercise RNA
Pancholy et al.[20]	521	+ Cath, + Exercise ECG and/or TI-201[b]	60	Higher HR, duration	TI-201 ischemia, coronary anatomy, death, MI[c]

[a]At least 30% of patients had prior MI.

[b]Patients with prior coronary artery bypass surgery were excluded.

[c]Patients who underwent revascularization early during follow-up (< 3 months) were excluded from analysis.

TI-201: thallium perfusion scintigraphy; Cath: cardiac catheterization; HR: heart rate; RPP: rate-pressure product; SBP: systolic blood pressure; MI: myocardial infarction; USAP: unstable angina pectoris; RNA: radionuclide angiography.

studies excluded patients with prior CABG surgery. Given these less stringent criteria, it is likely that many patients who were asymptomatic on exercise testing had no inducible myocardial ischemia rather than 'true silent ischemia'. These patients with no inducible ischemia (despite angiographic evidence of CAD), when analyzed together with those patients with 'true silent ischemia', would tend to bias the results in favor of showing less

Table 4.2 Studies suggesting that ischemia is less severe and/or the prognosis is better in silent versus symptomatic ischemia.

Author	Patients	Selection criteria	With silent ischemia (%)	Exercise variables (silent ischemia)	End-points
Bonow et al.[24]	131	+ Cath[a,b]	46	Not reported	Exercise RNA, coronary anatomy[c]
Travin et al.[21]	268	+ Exercise Tl-201[a]	N/A	N/A	Tl-201 ischemia, *early* CABG
Iskandrian and Hakki[25]	74	+ Cath[a,b]	58	Similar	Exercise RNA
Klein et al.[23]	117	+ Exercise ECG	75	Higher HR, RPP, duration	Tl-201 ischemia[c]
Hendler et al.[22]	152	+ Exercise ECG[a,b]	46	Higher HR, RPP, duration	Tl-201 ischemia, CABG
Kurata et al.[10]	471	Referral for Tl-201 study (only 37% had + Tl-201)	50	Higher RPP	Tl-201 ischemia, coronary anatomy

[a]Patients with prior coronary artery bypass surgery were excluded.

[b]Patients with recent (< 6 months) myocardial infarction were excluded.

[c]In subgroups with evidence of ischemia (e.g. + ECG and abnormal exercise RNA), end-points were similar in the silent and symptomatic groups.

Cath: cardiac catheterization; RNA: radionuclide angiography; Tl-201: thallium perfusion scintigraphy; CABG: coronary artery bypass grafting; HR: heart rate; RPP: rate-pressure product.

objective myocardial ischemia in asymptomatic patients and a better outcome.

The impact of patient selection is apparent in the study by Bonow et al.,[24] who examined the prognostic implications of silent myocardial ischemia as assessed by radionuclide angiography in 131 mildly symptomatic or asymptomatic patients with at least one coronary stenosis of ≥ 50% of the luminal diameter. Objective evidence of inducible myocardial ischemia was not an entry requirement. As one might expect in this low-risk and heterogeneous population, patients with angina during testing were more likely than those without angina to demonstrate ST-segment depression and a decrease in LVEF with exercise (61% versus 27%, respectively; $P < 0.001$), as well as a pattern of left main or three-vessel CAD on angiography (59% versus 25%, respectively; $P < 0.001$). However, when only those patients with objective evidence of inducible myocardial ischemia were analyzed, the presence or absence of angina was no longer predictive of the prognosis or the extent of CAD (Fig. 4.2). Thus, patient selection criteria can have an enormous impact on a study's conclusions.

Effects of end-point selection

Including the 'need for revascularization' as a study end-point tends to bias results in favor of showing more 'events' in the symptomatic group, because the decision to proceed with

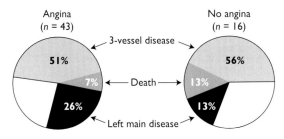

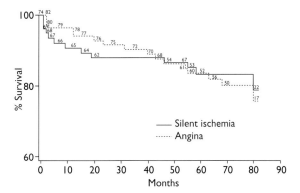

Figure 4.2 Both the anatomic extent of coronary artery disease and the death rate on medical therapy were similar in groups with and without exercise-induced angina when analysis was confined to those patients with objective evidence of inducible myocardial ischemia, defined by an exercise-induced decrease in ejection fraction and an abnormal ST-segment response. (Reproduced with permission from Bonow et al.[24])

Figure 4.3 In patients with objective evidence of inducible myocardial ischemia on thallium-201 perfusion imaging, there was no difference in survival between groups with (dashed line) and those without (solid line) exercise-induced angina, during a mean follow-up period of 5.2 years. (Reproduced with permission from Heller et al.[26])

revascularization is often driven by the presence of exercise-induced angina. To reduce this potential bias, Heller et al.[26] included angioplasty and bypass surgery as cardiac events only if they occurred more than 3 months after exercise Tl-201 testing. The cardiac event rates were very similar in the silent and symptomatic groups in this study, and the survival curves are shown in Fig. 4.3. The impact of end-point selection is also apparent in the study by Hendler et al.,[22] in which the cardiac event rates were defined as cardiac death, MI, revascularization for changing symptoms, or hospital admission for unstable angina. Despite the inclusion of the 'softer' end-points (unstable angina), events were not significantly different between the silent and symptomatic ischemia groups ($P = 0.065$) until revascularization for *any reason* was also included as an event. The difference between groups then became significant ($P = 0.021$).

Effect of post-test revascularization on prognosis

As already mentioned, the decision to perform revascularization may be driven by the presence of angina on exercise testing. Breitenbücher et al.[27] performed a retrospective 5-year follow-up study in 140 patients with unequivocal ischemia during exercise RNA, which was defined as a $\geq 10\%$ decrease in ejection fraction or a $\geq 5\%$ decrease in ejection fraction together with a distinct regional wall motion abnormality. Critical cardiac events (defined as cardiac death, MI, or unstable angina) tended to occur *more* frequently in the silent ischemia group (27%) than in the symptomatic ischemia group (16%) (Fig. 4.4), and the combined end-point of MI or death occurred significantly more frequently (22% versus 9%, respectively; $P < 0.05$) (Table 4.3). However, it is likely that the outcome of the study was influenced by the significantly higher incidence of revascularization procedures in symptomatic patients (34% versus 7% in the silent ischemia group; $P < 0.01$). Revascularization could have selectively influenced the 'natural history' of coronary disease in the symptomatic group.

Effect of exercise variables

In roughly half of the studies listed in Tables 4.1 and 4.2, the exercise duration, peak exercise

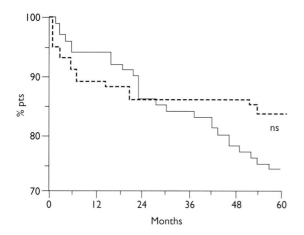

Figure 4.4 In patients with objective evidence of inducible myocardial ischemia on exercise radionuclide angiography there was no difference in survival between the 84 patients (pts) with (dashed line) and the 56 patients without (solid line) exercise-induced angina, during a mean follow-up period of 5 years. (Reproduced with permission from Breitenbücher et al.[27])

Table 4.3 Cardiac event rates in 140 patients with ischemia during exercise radionuclide angiography.

	Symptomatic group (n = 56)	Silent ischemia group (n = 84)
Critical events		
Unstable angina	5 (7%)	4 (5%)
Myocardial infarction (MI)	4 (7%)	12 (14%)
Sudden death	1 (2%)	7 (8%)
Combined death and nonfatal MI	5 (9%)	19 (22%)*
Revascularization procedures		
Coronary artery bypass grafting	19 (34%)	4 (5%)**
Coronary angioplasty	—	2 (2%)

Note: Ischemia was defined as an exercise-induced decline in ejection fraction of ≥ 10%, or a decline of ≥ 5% in the presence of a distinct regional wall motion abnormality. Follow-up averaged 52 months (range 6–69 months).

MI: myocardial infarction.

*$P < 0.05$; **$P < 0.01$ (silent ischemia versus symptomatic group).

(Adapted from Breitenbücher et al.[27])

heart rate, peak systolic blood pressure, and/or rate-pressure product (heart rate times systolic blood pressure) were noted to be significantly higher in the group with silent ischemia. This observation could be interpreted as proof that silent ischemia is less severe than symptomatic ischemia. Alternatively, it may simply imply that patients with silent ischemia lack an anginal warning system and may exercise longer than patients with symptomatic ischemia despite the presence of a similar degree of myocardial ischemia. This issue also remains unresolved.

DETECTION OF SILENT ISCHEMIA IN THE COMPLETELY ASYMPTOMATIC SUBJECT

Detection of silent myocardial ischemia in high-risk subgroups of asymptomatic persons could potentially improve long-term outcome, by justifying institution of aggressive lipid-lowering and other risk factor modifications *before*

cardiac events occur, and by selective use of elective revascularization procedures in those with particularly high-risk anatomy (for example, significant left main stenoses). Table 4.4 outlines seven studies utilizing nuclear imaging techniques for detecting the presence of silent ischemia in asymptomatic subjects.[35–41] A common theme in each of these studies is that the exercise electrocardiogram alone lacks sufficient diagnostic accuracy in this population with

Table 4.4 Detection of silent myocardial ischemia in completely asymptomatic subjects by nuclear testing.

Author	Patients	Selection criteria	Screening test	Results
Fleg et al.[40]	407	Volunteers (≥ 40 years old)	Exercise ECG Exercise planar Tl-201	Cardiac events in 48% if both tests +
Uhl et al.[36]	191	Aircrewmen with + exercise ECG	Exercise planar Tl-201	Tl-201: sens. = 95%; spec. = 91% PPV of exercise ECG = 21%
Becker et al.[38]	83	Siblings of CAD patients	Exercise SPECT Tl-201	+ Tl-201 scan in 23% of siblings, correlated with no. of CAD risk factors
Massie et al.[37]	226	Hypertensive men with ≥ 1 more CAD risk factor	Exercise ECG Ambulatory ECG Exercise (dipyridamole) Tl-201	Tl-201: sens = 90%; spec. = 79% Exercise ECG: Spec. = 14% Ambulatory ECG: Spec. = 57%
Uhl et al.[39]	32	Aircrewmen with + exercise ECG	Exercise planar Tl-201 Bicycle RNA	Tl-201: sens. = 92%; spec. = 95% RNA (global): sens. = 85%; spec. = 85% RNA (regional): sens. = 62%; spec. = 95%
Guiney et al.[35]	35	+ Exercise ECG	Exercise planar Tl-201	Tl-201: sens. = 89%; spec. = 88%; PPV = 73%; NPV = 96% Exercise ECG: PPV = 26%
Mouratidis et al.[41]	54	Familial hyper-cholesterolemia	Exercise ECG Exercise SPECT Tl-201	+ Tl-201 in 75% homozygotes, 22% heterozygotes Exercise ECG, FH of CAD, and cholesterol level were not predictive of Tl-201 ischemia

Tl-201: thallium perfusion scintigraphy; sens.: sensitivity; spec.: specificity; PPV: positive predictive value; CAD: coronary artery disease; SPECT: single-photon emission computed tomography; RNA: radionuclide angiography; NPV: negative predictive value; FH: family history.

Gated SPECT Sestamibi

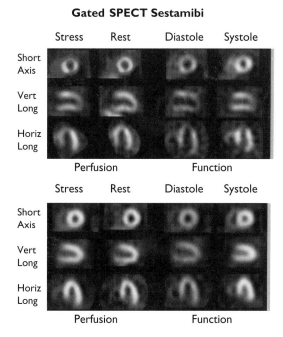

Figure 4.5 The ability of myocardial perfusion imaging to identify false-negative (upper panel) and false-positive (lower panel) ST-segment responses to exercise is demonstrated in these SPECT technetium-99m sestamibi images. In the upper panel, the finding of a reversible perfusion defect in the left anterior descending coronary distribution (with anteroseptal and anteroapical hypokinesis on ECG-gated images) was noted in the absence of ST depression. In the lower panel, normal perfusion and normal regional systolic function is seen in a patient with > 1 mm of ST depression.

a relatively low pretest probability of CAD. Diamond et al.[42] have pointed out that in subjects with only a 10% pretest likelihood of CAD, finding 1.0 mm of ST depression at peak exercise increases the likelihood of CAD to only 35%. This highlights the importance of the pretest probability of disease in determining the predictive accuracy of any test (Bayes' theorem). The rationale for using exercise radionuclide imaging to detect ischemia is based on superior sensitivity and specificity compared with the exercise ECG, and the ability to localize the

anatomic site of ischemia and to measure quantitatively both the extent and severity of ischemia. Exercise Tl-201 imaging has proven to be very useful in distinguishing true-positive from false-positive exercise ECG responses.[35-37] Figure 5 shows an example of technetium-99m sestamibi studies in patients with false-negative (upper panel) and false-positive (lower panel) ECG responses to exercise. In the upper panel, an obvious regional reduction in activity is seen in the distribution of the left anterior descending coronary artery (LAD), with nearly complete reversibility seen on resting images, implying ischemic and viable myocardium in this region. On ECG-gated images, hypokinesis is present in the LAD zone. Despite this convincing evidence of inducible ischemia, this patient had neither angina nor ST depression with exercise. In the lower panel, there is normal homogeneous tracer uptake in all myocardial segments, both at rest and during stress, with normal regional systolic thickening on gated images. This patient had >1 mm of ST depression at a high level of exercise (>12 metabolic equivalents (METs)), a normal blood pressure response to exercise, and no angina. On the basis of this normal perfusion study, this patient can be spared the risks of coronary angiography.

Becker et al.[38] performed exercise single-photon emission computed tomography imaging in asymptomatic siblings of patients with CAD. Interestingly, although 23% of siblings demonstrated an abnormal SPECT Tl-201, only 4% had angina on the treadmill. As expected, the frequency of an abnormal scan increased with age (in men) and increased in relation to the number of coronary risk factors (as shown in Fig. 4.6). Uhl et al.[39] compared the accuracy of exercise planar Tl-201 perfusion imaging with bicycle radionuclide angiography in a group of aircrewmen with abnormal exercise ECG responses. While both nuclear techniques were far superior to the exercise ECG alone, Tl-201 perfusion imaging was more sensitive (92%) than either global (85%) or regional (62%) systolic dysfunction by radionuclide angiography, with comparable specificity.

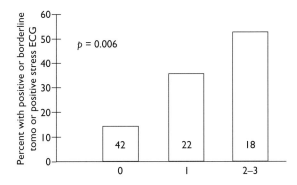

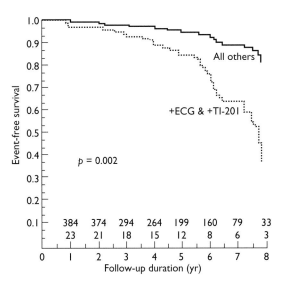

Figure 4.6 Prevalence of abnormal exercise SPECT thallium-201 studies in asymptomatic siblings of patients with coronary artery disease relates to the number of coronary risk factors present. Numbers in bars represent the number of participants in each category. (Reproduced with permission from Becker et al.[38])

Figure 4.7 Plot of event-free survival in asymptomatic subjects with concordant positive ECG and thallium-201 results versus all other patient subgroups. A concordant positive result predicted a 3.6-fold risk for a coronary event, independent of conventional risk factors. Numbers along the x axis indicate the number of persons at risk for each year in the all-others (top) and the concordant positive ECG and thallium (bottom) groups, respectively. (Reproduced with permission from Fleg et al.[40])

These findings are consistent with the ischemic cascade theory in which flow heterogeneity occurs earlier than systolic dysfunction.

As part of the Baltimore Longitudinal Study on Aging, Fleg et al.[40] defined the prevalence of exercise-induced silent ischemia in 407 asymptomatic volunteers. When myocardial ischemia was defined as a concordant presence of ST depression and a Tl-201 perfusion defect, the prevalence increased sevenfold with age, from 2% in the fifth and sixth decades to 15% in the ninth decade ($P < 0.01$). A plot of event-free survival is shown in Fig. 4.7. Those asymptomatic subjects with both ST depression and a Tl-201 perfusion defect were significantly more likely to have a cardiac event, with a cumulative event rate of 48%. It should be pointed out that of the 20 patients who died ($n = 7$) or experienced a nonfatal MI ($n = 13$) during follow-up, 65% had a normal Tl-201 scan on initial screening. In addition, the cardiac events in this study included the relatively 'soft' endpoint of angina, which accounted for half of the cardiac events.

Figure 4.8 provides a rational approach to screening for silent myocardial ischemia in asymptomatic subjects. Identification of clinically high-risk subgroups is the first (and perhaps the most important) step. Appropriate subgroups might include those with a strong family history of early CAD, familial hypercholesterolemia (even with no family history of early CAD), multiple CAD risk factors, or subjects with occupations in which an acute complication of CAD might pose an immediate risk to the safety of others (airline pilots, for example). The exercise ECG may be appropriate as the initial screening test in subjects with a normal baseline ECG (despite the limitations described above). Those subjects with a normal blood pressure and ECG response to very high-level exercise can avoid the need for further testing, and those with an abnormal blood pressure and ECG response to low-level

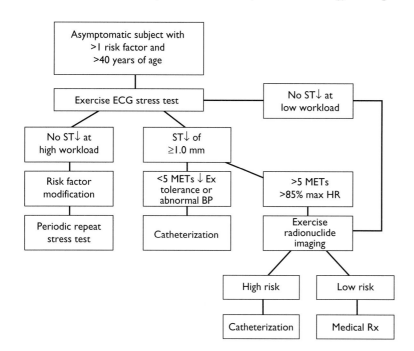

Figure 4.8 Approach to screening for silent coronary artery disease in asymptomatic subjects. ST ↓: ST depression; Ex: exercise; Abn'l BP: abnormal blood pressure response; HR: heart rate. (Reproduced with permission from Beller GA. Role of nuclear cardiology in evaluating the total ischemic burden in coronary artery disease. *Am J Cardiol* 1987; **59**: 31C–38C.)

exercise (< 5 METs) could probably be assumed to have significant CAD and forgo confirmatory radionuclide imaging. If the exercise level is limited or the ECG response is abnormal at a high exercise level with a normal blood pressure response, then radionuclide perfusion imaging is recommended. Of course, not all subjects with evidence of CAD on perfusion scintigraphy require coronary angiography. Subjects with evidence of ischemia involving a single coronary artery distribution (excluding the proximal LAD artery) and reasonable exercise tolerance are at relatively low risk, and aggressive risk factor modification might be more appropriate in the absence of symptoms.

SILENT ISCHEMIA IN SYMPTOMATIC PATIENTS WITH KNOWN CORONARY ARTERY DISEASE

In this population, myocardial perfusion imaging has been clearly demonstrated to add important incremental information to the routine exercise ECG. Perfusion imaging with

Tl-201 (a) is more sensitive and specific for myocardial ischemia, (b) can define the anatomic site, extent, and severity of ischemia, (c) detects ischemia even in the presence of baseline ECG abnormalities, and (d) has relatively preserved sensitivity even at relatively lower levels of exercise.[3,43] In contrast, the magnitude of ST depression on symptom-limited exercise testing does not correlate with the extent of myocardial ischemia as assessed by quantitative Tl-201 scintigraphy.[44]

There have been several approaches to the assessment of patients with stable coronary artery disease. Jiang et al.[45] found that mental-stress-induced myocardial ischemia (by radionuclide ventriculography) in patients with documented CAD was associated with significantly higher rates of subsequent cardiac events (*P* < 0.05). Exercise and ambulatory ECG were not significant predictors of cardiac events in this study. Younis et al.[2] demonstrated the prognostic importance of silent myocardial ischemia as detected by dipyridamole Tl-201 imaging in asymptomatic patients with CAD

Table 4.5 Dipyridamole thallium imaging predicts cardiac events in asymptomatic patients with coronary artery disease.

Thallium pattern	No. (%)	Free from any cardiac event at 24 months (%)	Free from death or MI at 24 months (%)
Normal	36 (34)	93 ± 5	100
Fixed defect	24 (22)	67 ± 13	93 ± 7
Reversible defect	27 (25)	21 ± 10*	65 ± 15*
Combined defects	20 (19)	44 ± 11*	58 ± 12*

Note: Cardiac events include cardiac death, nonfatal myocardial infarction (MI), unstable angina pectoris, occurrence of functional class III or IV angina, or the need for revascularization. Events reported as mean ± standard error.
*$P < 0.001$.
(Adapted from Younis et al.[2])

(Table 4.5). In this study, the finding of Tl-201 redistribution (by stepwise logistic regression analysis) was the only significant predictor of a cardiac event. Thus, myocardial perfusion imaging is a powerful tool in the assessment of prognosis in patients with known CAD, and is superior to exercise or ambulatory ECG in this regard.

SILENT ISCHEMIA IN ACUTE CORONARY SYNDROMES

Unstable angina

In the clinical setting of unstable angina, Nagy et al.[46] reported the finding of asymptomatic hypoperfusion at rest (by Rb-82 PET imaging) accompanied by ST depression, which normalized after administration of sublingual nitroglycerin. Samman et al.[47] reported similar asymptomatic transient resting hypoperfusion using technetium-99m sestamibi imaging. These observations support the contention that the pathophysiology of unstable angina involves transient regional hypoperfusion (presumably due to atherosclerotic plaque rupture and thrombus formation), and that at least some of these episodes occur without symptoms.

Several approaches have been proposed for risk stratification in patients with unstable angina. Marmur et al.[48] compared 24-hour Holter ST-segment monitoring, quantitative exercise Tl-201 tomography, and cardiac catheterization in patients with medically stabilized unstable angina. The exercise Tl-201 studies were performed 5 ± 2 days after admission, and at least 24 hours after the last episode of anginal pain. Patients with a favorable outcome at 6 months were distinguished from those with an unfavorable outcome by a higher maximum rate-pressure product, a smaller redistribution Tl-201 defect size (expressed as a percentage of the total myocardium), and a smaller number of vessels with at least 50% stenoses. Figure 4.9 shows the relationship between Tl-201 redistribution defect size and outcome. By multiple logistic regression analysis, a history of previous MI was the most powerful predictor of outcome, while in patients without MI, Tl-201 redistribution defect size was the only predictor. In contrast, no significant difference between favorable and unfavorable outcome groups was detected by duration of ST-segment shift on Holter monitoring, exercise duration on the Bruce protocol, exercise-induced ST depression, or contrast left ventriculography.

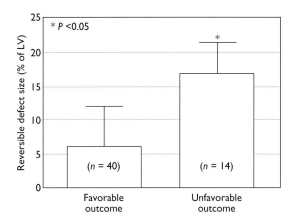

Figure 4.9 In patients with medically stabilized unstable angina, the reversible defect size on exercise thallium-201 tomography (expressed as a percentage of the total myocardium) correlated with the clinical outcome at 6 months. (Adapted from Marmur JD et al.[48] (The American College of Physicians is not responsible for the accuracy of the translation))

These results suggest that exercise Tl-201 imaging can be used to risk-stratify patients with medically stabilized unstable angina, and that Tl-201 imaging is superior to ambulatory ECG monitoring for this purpose. As medical treatments for unstable angina continue to improve, most patients can now be stabilized. In these patients, it is reasonable to withhold early invasive evaluation, and to pursue angiography only in those patients with high-risk findings on radionuclide exercise testing. Patients whose symptoms are refractory to aggressive medical management should promptly undergo coronary angiography.

Myocardial infarction

Silent ischemia is frequently observed following MI, particularly if the ischemia is localized to the infarct borderzone,[11] where ischemic injury to the sympathetic nerves may play an important pathophysiologic role. In the study by Gasperetti et al.[31] (Table 4.1), the patients with silent ischemia had a significantly higher prevalence of recent MI (within 10 days of testing)

than the group with symptomatic ischemia (31% versus 7%; $P < 0.01$). Kayden et al.[49] noted frequent episodes of silent LV dysfunction using the VEST device in 12 of 33 patients following thrombolytic therapy for MI. At follow-up over 21 ± 3 months, those patients with transient silent LV dysfunction (defined as a 5% decrease in ejection fraction lasting ≥ 1 minute) had significantly more cardiac events (death, recurrent MI, unstable angina) than those patients without transient left ventricular dysfunction ($P < 0.01$). The systolic function response to submaximal supine bicycle exercise was not a useful predictor of events in this study, although Corbett et al.[50] found that exercise LV function by RNA was predictive of subsequent cardiac events during 6 months of follow-up.

Nevertheless, exercise or pharmacologic stress myocardial perfusion imaging is the predominant method of detecting silent myocardial ischemia after infarction.[51] The superiority of Tl-201 perfusion imaging over exercise ST-segment monitoring alone was demonstrated by Gibson et al.[52] The results of this study are summarized in Table 4.6. The presence or absence of Tl-201 redistribution predicted cardiac events in all subgroups of patients, including those with no exercise-induced angina or ST depression, those with painless ST depression, and those with angina. The rate of death or recurrent infarction for patients with exercise-induced angina and Tl-201 redistribution was 24%, a rate identical to that for patients with Tl-201 redistribution and no angina or ST depression. Thus, the absence of angina and ST depression cannot reliably exclude the presence of residual myocardial ischemia and an increased risk for subsequent cardiac events. Tl-201 scintigraphy is both more sensitive and more specific for identifying these high-risk postinfarction patients than is exercise ECG alone.

The present authors recommend performing exercise myocardial perfusion imaging as the risk stratification procedure of choice following uncomplicated MI. In those patients who are unable to exercise, pharmacologic stress can be substituted for exercise. Patients with evidence

Table 4.6   Cardiac events in 190 patients following myocardial infarction (MI) based on predischarge exercise Tl-201 results.

Event	No ST depression or angina		Painless ST depression		Angina ± ST depression	
	No Rd (%)	RD (%)	No Rd (%)	Rd (%)	No Rd (%)	Rd (%)
Death (n = 15)	0	10*	4	15	10	14
MI (n = 17)	2	18**	4	5	0	14
Death or MI (n = 30)	2	24**	9	20	10	24
Death, MI, or USAP (n = 69)	16	43**	22	55*	20	57***

Rd: thallium redistribution by quantitative criteria; USAP: unstable angina pectoris.
*P< 0.05; **P< 0.01; ***P ≤ 0.09 compared with no thallium redistribution.
(Adapted from Gibson et al.[52])

of residual ischemia within the infarct zone, or ischemia in other coronary artery territories should be referred for coronary angiography and revascularization.

SILENT ISCHEMIA FOLLOWING CORONARY REVASCULARIZATION PROCEDURES

After successful balloon angioplasty, restenosis occurs in approximately one-third of patients, typically within the following 6 months. Stuckey et al.[53] studied the predictive value of quantitative exercise Tl-201 scintigraphy early (2.2 ± 1.2 weeks) after angioplasty in 68 asymptomatic patients. Although the occurrence of recurrent angina was more likely when Tl-201 redistribution was present (specificity = 91%), the sensitivity of Tl-201 redistribution was only 39%, perhaps because many of the restenosis events occurred later than 2 weeks after the procedure. In addition, the ability to predict the recurrence of angina (as opposed to harder endpoints) is of only questionable clinical value.

Silent ischemia is even more frequently noted after coronary bypass surgery,[11,12] and it is likely that surgical disruption of innervation plays a pathophysiologic role.

Routine follow-up exercise myocardial perfusion imaging is probably not necessary in all patients who are asymptomatic following angioplasty or bypass surgery. However, in subgroups with severe but predominantly silent myocardial ischemia prior to revascularization, periodic perfusion imaging may be considered.

SILENT ISCHEMIA IN ISCHEMIC CARDIOMYOPATHY

The clinical syndrome of chronic LV systolic dysfunction due to chronic CAD is termed ischemic cardiomyopathy, and it represents an often-overlooked example of severe silent ischemia. Although an in-depth discussion of this rapidly evolving field of clinical and basic research is beyond the scope of this chapter, suffice it to say that the syndrome of ischemic cardiomyopathy easily meets the criteria for silent ischemia. It is common for patients with this syndrome to present with exertional heart failure symptoms, and often there are no symptoms whatsoever at rest. Resting regional myocardial ischemia can be demonstrated either by rest-redistribution thallium-201 imaging or by quantitation of blood flow using N-13 ammonia or O-15 water PET. Preserved glucose utilization (by 18-F-fluorodeoxyglucose PET) in areas of hypoperfusion implies that viable myocardium exists, and the improvement in systolic function after revascularization confirms that the reversible dysfunction was ischemic in etiology. Whether the mechanism of chronic/reversible ischemic dysfunction is that of myocardial hibernation (an adaptive decrease in systolic function in the setting of reduced resting blood flow) or repetitive myocardial stunning (with normalization of myocardial blood flow between ischemic insults), either of these mechanisms implies the presence of silent myocardial ischemia.

SUMMARY AND CONCLUSIONS

Silent myocardial ischemia is quite prevalent among patients presenting with a variety of acute and chronic coronary syndromes. Silent ischemia is detected with greater sensitivity and specificity with stress radionuclide imaging than by exercise ECG testing alone—in totally asymptomatic subjects, in patients with known coronary artery disease and stable angina, in patients with acute coronary syndromes (unstable angina and MI), in patients who have undergone coronary revascularization procedures, and in patients with chronic ischemic LV dysfunction (ischemic cardiomyopathy). In patients unable to exercise, pharmacologic stress imaging adds important prognostic information as well.

Although data are conflicting, the severity of silent ischemia and the prognostic importance are probably similar to that of symptomatic ischemia, especially in those patients with objective evidence of inducible myocardial ischemia.

Nuclear cardiology techniques are uniquely capable of detecting, localizing, and quantitating the extent and severity of silent myocardial ischemia. Thus, nuclear techniques will continue to play a leading role in the evaluation of silent myocardial ischemia in the future.

REFERENCES

1. Beller GA. *Clinical Nuclear Cardiology* (Philadelphia, PA: WB Saunders, 1995).
2. Younis LT, Byers S, Shaw L, Barth G, Goodgold H, Chaitman BR. Prognostic importance of silent myocardial ischemia detected by intravenous dipyridamole thallium myocardial imaging in asymptomatic patients with coronary artery disease. *J Am Coll Cardiol* 1989; **14**: 1635–41.
3. Heller GV, Ahmed I, Tilkemeier PL, Barbour MM, Garber CE. Comparison of chest pain, electrocardiographic changes and thallium-201 scintigraphy during varying exercise intensities in men with stable angina pectoris. *Am J Cardiol* 1991; **68**: 569–74.
4. Upton MT, Rerych SK, Newman GE, Port S, Cobb FR, Jones RH. Detecting abnormalities in left ventricular function during exercise before angina and ST-segment depression. *Circulation* 1980; **62**: 341–9.
5. Kayden DS, Remetz MS, Cabin HS et al. Validation of continuous radionuclide left ventricular functioning monitoring in detecting silent myocardial ischemia during balloon angioplasty of the left anterior descending coronary artery. *Am J Cardiol* 1991; **67**: 1339–43.
6. Imbriaco M, Cuocolo A, Pace L et al. Ambulatory monitoring of left ventricular function during cardiopulmonary exercise tests in normal sedentary subjects. *J Nucl Med* 1995; **36**: 564–8.
7. Langer A, Freeman MR, Josse RG, Armstrong PW. Metaiodobenzylguanidine imaging in diabetes mellitus: assessment of cardiac sympathetic denervation and its relation to autonomic dysfunction and silent myocardial ischemia. *J Am Coll Cardiol* 1995; **25**: 610–18.
8. Shimonagata T, Ishida Y, Hayashida K, Takamiya M, Uehara T, Nishimura T. Scintigraphic assessment of silent myocardial ischaemia after early infarction using myocardial SPET imaging with ^{201}Tl and ^{123}I-MIBG. *Nucl Med Commun* 1995; **16**: 893–900.

9. Shakespeare CF, Page CJ, O'Doherty MJ et al. Regional sympathetic innervation of the heart by means of metaiodobenzylguanidine imaging in silent ischemia. *Am Heart J* 1993; **125**: 1614–22.

10. Kurata C, Sakata K, Taguchi T, Kobayashi A, Yamazaki N. Exercise-induced silent myocardial ischemia: evaluation by thallium-201 emission computed tomography. *Am Heart J* 1990; **119**: 557–67.

11. Ribeiro P, Shea M, Deanfield JE et al. Different mechanisms for the relief of angina after coronary bypass surgery: physiological versus anatomical assessment. *Br Heart J* 1984; **52**: 502–9.

12. Williams KA, Taillon LA, Carter JE. Asymptomatic and electrically silent myocardial ischemia during upright leg cycle ergometry and treadmill exercise (clandestine myocardial ischemia). *Am J Cardiol* 1993; **72**: 1114–20.

13. Deanfield JE, Shea M, Kensett M et al. Silent myocardial ischaemia due to mental stress. *Lancet* 1984; **2**: 1001–5.

14. Rozanski A, Bairey CN, Krantz DS et al. Mental stress and the induction of silent myocardial ischemia in patients with coronary artery disease. *N Engl J Med* 1988; **318**: 1005–12.

15. Bairey CN, Krantz DS, Rozanski A. Mental stress as an acute trigger of ischemic left ventricular dysfunction and blood pressure elevation in coronary artery disease. *Am J Cardiol* 1990; **66**: 28G–31G.

16. Blumenthal JA, Jiang W, Waugh RA et al. Mental stress-induced ischemia in the laboratory and ambulatory ischemia during daily life: association and hemodynamic features. *Circulation* 1995; **92**: 2102–8.

17. Zaret BL, Kayden DS. Ambulatory monitoring of left ventricular function: a new modality for assessing silent myocardial ischemia. *Adv Cardiol* 1990; **37**: 105–16.

18. Burg MM, Jain D, Soufer R, Kerns RD, Zaret BL. Role of behavioral and psychological factors in mental stress-induced silent left ventricular dysfunction in coronary artery disease. *J Am Coll Cardiol* 1993; **22**: 440–8.

19. Mahmarian JJ, Pratt CM, Cocanougher MK, Verani MS. Altered myocardial perfusion in patients with angina pectoris or silent ischemia during exercise as assessed by quantitative thallium-201 single-photon emission computed tomography. *Circulation* 1990; **82**: 1305–15.

20. Pancholy SB, Schalet B, Kuhlmeier V, Cave V, Heo J, Iskandrian AS. Prognostic significance of silent ischemia. *J Nucl Cardiol* 1994; **1**: 434–40.

21. Travin MI, Flores AR, Boucher CA, Newell JB, LaRaia PJ. Silent versus symptomatic ischemia during a thallium-201 exercise test. *Am J Cardiol* 1991; **68**: 1600–8.

22. Hendler AL, Greyson ND, Robinson MG, Freeman MR. Patients with symptomatic ischemia have larger thallium perfusion abnormalities and more adverse prognosis than patients with silent ischemia. *Can J Cardiol* 1992; **8**: 814–18.

23. Klein J, Chao SY, Berman DS, Rozanski A. Is 'silent' myocardial ischemia really as severe as symptomatic ischemia? The analytical effect of patient selection biases. *Circulation* 1994; **89**: 1958–66.

24. Bonow RO, Bacharach SL, Green MV, LaFreniere RL, Epstein SE. Prognostic implications of symptomatic versus asymptomatic (silent) myocardial ischemia induced by exercise in mildly symptomatic and in asymptomatic patients with angiographically documented coronary artery disease. *Am J Cardiol* 1987; **60**: 778–83.

25. Iskandrian AS, Hakki AH. Left ventricular function in patients with coronary heart disease in the presence or absence of angina pectoris during exercise radionuclide ventriculography. *Am J Cardiol* 1984; **53**: 1239–43.

26. Heller LI, Tresgallo M, Sciacca RR, Blood DK, Seldin DW, Johnson LL. Prognostic significance of silent myocardial ischemia on a thallium stress test. *Am J Cardiol* 1990; **65**: 718–21.

27. Breitenbücher A, Pfisterer M, Hoffmann A, Burckhardt D. Long-term follow-up of patients with silent ischemia during exercise radionuclide angiography. *J Am Coll Cardiol* 1990; **15**: 999–1003.

28. Bech J, Pedersen FH, Madsen BK, Jacobsen I, Madsen JK. Changes in left ventricular ejection fraction during transient myocardial ischemia in patients with angina pectoris and silent ischaemia. *Dan Med Bull* 1994; **41**: 231–3.

29. Bandu I, Friedman HS, Raggi P et al. Symptoms of patients with silent ischemia as detected by thallium stress testing. *Chest* 1994; **105**: 1009–12.

30. Hecht HS, Shaw RE, Bruce T, Myler RK. Silent ischemia: evaluation by exercise and redistribution tomographic thallium-201 myocardial imaging. *J Am Coll Cardiol* 1989; **14**: 895–900.

31. Gasperetti CM, Burwell LR, Beller GA. Prevalence of and variables associated with silent

myocardial ischemia on exercise thallium-201 stress testing. *J Am Coll Cardiol* 1990; **16**: 115–23.

32. Reisman S, Berman DS, Maddahi J, Swan HJC. Silent myocardial ischemia during treadmill exercise: thallium scintigraphic and angiographic correlates. *J Am Coll Cardiol* 1985; **5**: 406 (abst).

33. Cohn PF, Brown EJ, Wynne J, Holman BL, Atkins HL. Global and regional left ventricular ejection fraction abnormalities during exercise in patients with silent myocardial ischemia. *J Am Coll Cardiol* 1983; **1**: 931–3.

34. Assey ME, Walters GL, Hendrix GH, Carabello BA, Usher BW, Spann JF. Incidence of acute myocardial infarction in patients with exercise-induced silent myocardial ischemia. *Am J Cardiol* 1987; **59**: 497–500.

35. Guiney TE, Pohost GM, McKusick KA, Beller GA. Differentiation of false- from true-positive ECG responses to exercise stress by thallium 201 perfusion imaging. *Chest* 1981; **80**: 4–10.

36. Uhl GS, Kay TN, Hickman JR. Computer-enhanced thallium scintigrams in asymptomatic men with abnormal exercise tests. *Am J Cardiol* 1981; **48**: 1037–43.

37. Massie BM, Szlachcic Y, Tubau JF, O'Kelly BF, Ammon S, Chin W. Scintigraphic and electro-cardiographic evidence of silent coronary artery disease in asymptomatic hypertension: a case–control study. *J Am Coll Cardiol* 1993; **22**: 1598–606.

38. Becker LC, Becker DM, Pearson TA, Fintel DJ, Links J, Frank TL. Screening of asymptomatic siblings of patients with premature coronary artery disease. *Circulation* 1987; **75** (suppl II): 14–17.

39. Uhl GS, Kay TN, Hickman JR. Comparison of exercise radionuclide angiography and thallium perfusion imaging in detecting coronary artery disease in asymptomatic men. *J Cardiac Rehabil* 1982; **2**: 118–24.

40. Fleg JL, Gerstenblith G, Zonderman AB et al. Prevalence and prognostic significance of exercise-induced silent myocardial ischemia detected by thallium scintigraphy and electro-cardiography in asymptomatic volunteers. *Circulation* 1990; **81**: 428–36.

41. Mouratidis B, Vaughan-Neil EF, Gilday DL et al. Detection of silent coronary artery disease in adolescents and young adults with familial hypercholesterolemia by single-photon emission computed tomography thallium-201 scanning. *Am J Cardiol* 1992; **70**: 1109–12.

42. Diamond GA, Staniloff HM, Forrester JS, Pollock BH, Swan HJC. Computer-assisted diagnosis in the noninvasive evaluation of patients with suspected coronary artery disease. *J Am Coll Cardiol* 1983; **1**: 444–55.

43. Esquivel L, Pollock SG, Beller GA, Gibson RS, Watson DD, Kaul S. Effect of the degree of effort on the sensitivity of the exercise thallium-201 stress test in symptomatic coronary artery disease. *Am J Cardiol* 1989; **63**: 160–5.

44. Taylor AJ, Sackett MC, Beller GA. The degree of ST-segment depression on symptom-limited exercise testing: relation to the myocardial ischemic burden as determined by thallium-201 scintigraphy. *Am J Cardiol* 1995; **75**: 228–31.

45. Jiang W, Babyak M, Krantz DS et al. Mental stress-induced myocardial ischemia and cardiac events. *JAMA* 1996; **275**: 1651–6.

46. Nagy B, Grella R, Garza D, Van Tosh A, Horowitz SF. Silent myocardial ischemia during PET. *J Nucl Med* 1995; **36**: 1034–6.

47. Samman B, Hahn SD, Messinger DE, Heller GV. Spontaneous silent myocardial ischemia assessed by technetium-99m-sestamibi imaging. *J Nucl Med* 1993; **34**: 134–6.

48. Marmur JD, Freeman MR, Langer A, Armstrong PW. Prognosis in medically stabilized unstable angina: early Holter ST-segment monitoring compared with predischarge exercise thallium tomography. *Ann Intern Med* 1990; **113**: 575–9.

49. Kayden DS, Wackers FJT, Zaret BL. Silent left ventricular dysfunction during routine activity after thrombolytic therapy for acute myocardial infarction. *J Am Coll Cardiol* 1990; **15**:1500–7.

50. Corbett JR, Dehmer GJ, Lewis SE et al. The prognostic value of submaximal exercise testing with radionuclide ventriculography before hospital discharge in patients with recent myocardial infarction. *Circulation* 1981; **64**: 535–44.

51. Gibson RS, Watson DD, Craddock GB et al. Prediction of cardiac events after uncomplicated myocardial infarction: a prospective study comparing predischarge exercise thallium-201 scintigraphy and coronary angiography. *Circulation* 1983; **68**: 321–36.

52. Gibson RS, Beller GA, Kaiser DL. Prevalence and clinical significance of painless ST segment depression during early postinfarction exercise testing. *Circulation* 1987; **75**: (suppl II): 36–9.

53. Stuckey TD, Burwell LR, Nygaard TW, Gibson RS, Watson DD, Beller GA. Quantitative exercise thallium-201 scintigraphy for predicting angina recurrence after percutaneous transluminal coronary angioplasty. *Am J Cardiol* 1989; **63**: 517–21.

5

Unrecognized myocardial infarction

William B Kannel

Coronary heart disease often progresses with little warning from an inapparent or asymptomatic state to abrupt lethal outcome. One in six coronary attacks presents with sudden death as the first, last, and only symptom.[1] Only one in five myocardial infarctions is preceded by angina pectoris of any duration. Half of all coronary fatalities are sudden deaths and half of these occur in persons without known coronary disease.

Although these attacks seem to occur unforeseen, they are more often than not heralded by an ominous coronary risk profile and signs of presymptomatic ischemic myocardial involvement. There is actually a large reservoir of advanced silent coronary disease in the general population from which most of these apparently unheralded coronary attacks evolve. Some 2–30% of the asymptomatic general population are reported to have a compromised coronary circulation that can be detected by an exercise electrocardiogram (ECG) or ambulatory monitoring.[2,3] Also, 20% of persons surviving a myocardial infarction without residual symptoms have a positive ischemic exercise ECG test indicating the existence of residual myocardial ischemia. Even in persons with angina, ambulatory monitoring indicates that three of four transient ischemic episodes during the day occur in the absence of pain[4,5] and the more these asymptomatic episodes are present the worse the prognosis.[6,7]

There is at present no accepted classification of this silent phase of coronary disease. A number of varieties may be considered including: the adverse coronary risk profile suggesting accelerated atherogenesis; angiographically demonstrated asymptomatic severe coronary artery disease; a positive exercise test; and the asymptomatic post-MI (myocardial infarction) state. Silent coronary disease may also be manifested by common ECG abnormalities such as left ventricular hypertrophy, intraventricular conduction disturbances and nonspecific repolarization abnormality. More specifically, it may be indicated by development of ECG features of MI on a routine ECG. A substantial proportion of actual myocardial infarctions are silent, or so atypical that they go unrecognized.[8] These silent or unrecognized myocardial infarctions constitute a substantial part of potentially lethal, inapparent coronary disease.

INCIDENCE

The incidence of MI increases sharply with advancing age, with a marked male predominance. Women lag men in incidence by about 20 years, but the gap in incidence closes with advancing age. Myocardial infarction incidence reaches substantial proportions beyond age 45 years in men and age 55 years in women. In men, the annual MI rate under age 65 years (6 per 1000) more than doubled to 13 per 1000 after that age (Fig. 5.1). Of the MIs that occurred in the Framingham Study over 36 years of follow-up, 36% were discovered only because of the appearance of diagnostic evidence on routine ECGs obtained every two years (Table

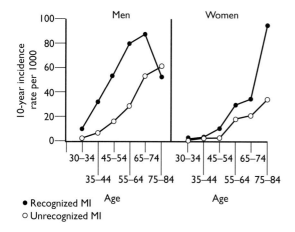

- ● Recognized MI
- ○ Unrecognized MI

Figure 5.1 Incidence of recognized and unrecognized myocardial infarction by age and sex. Framingham Study, 30-year follow-up.

5.1). The proportion of MIs that went unrecognized was greater in women than men, particularly under age 65 years, when almost half of all MIs in women were undetected prior to routine biennial ECG examination. The fraction of MIs unrecognized tended to increase with age in men, whereas in women the proportion undetected tended to decline (Table 5.1).

There is a likelihood that the incidence of unrecognized MIs is underestimated in these population-based data because it has been noted that 10% of anterior and 25% of inferior MIs detected on ECG examination revert to a nondiagnostic ECG pattern within two years of the onset of the MI. Also, some unrecognized MIs may result in a sudden death before they can be discovered.

About half of the unrecognized MIs in men are completely silent, whereas only one-third are in women.[9,10] The rest are atypical, so that neither the patient nor attending physician even considers the possibility. Some of these are attributed to gallstones, hiatus hernia, cervical arthritis, or peptic ulcer.[9,11] The ECG location of the MI is no different in unrecognized than in symptomatic MI, suggesting that an unusual pain referral pattern is an unlikely explanation for the atypical symptoms.

Long-term angina pectoris precedes MI about 20% of the time. However, when the MI is silent or unrecognized only 5% are preceded by long-term angina. Likewise, following MI, only about 14% of patients with unrecognized MIs experience angina whereas 23% of men and 17% of women with recognized MIs do so (Table 5.2). This suggests that persons prone to silent or unrecognized MIs manifest ischemia without experiencing pain. However, this has never been adequately tested. The Framingham Study examined the occurrence of silent ischemia on ambulatory ECG monitoring

Table 5.1 Percentage of myocardial infarctions that are unrecognized. Framingham Study, 36-year follow-up.

Age	Men	Women	Total
35–64	27	48	33
65–94	42	37	40
Total	33	38	36

Table 5.2 Risk of angina pectoris according to type of myocardial infarction. Framingham Study, 30-year follow-up.

Type of myocardial infarction (MI)	10-year incidence (%)	
	Men	Women
Unrecognized MI	14.2	13.9
Recognized MI	23.4	16.8
Risk ratio (unrecog./recog.)	0.5	0.7

following unrecognized MI compared with controls matched by age, sex and the major cardiovascular risk factors. Twice as many patients with unrecognized MI as controls (15.4% versus 7.7%) had ambulatory ECG evidence of silent ischemia, but the sample size was too small for any confidence in the estimate.[12]

It is likely, however, that unrecognized MI is only one manifestation of a broader, more extensive syndrome of silent myocardial ischemia which occurs both in persons with and without overt coronary heart disease.

UNEXPLAINED GRADUAL-ONSET Q-WAVES

Abnormal Q-waves usually indicate previous MI but similar changes can be due to positional variants, impaired ventricular conduction, ventricular hypertrophy and noncoronary heart disease.[13] ECG tracings suspected of representing MI were encountered in the Framingham Study which, upon comparison with routinely obtained prior ECGs, failed to reveal an abrupt change, but rather a gradual evolution of increasingly prominent Q-waves.[14] These have been compared with unrecognized MIs in which the Q-waves appeared abruptly between a biennial examination.

Compared with persons with abruptly appearing unrecognized MIs, those with gradual-onset Q-waves had only 40% of the risk of a true unrecognized MI for coronary death or MI, and a trend toward a lower risk of overall mortality. When compared with normal subjects, adjusting for age and risk factors, those with gradual-onset Q-waves suggesting MI had no different CHD mortality and overall mortality rates. Hence, it is important to distinguish these gradual-onset Q-waves from true, unrecognized MIs by obtaining prior ECG tracings.

RISK FACTORS

A poor cardiovascular risk profile predicts unrecognized MIs as well as symptomatic MIs.[8–10] Two risk factors—hypertension and

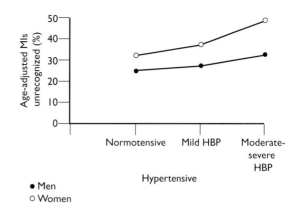

Figure 5.2 Proportion of myocardial infarctions unrecognized by hypertensive status. Framingham Study, 34-year follow-up.

diabetes—are associated with a distinct tendency to have unrecognized MIs. The incidence of both unrecognized and recognized MIs increases with the severity of hypertension, but the fraction of infarctions that go undetected is much greater in hypertensive than normotensive persons.[15] Among persons with moderate to severe hypertension (>160/95 mmHg), 48% of MIs in women and 32% in men went unrecognized (Fig. 5.2). The proportion of MIs that go unrecognized increases with the severity of the blood pressure elevation. This is puzzling, because one would expect more symptomatic infarctions in hypertensive persons, and they are usually under closer medical supervision. This predisposition to silent or unrecognized MIs persists on excluding possible confounding factors such as diabetes, left ventricular hypertrophy and antihypertensive treatment (Fig. 5.3). In all instances, the fraction of unrecognized MIs is substantially higher in women than in men.

Diabetes is a recognized cause of silent MI. This was confirmed in the Framingham Study, but only for men (Fig. 5.4). Whereas in men the proportion of MIs unrecognized was more than double that in nondiabetic patients (39% versus

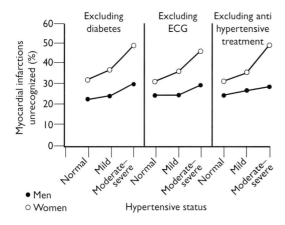

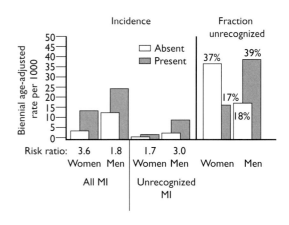

Figure 5.3 Proportion of myocardial infarctions unrecognized by hypertensive status excluding confounders. Framingham Study, 34-year follow-up.

Figure 5.4 Unrecognized myocardial infarction and glucose intolerance in subjects aged 35–84 years. Framingham Study, 26-year follow-up.

18%), in women the opposite applies. Women with diabetes have a risk ratio of 3.6 for all MIs, which is twice that of male persons with diabetes. For unrecognized MIs the risk ratio is only 1.7 comparing women with and without diabetes (Fig. 5.4). It has been suggested that decreased sensitivity to pain may be an important factor in unrecognized

MI in general, and in persons with diabetes in particular.[16,17] If so, this would appear to apply only in men.

PROGNOSIS

Mortality following MI is substantial whether it is recognized or unrecognized. Of persons

Table 5.3   Mortality (%) following initial recognized versus unrecognized myocardial infarction (MI) and 30-day survival. Framingham Study, 36-year follow-up.

| Years of follow-up | Age 35–64 | | | | Age 65–94 | | | |
| | Recognized MI | | Unrecognized MI | | Recognized MI | | Unrecognized MI | |
	Men	Women	Men	Women	Men	Women	Men	Women
1–2	7	15	8	2	24	22	18	23
3–4	14	21	20	8	43	49	40	46
5–8	32	33	44	23	67	68	63	62
9–12	45	55	63	39	80	79	84	74
13–16	58	79	76	44	90	89	90	84
17–20	71	90	91	62	—	—	96	91

Table 5.4   Age-adjusted risk of mortality following recognized and unrecognized myocardial infarction (MI) at 10 years. Framingham Study, 30-year follow-up.

Cardiovascular causes	Recognized				Unrecognized			
	10-year rate (%)		Risk ratio		10-year rate (%)		Risk ratio	
	Men	Women	Men	Women	Men	Women	Men	Women
Cardiovascular disease	29	29	3.2	5.9	38	21	3.5	4.1
Coronary disease	26	22	4.1	8.9	26	20	3.8	7.5
Sudden death	12	5	4.5	5.9	10	5	3.3	6.5

under age 65 years, 45% of men and 55% of women with recognized MIs are dead within 10 years. The corresponding rates for men and women with unrecognized MIs are 63% and 39%, respectively (Table 5.3). For MI victims over age 65 years, about 80% of either sex will die within 10 years whether the MI is recognized or unrecognized. This constitutes a death rate 2.5 times that of the general population of the same age composition. In both sexes cardiovascular, coronary, and sudden death mortality were also comparable for unrecognized and recognized MIs (Table 5.4). In both cases the risk ratios, adjusted for age, were substantially greater in women.

Cardiovascular events are also substantially increased following unrecognized MI, with risk ratios almost as large as for recognized MIs (Table 5.5). At 10-year follow-up the risk of a major cardiovascular event is increased about 3.6-fold in men with a recognized MI and 2.4-fold in those sustaining an unrecognized MI. For women, the risk ratios are 4.8 and 3.2, respectively, compared with the general population of the same age. Absolute risk and risk ratios for cardiac failure are similar in persons with recognized and unrecognized MIs, suggesting that the amount of myocardial damage sustained is little different in these two types of MI (Fig. 5.5).

Risk of recurrent MI and angina are lower in persons with unrecognized MIs than in those who sustain recognized MIs. Furthermore, in persons with unrecognized MIs, the subsequent recurrent event is less likely to be unrecognized or silent than the first attack. About half the recurrent MIs are fatal whether the prior MI is silent or symptomatic.

Table 5.5   Risk of cardiovascular events following recognized and unrecognized myocardial infarction (MI). Framingham Study, 30-year follow-up.

Type of MI	Myocardial infarction		Stroke		Cardiac failure	
	Men	Women	Men	Women	Men	Women
Recognized MI	2.8	8.3	2.4	5.9	3.7	7.6
Unrecognized MI	2.0	4.3	3.6	2.3	4.6	4.8

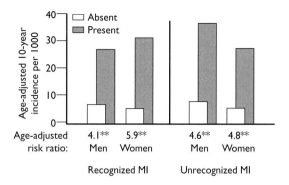

Figure 5.5 Risk of cardiac failure by recognized versus unrecognized myocardial infarction in subjects aged 35–94 years (**$P<0.01$). Framingham Study, 30-year follow-up.

PATHOGENESIS

The reasons for the occurrence of ischemic episodes in the absence of pain remain unclear. For transient, short-term ischemic episodes, it may be only a function of the duration of the ischemia, but this would not apply for silent MIs. It is not known why ischemia sufficient to produce an infarction occurs without symptoms in some persons, with atypical symptoms in others and with severe symptoms in most. Denial probably plays a role, as patients with unrecognized MIs appear to visit doctors less frequently than those who have symptomatic infarctions. There is some evidence suggesting that patients who have unrecognized MIs tend not to express ischemia with pain as indicated by less associated angina. They may have a higher pain threshold.[12] It is possible that the extent of ischemic involvement or the rapidity of its evolution may not be as pronounced in painless infarctions. Pain may only be the tip of the dangerous iceberg of MI.

PREVENTIVE IMPLICATIONS

There is little indication that the incidence of unrecognized MIs or the proportion that go undetected has decreased over the past several decades. Increased awareness and improved diagnosis of silent coronary disease have not made this a less common feature of coronary heart disease.[18] Clearly, closer monitoring of candidates for MI, particularly those with diabetes or hypertension, is needed. Unrecognized MI is a common and potentially lethal condition that warrants greater attention. This can be implemented by periodic ECG monitoring of persons with a poor multivariate risk profile. Earlier detection of ischemia may be achieved by exercise ECG and ambulatory monitoring of such persons.

Because of the serious prognosis of unrecognized MI, preventive management should be the same as that given to survivors of symptomatic infarctions, including aspirin, angiotensin converting enzyme (ACE) inhibitors, beta-blockers, and even revascularization when there is indication of frequent transient ischemic episodes on ambulatory monitoring or easily induced ischemia on the treadmill.

Because cardiac failure risk is substantial in patients with unrecognized MIs, control of blood pressure, ACE inhibitors, and treatment of dyslipidemia would appear indicated. Quitting cigarette smoking deserves a high priority because it may halve the risk of a recurrent MI. Weight reduction can improve insulin sensitivity and lessen the burden of all the major contributors to accelerated atherogenesis. The role of surgery or angioplasty for silent MI is controversial because there are no symptoms to relieve, but it may well be indicated if there is left main or three-vessel disease and impaired left ventricular function.

Patients who are high-risk candidates for coronary disease need to be monitored by ECG examinations for the occurrence of unrecognized MIs and then carefully followed for signs of cardiac failure, evidence of frequent silent transient ischemic events on ambulatory monitoring, and evidence of deteriorating left ventricular function on echocardiographic examination.

ACKNOWLEDGMENT

This chapter was supported by NIH, NHLBI Grant No. NO1–HC–38038, Astra USA, Inc. Visiting Scientist Program.

REFERENCES

1. Gordon T, Kannel WB. Premature mortality from coronary heart disease. The Framingham Study. *JAMA* 1971; **215**: 1617–25.

2. Selwyn AP, Shea M, Deanfield JE, Wilson R, Horlock P, O'Brien H. Character of transient ischemia in angina pectoris. *Am J Cardiol* 1986; **58**: 21B–25B.

3. Quyyumi AA, Wright C, Fox K. Ambulatory electrocardiographic ST-segment changes in healthy volunteers. *Br Heart J* 1983; **50**: 460–4.

4. Cecchi AC, Dobelli EV, Marchi F, Pucci P, Santoro GM, Faxxi PF. Silent myocardial ischemia during ambulatory electrocardiographic monitoring in patients with effort angina. *J Am Coll Cardiol* 1983; **1**: 934–9.

5. Deanfield JE, Shea M, Ribiero P et al. Transient ST-segment depression as a marker of myocardial ischemia during daily life. *Am J Cardiol* 1984; **54**: 1195–200.

6. Rocco MB, Nabel EG, Campbell S et al. Prognostic importance of myocardial ischemia detected by ambulatory monitoring in patients with coronary disease. *Circulation* 1988; **78**: 877–84.

7. Gottlieb SO, Weisfeldt ML, Ouyang P, Mellits ED, Gerstenblith G. Silent ischemia as a marker for early unfavorable outcomes in patients with unstable angina. *New Engl J Med* 1986; **314**: 1214–19.

8. Kannel WB, Abbott RD. Incidence and prognosis of unrecognized myocardial infarction. An update from the Framingham Study. *New Engl J Med* 1984; **311**: 1144–7.

9. Kannel WB, Dannenberg AL, Abbott R. Unrecognized myocardial infarction: the Framingham Study. *Am Heart J* 1985; **109**: 581–5.

10. Margolis JR, Kannel WB, Feinleib M et al. Clinical features of unrecognized myocardial infarction—silent and asymptomatic: eighteen-year follow-up: the Framingham Study. *Am J Cardiol* 1973; **32**: 1–7.

11. Koonlawee N, Intarachot V, Singh P, Josephson MA, Singh BN. Characteristics and clinical significance of silent myocardial ischemia in unstable angina. *Am J Cardiol* 1986; **58**: 26B–33B.

12. Hands ME, Sia B, Shook TL et al. Silent myocardial ischemia in asymptomatic survivors of unrecognized myocardial infarction and matched controls. *Am Heart J* 1988; **116**: 1488–92.

13. Goldberger AL. Normal and non-infarct Q-waves. *Cardiol Clin* 1987; **5**: 357.

14. Murabito JM, Larson MG, Lin S-T, Evans JC, Levy D. Unexplained gradual-onset Q-wave patterns. A case series from the Framingham Study. *J Electrocardiol* 1995; **28**: 267–75.

15. Kannel WB, Dannenberg AL, Abbott RD. Unrecognized myocardial infarction and hypertension. The Framingham Study. *Am Heart J* 1985; **109**: 581–5.

16. Droste C, Roskamon H. Experimental pain measurement in patients with asymptomatic myocardial ischemia. *J Am Coll Cardiol* 1983; **1**: 940–5.

17. Bradley RF, Schonfeld A. Diminished pain in diabetic patients with acute myocardial infarction. *Geriatrics* 1962; **17**: 322–6.

18. Armstrong WF, Jordan JW, Morris SN, McHenry PL. Prevalence and magnitude of ST-segment and T-wave abnormality in normal men during continuous ambulatory electrocardiography. *Am J Cardiol* 1982; **49**: 1638–42.

6

The prognostic significance of silent myocardial ischemia

Peter H Stone and Andrew P Selwyn

INTRODUCTION

The appreciation that episodes of myocardial ischemia frequently occur during daily life, are usually asymptomatic, and can be readily detected in patients using ambulatory ECG (AECG) monitoring has led to great interest in exploring their significance in the management of patients with coronary artery disease (CAD). Episodes of myocardial ischemia occur in 25–50% of patients who exhibit coronary syndromes, from chronic stable angina to acute syndromes of unstable angina and myocardial infarction, and the vast majority of such episodes are asymptomatic.[1–4] Patients who exhibit asymptomatic ischemic episodes during routine daily activities have more adverse coronary events than patients who do not exhibit such episodes in each of the coronary syndromes, and the purpose of this chapter is to review current understanding of the prognostic significance of such ischemia in patients with stable CAD.

PATHOPHYSIOLOGY OF DAILY LIFE ISCHEMIA IN PATIENTS WITH STABLE CAD

Myocardial ischemia may occur either from an episodic increase in myocardial O_2 demand, identified most conveniently by the heart rate and systolic blood pressure, or from an episodic decrease in myocardial O_2 supply. Ischemia due to a decrease in O_2 supply is related to either coronary artery vasoconstriction, transient

platelet aggregation or both. Transient platelet aggregation in the setting of coronary atherosclerosis is a common cause of transient ischemia in patients with acute coronary syndromes, but has been shown not to contribute to ischemia in patients with stable angina.[5] Actual identification of the presence of episodic coronary vasoconstriction has been elusive in patients with stable CAD, and most approaches to understanding the role of vasoconstriction have been deductive, based on the 'heart rate threshold' (HR threshold) at which ischemia (typically ≥1.0 mm ST-segment depression) occurs. If the HR threshold for ischemia varies within a given patient with stable CAD, it is deduced that intermittent coronary vasoconstriction is likely responsible, that is, when transient vasoconstriction is present, ischemia occurs at a lower HR threshold, and when vasoconstriction is relieved, or vasodilatation occurs, ischemia develops at a higher HR threshold. The pattern of heart rate activity preceding an ischemic episode may also suggest whether the episode is due to an increase in O_2 demand (indicated by an increase in heart rate ≥5 bpm before the episode) or to a decrease in O_2 supply (indicated by the absence of an increase in heart rate preceding the episode).

The fact that daily life ischemia as identified by AECG monitoring occurs at the HR threshold 10–20% lower than the HR threshold for ischemia during an exercise treadmill test

(ETT)[6,7] has suggested that episodes of daily life ischemia may at least in part be related to intermittent coronary vasoconstriction. There is also substantial variability in the HR threshold for ischemia throughout the day within a given patient,[8] supporting the role of varying degrees of coronary vasoconstriction throughout the day contributing to ischemia. Andrews et al.[9] related the minute-by-minute heart rate profile of stable coronary patients to the episodes of daily life ischemia and found that only 20% of ischemic episodes occurred in the absence of a heart rate increase, which would be the case if vasoconstriction were the primary pathophysiologic mechanism, and that approximately 80% of ischemic episodes were preceded by an increase in heart rate. Furthermore, Andrews and colleagues found that the likelihood of developing ischemia throughout the day was proportional to the magnitude and duration of the heart rate increase and the baseline heart rate before the increases in heart rate. Thus, the vast majority of daily life ischemia is preceded by some evidence of an increase in myocardial O_2 demand. Therefore, it is interesting to note that therapies directed at reducing O_2 demand, such as beta-blockers, which are so effective at reducing daily life ischemia,[10] are also most effective at improving prognosis.

Understanding the pathophysiology of ischemia in stable coronary disease is complicated by the current appreciation that many routine daily activities can both increase myocardial demand *and* provoke coronary vasoconstriction: mental stress,[11–13] physical stress,[14,15] cigarette smoking,[16] and exposure to cold.[17] Furthermore, other important pathophysiologic considerations may influence the development of myocardial ischemia, such as hypercholesterolemia and the hormonal milieu in postmenopausal women. Elevated serum low-density lipoprotein (LDL) cholesterol,[18] particularly oxidized LDL cholesterol,[19,20] and estrogen deprivation[21] create, and may exacerbate, the endothelial dysfunction that is responsible for atherosclerosis and perhaps for episodic vasoconstriction as well. These pathophysiologic and mechanistic considerations are

important since pharmacologic treatment is often quite different, based on the culprit mechanism, and these treatment options may also have important implications for prognosis.

The complex inter-relationship between the atherosclerotic plaque, endothelial function, and alterations in myocardial O_2 demand precludes a simplistic approach to understanding the prognostic significance of daily life ischemia, and the prognostic effects of decreasing or preventing episodes of daily life ischemia. The presence of daily life ischemia and its decrease or prevention by pharmacologic therapy may, in fact, only represent an epiphenomenon in terms of prognosis. Beta-adrenergic blockers or HMG Co-A-reductase inhibitors, for example, may reduce episodes of myocardial ischemia during daily life, but the beneficial prognostic effect of their administration may be related solely to prevention of plaque rupture and the subsequent complications (for example, thrombus formation and possible vasoconstriction) and not to the reduction in daily life ischemia per se. Treatment of the marker of high risk (that is, daily life ischemia) may be a useful sign, but may not necessarily be synonymous with treatment of the high-risk process itself (the atherosclerotic plaque).

PROGNOSTIC SIGNIFICANCE OF THE PRESENCE OF DAILY LIFE ISCHEMIA

Most studies have demonstrated that the presence of ischemia during AECG monitoring of routine daily life activities is associated with an adverse cardiac prognosis (Table 6.1).[2,9,13,22–27] Rocco et al.,[22] for example, found that among 86 patients with stable CAD who were monitored off antianginal medications, the 49 (57%) who had ≥ one episode of daily life ischemia had a significantly worse cardiac event rate after 12.5 ± 7.5 months compared with the 37 patients who did not have such ischemia (Fig. 6.1). Yeung et al.[13] confirmed the long-term prognostic significance (37 ± 17 months' follow-up) of daily life ischemia detected off medications in these same patients and also suggested that

Table 6.1 Observational studies defining the incidence and prognostic significance of daily life ischemia

Authors, year	No. patients	Incidence of AECG ischemia (%)	End points	Mean follow-up (months)	Event rates (%) With AECG ischemia	Without ischemia	P-value	Comments
Rocco et al., 1988[22]	86	57	Death, MI, UA, revasc.	12.5	40	3	0.003	Patients monitored once off Rx
Tzivoni et al., 1988[23]	118	33	Cardiac death, MI, UA, revasc.	28	51	20	<0.001	All patients with previous MI
Hedblad et al., 1989[24]	394	25	Cardiac death & nonfatal MI	43	15	3	<0.001	
Deedwania and Carbajal, 1990[2]	107	43	Cardiac death	23	24	8	0.02	Monitored on Rx
Raby et al., 1990[27]	176	18	Cardiac death, nonfatal MI	20	38	7	<0.0001	Patients with peripheral vascular disease
Yeung et al., 1991[13]	138	59	Death, MI, revasc.	37	56	42	0.02	Monitored off Rx
Deedwania and Carbajal, 1991[25]	86	45	Cardiac death	24	23	4	<0.008	Monitored on Rx which controlled symptoms
Quyyumi et al., 1993[31]	116	39	MI, UA, revasc.	29	13	15	NS	Very low-risk patients
Moss et al., 1993[32]	936	5	Cardiac death, nonfatal MI, or UA	23	27	24	NS	Very low-risk patients
deMarchena et al., 1994[28]	50	32	Cardiac death, MI, UA, revasc.	10	56	21	<0.02	All patients monitored on Rx which controlled symptoms
Madjlessi-Simon et al., 1996[30]	331	27	Death, MI, revasc., or worsening angina	21	33	17	0.004	All patients initially treated with a beta-blocker

AECG: ambulatory ECG; MI: myocardial infarction; UA: unstable angina; revasc.: revascularization; Rx: anti-anginal medication

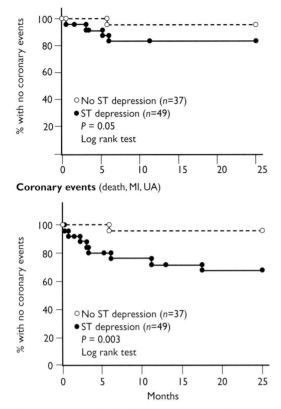

Coronary events (death, MI, UA)

Coronary events (death, MI, UA, revascularization)

Figure 6.1 Kaplan–Meier curves comparing the probability of not experiencing (top panel) an acute ischemic event (death, myocardial infarction, unstable angina) and (bottom panel) progressive ischemic event (acute events or revascularization for worsening symptoms) during follow-up for the 37 patients without ST-segment depression (O—O) and the 49 patients with ST-segment depression (●—●) as detected by ambulatory monitoring. (Reproduced with permission from Rocco et al.[22])

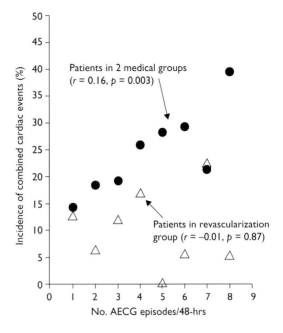

Figure 6.2 Relationship between AECG ischemic episodes at the qualifying visit and incidence of combined cardiac events (death, MI, coronary revascularization procedure, or hospitalization for an ischemic event) between week 12 and 1 year. Patients in the two medical groups are indicated by closed circles and patients in the revascularization group are indicated by open triangles. The r values represent the correlation between the number of AECG ischemic episodes and the incidence of combined cardiac events in the respective groups. (Reproduced with permission from Stone et al.[29])

patients showing no evidence of ischemia while on medication exhibited an event rate similar to that of patients who exhibited ischemia while off medication. Deedwania and Carbajal[2,25] and deMarchena et al.[28] also demonstrated that detection of daily life ischemia in patients whose symptoms are adequately controlled on antianginal medications had a significantly worse prognosis than patients without daily life ischemia.

In the Asymptomatic Cardiac Ischemia Pilot (ACIP) Study, there was a highly significant linear association between the number of ischemic episodes present on the qualifying AECG off medications and the subsequent 1-year incidence of death, MI, PTCA, CABG, or an ischemic event requiring hospitalization in patients treated medically (p=0.003) (Fig. 6.2).[29]

In some studies that compared the significance of ischemia detected by AECG, ETT, as well as angiographic and clinical variables, the presence of daily life ischemia, detected by AECG monitoring, has been the most powerful predictor of cardiac mortality in follow-up to 2 years ($P=0.003$),[13,25] and of all cardiac events (death, myocardial infarction (MI), percutaneous transluminal coronary angioplasty (PTCA), or coronary artery bypass grafting (CABG)) for up to 5 years ($P=0.009$).[13] Madjlessi-Simon et al.[30] found that the presence of transient ischemia, the number of coronary stenoses, and beta-blocker withdrawal were the only significant prognostic factors of cardiac events. The value of the prognostic information from most studies of AECG monitoring has been limited, however, by performance of AECG monitoring at only one point in time in the long-term natural history of CAD, either when the patients were withdrawn from all antianginal medications,[22] or while they were on antianginal therapy.[2,28,30] It is unknown whether more prognostic information would be derived from serial AECG monitoring of these patients at different points in their natural history.

There have been two observational studies that indicated no prognostic significance of daily life ischemia,[31,32] but these studies are limited by exclusion of high- or medium-risk patients. Quyyumi et al.[31] focused only on very low-risk patients and excluded patients with two- or three-vessel disease and a positive exercise test, three-vessel disease associated with left ventricular dysfunction, and left main disease. Moss et al.[32] included only patients who were clinically stable a mean of 2.7 months following an acute MI or unstable angina and excluded those who had a revascularization procedure after their index event.

A fundamental problem with virtually all the previous prognosis studies is that the event rates for 'hard end points', such as cardiac death or MI, are very low in these stable patients and, consequently, essentially all the studies have relied upon much less meaningful end points, such as revascularization procedures, worsening angina, or unstable angina, to obtain statistical power. Even though the AECG monitoring results may not have been made available to the treating

physicians, and may not have therefore influenced the decisions to consider revascularization or to hospitalize with progressive angina, the presence of AECG ischemia is highly correlated with a strongly positive exercise treadmill test.[7] Since treating physicians knew the results of their patients' exercise test, they may have made more aggressive treatment decisions which would exert a bias towards more revascularization procedures and more hospitalizations in those patients with daily life ischemia.

CLINICAL TRIALS TO ASSESS THE EFFECT OF ANTI-ISCHEMIA STRATEGY ON THE PROGNOSTIC SIGNIFICANCE OF DAILY LIFE ISCHEMIA

The ability of anti-ischemic therapies to improve the adverse prognosis associated with AECG ischemia has been inadequately studied (Table 6.2). The studies investigating pharmacologic treatment have been limited and no prior studies have investigated the effect of revascularization to improve AECG ischemia and consequently to improve prognosis. Pepine et al.[33] studied 306 patients with ischemia detected both by ETT and by AECG and found that those patients treated with atenolol had improved event-free survival and increased time to the occurrence of a first adverse event compared with those patients treated with placebo. The most powerful univariate and multivariate correlate of event-free survival was the absence of AECG ischemia after 4 weeks of treatment.[33] The control group, however, received no antianginal therapy, and the study consequently does not address the question of the incremental value of treating asymptomatic ischemia detected by AECG monitoring in addition to treating symptomatic ischemia. The Total Ischemic Burden Bisoprolol Study (TIBBS)[26] indicated that patients with six or more episodes of AECG ischemia/48 hours at baseline had an event rate (death, MI, unstable angina or revascularization) of 32.5% compared with 25.0% for patients with two to six episodes and 13.2% for patients with fewer than two

Table 6.2 Clinical trials to assess effect of anti-ischemic strategies on prognostic significance of daily life ischemia

Authors, year	No. patients	End points	Follow-up	Event rate by treatment group	P
Pepine et al., 1994[33]	306	Death, MI, UA, worsening angina, or revascularization	1 year	25% placebo 11% atenolol	0.001
Rogers et al., 1995[36]	558	Death, MI, revascularization, hospital admission	1 year	32% angina-guided medical strategy 31% ischemia-guided medical strategy 18% revascularization strategy	0.003
Dargie et al., 1996[34]	682	Cardiac death, nonfatal MI, and UA	2 years	13% atenolol 11% nifedipine 8% combination	NS
		Revascularization, worsening angina		8% atenolol 9% nifedipine SR 3% combination	NS
von Armin et al., 1996[26]	520	Death, MI, UA, or revascularization	1 year	32% for non-100% responders 18% for 100% responders	0.008
				33% for nifedipine 22% for bisoprolol	0.03

MI: myocardial infarction; UA: unstable angina.

episodes ($P < 0.001$). Patients whose AECG ischemia was entirely abolished by bisoprolol or nifedipine had a 17.5% event rate at 1 year compared with 32.3% for those patients who had at least one episode of residual ischemia ($P = 0.008$). The Total Ischaemic Burden European Trial (TIBET)[34] found no difference in the occurrence of cardiac events after an average of 2 years in patients treated with fixed doses of either atenolol, nifedipine, or the combination (Fig. 6.3), but there was no parallel placebo group to determine whether patients on anti-ischemic therapy had a better outcome than patients without therapy. There was also no dose titration to determine the incremental benefit of escalation of anti-ischemic therapy, and there

was substantial withdrawal (up to 40%) of assigned medication over the 3-year follow-up.

The Asymptomatic Cardiac Ischemia Pilot (ACIP) study was designed to determine the feasibility of performing a large-scale clinical trial to assess the prognostic significance of daily life ischemia.[35] In the pilot study, 558 patients with coronary anatomy amenable to revascularization, one or more episodes of daily life ischemia on a 48-hour AECG, and ischemia on an ETT were randomized to one of three treatment strategies: (1) medication to suppress angina alone (angina-guided strategy, $n = 183$); (2) medication to suppress both angina and daily life ischemia (ischemia-guided strategy, $n = 183$); or (3) revascularization strategy (angioplasty or bypass

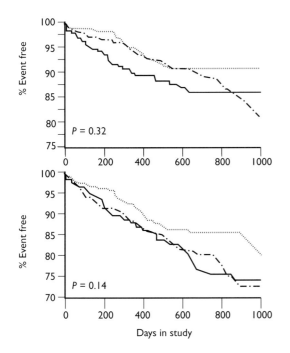

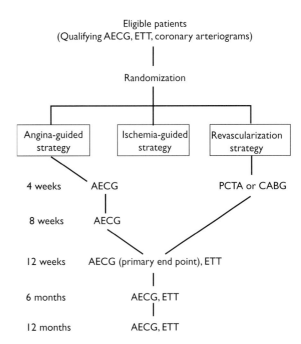

Figure 6.3 Kaplan–Meier survival curves showing percentage of subjects event-free by days in study, for the three arms, for hard end points (a) and hard+soft end points (b). ⎯⎯: atenolol; ⎯ · ⎯ · ⎯: nifedipine; ....: combination. (Reproduced with permission from Dargie et al.[34])

Figure 6.4 Sequence of testing for ischemia in the ACIP study from entry through 1-year follow-up. AECG: ambulatory electrocardiogram; CABG: coronary artery bypass surgery; ETT: treadmill exercise test (or equivalent); PTCA: percutaneous coronary angioplasty. (Reproduced with permission from Rogers et al.[36])

surgery, $n = 192$).[3] Patients were evaluated with serial AECGs and medication was titrated to reduce anginal symptoms (all patients) and to eliminate daily life ischemia (ischemia-guided strategy patients) (Fig. 6.4). The percentage of patients free of daily life ischemia on AECG monitoring through 1 year of follow-up is shown in Fig. 6.5.[36] At the 12-week, 6-month, and 1-year follow-up, daily life ischemia was suppressed in each of the three treatment groups, but was more often completely suppressed in patients assigned to revascularization ($P < 0.001$ at each follow-up interval).[36]

Although not powered to be a prognosis study, the ACIP pilot study nevertheless provides important suggestions concerning the prognostic value of treating daily life ischemia.[36] While the number of fatal events was small, the percentage of patients who died during the 1-year follow-up was significantly lower for patients assigned to the revascularization strategy (0%) than for those assigned to the angina-guided strategy (4.4%; $P = 0.003$) (Fig. 6.6).[36] The ischemia-guided strategy patients had an intermediate mortality rate (1.6%) between the revascularization strategy and the angina-guided strategy. There was no difference in mortality rate between the revascularization and the ischemia-guided strategies. Similar results were found combining the end points of death or MI.[36] The incidence of either death, MI, or non-protocol revascularization

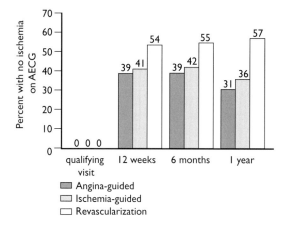

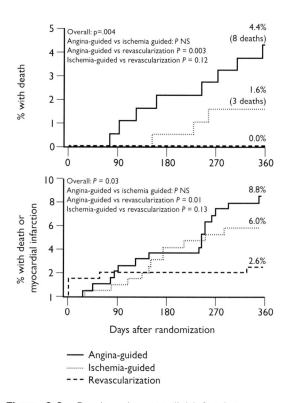

Figure 6.5 Percentage of patients free of ischemia on the ambulatory electrocardiogram (AECG). By definition, all patients had one or more episodes of asymptomatic ischemia on 48-hour ambulatory ECG monitoring at the baseline qualifying visit. At 12-week (primary outcome), 6-month and 1-year follow-up, ischemia on the ambulatory ECG was suppressed in each of the three treatment groups but was more often completely suppressed in patients assigned to revascularization (overall comparison and pairwise comparisons of revascularization strategy versus each of the other two arms, P < 0.001 at each follow-up interval; angina-guided versus ischemia-guided strategy, P = nonsignificant at each follow-up interval). (Reproduced with permission from Rogers et al.[36])

Figure 6.6 Death and myocardial infarction. Although the number of fatal events was small, the percentage of patients who died during the 1-year follow-up was significantly lower for patients assigned to the revascularization strategy than for those assigned to the angina-guided strategy, but not for those assigned to the ischemia-guided strategy (top). The mortality rate was similar between the angina-guided and ischemia-guided strategies. The combination of death or myocardial infarction was significantly less common among patients assigned to the revascularization strategy than among those assigned to the angina-guided but not the ischemia-guided strategy (bottom). (Reproduced with permission from Rogers et al.[36])

was less common with revascularization than with either of the two medical strategies, but there was no significant difference between the two medical strategies (Fig. 6.7). Medical titration in the ischemia-guided strategy patients was not aggressive enough to eradicate ischemia,[33] however, and a better prognostic effect might have been achieved if the medical regimen had been more effective.

Nevertheless, in the two medical groups in ACIP there was a trend associating greater reduction in AECG ischemia at 12 weeks with an improved subsequent prognosis (p=0.04).[29] This trend was evident primarily in the AECG-ischemia-guided group (p=0.06) compared to the angina-guided group (p=0.32).[29] These observations consitute the first suggestion that

AECG-guided treatment of ischemia enhances prognosis in patients with stable coronary disease. There was not uniform consistency regarding the benefit of reducing the frequency of AECG ischemia in ACIP, however, and the results only provide a hypothesis for future investigation.

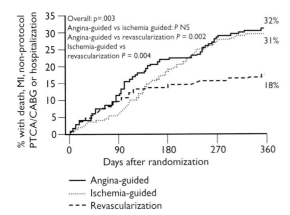

Figure 6.7 Death, myocardial infarction (MI), non-protocol angioplasty (PTCA) or bypass surgery (CABG) or hospital admission. The composite secondary outcome was significantly less common among patients assigned to the revascularization strategy than among those assigned to the other two treatment strategies. (Reproduced with permission from Rogers et al.[36])

In contrast to the observations in the two medical groups in ACIP, in the revascularization group there was no association between the number of AECG ischemic episodes at baseline and the incidence of subsequent cardiac events, nor in the change in ischemic episodes from the baseline to the week 12 AECG (Fig. 7.2).[29] These observations suggest that revascularization is effective in lowering the incidence of subsequent cardiac events in all patients, regardless of the number of ischemic episodes present prior to revascularization. The lack of relationship between the change in ischemic episodes and improvement in clinical events in this group may indicate that the clinical benefit resulting from revascularization may not be due to suppression of ischemia per se, but instead to an improvement in the underlying anatomic substrate that is responsible for the subsequent development of cardiac events.

Of note, recent studies have suggested that therapies directed at improving coronary endothelial function and atherogenesis itself may also improve the incidence of daily life ischemia. The HMG Co-A-reductase inhibitors (statins) have been found to exert a marked effect on lowering morbidity and mortality in patients with coronary disease, particularly those with increased total cholesterol and LDL cholesterol at study entry.[37–39] Quantitative coronary angiographic studies have shown that there is little regression of the bulk atherosclerotic obstruction per se from lowering serum lipids,[40,41] indicating that the prognostic benefit of lipid lowering is most likely due to prevention of plaque rupture, and restoration of a more healthy coronary arterial endothelium.[42] Consistent with this hypothesis are the recent findings that marked lipid lowering is associated with a marked reduction in the number and duration of daily life ischemic episodes.[43,44] In the REGRESS study of 768 male patients with documented coronary disease,[43] daily life ischemia was found in 28% at baseline, and in 19% after 2-year treatment with pravastatin 40 mg q.d. (P = 0.02). Total cholesterol dropped in these patients from 233 to 189 mg/dl and LDL cholesterol from 166 to 125 mg/dl. In contrast, the placebo group had no change in serum lipids and there was no observed reduction in daily life ischemia. At baseline there was a mean of 5.15 ± 5.99 episodes/48-hour monitoring in the patients who had daily life ischemia and this decreased by 1.23 ± 0.25 episodes in the pravastatin group and 0.53 ± 0.25 episodes in the placebo group (P = 0.047). The total duration of ischemia decreased from 80 ± 12 minutes to 42 ± 10 minutes in the pravastatin group (P = 0.017), and from 60 ± 13 minutes to 51 ± 9 minutes in the placebo group (P = 0.56). Interestingly, there were no differences in the number of clinical events between patients with and without ischemia. There is no mention concerning the event rates in patients who experienced a decrease in daily life ischemia compared with those without a change.

Andrews et al.[44] have shown that therapeutic lowering of serum LDL cholesterol using statins

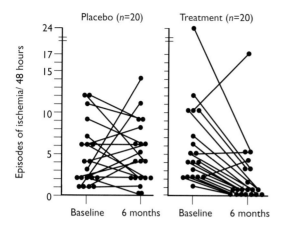

Figure 6.8 Data show patient-by-patient effect of cholesterol-lowering over 6 months on the number of episodes of ischemic ST-segment depression in patients with coronary disease. Two of 20 in the placebo group versus 13 of 20 in the treatment group show resolution of ischemia. (Reproduced with permission from Andrews et al.[44])

in coronary patients with asymptomatic daily life ischemia resulted in resolution of ischemia in 13 of 20 treated patients over 6 months. In contrast, only two of 20 patients in a placebo group showed resolution of ischemia over the same time ($P = 0.05$) (Fig. 6.8).

SUMMARY AND CONCLUSIONS

Episodes of asymptomatic ischemia identified by AECG monitoring during routine daily life activities are associated with an adverse cardiac prognosis in patients with stable coronary

disease, especially in those patients who have a positive exercise test and are known to have at least moderate risk. The independent prognostic significance of asymptomatic daily life ischemia remains to be determined. Although there is a statistically significant association between a positive exercise test, an established indicator of cardiac risk, and the frequency of daily life ischemia by AECG,[7] the strength of the association is very weak[7] and one would anticipate that those tests provide complementary prognostic information. Exercise testing and AECG monitoring assess different manifestations of coronary disease.[7,45] In small observational studies the presence of daily life ischemia exerts an independent prognostic effect above and beyond that associated with a positive exercise test, but these findings must be confirmed in a large-scale clinical trial with sufficient power to identify a benefit using reliable and accepted end points such as cardiac death and MI. It seems likely that daily life ischemia indicates increased risk because of its association with 'active coronary lesions', as well as severe lesions. Therefore, large-scale randomized trials that aim to benefit patients with daily life ischemia should select therapies that improve the dysfunctional cell biology that characterizes atherosclerotic coronary lesions, as well as therapies to improve the myocardial O_2 supply : demand balance.

ACKNOWLEDGMENT

We are grateful to John A Loring for help in the preparation of the manuscript.

REFERENCES

1. Gottlieb SO, Weisfeldt ML, Ouyang P, Mellits ED, Gerstenblith G. Silent ischemia predicts infarction and death during 2 year follow-up of unstable angina. *J Am Coll Cardiol* 1987; **10**: 756–60.
2. Deedwania PC, Carbajal EV. Silent ischemia during daily life is an independent predictor of mortality in stable angina. *Circulation* 1990; **81**: 748–56.
3. Pepine CJ, Geller NL, Knatterud GL et al. for the ACIP Investigators. The Asymptomatic Cardiac Ischemia Pilot (ACIP) study: design of a randomized clinical trial, baseline data and implications for a long-term outcome trial. *J Am Coll Cardiol* 1994; **24**: 1–10.
4. Gill JB, Cairns JA, Roberts RS et al. Prognostic

importance of myocardial ischemia detected by ambulatory monitoring early after acute myocardial infarction. *N Engl J Med* 1996; **334**: 65–70.

5. Willich SN, Sintonen SP, Bhatia SJS et al. Suppression of silent ischemia by metoprolol without alteration of morning increase of platelet aggregability in patients with stable coronary artery disease. *Circulation* 1989; **79**: 557–65.

6. Deanfield JE, Selwyn AP, Chierchia S et al. Myocardial ischemia during daily life in patients with stable angina: its relation to symptoms and heart rate changes. *Lancet* 1983; **ii**: 753–8.

7. Stone PH, Chaitman B, McMahon RP et al. for the ACIP Investigators. The relationship between exercise-induced and ambulatory ischemia in patients with stable coronary disease. The Asymptomatic Cardiac Ischemia Pilot (ACIP) Study. *Circulation* 1996; **94**: 1537–44.

8. Banai S, Moriel M, Benhorin J, Gavish A, Stern S, Tzivoni D. Changes in myocardial ischemia threshold during daily activities. *Am J Cardiol* 1990; **66**: 1403–6.

9. Andrews TC, Fenton T, Toyosaki N et al. for the Angina and Silent Ischemia Study Group (ASIS). Subsets of ambulatory myocardial ischemia based on heart rate activity: circadian distribution and response to anti-ischemic medication. *Circulation* 1993; **88**: 92–100.

10. Stone PH, Gibson RS, Glasser SP et al. and the ASIS Study Group. Comparison of propranolol, diltiazem, and nifedipine in the treatment of asymptomatic ischemia in patients with stable angina. Differential effects on asymptomatic ischemia, exercise performance, and anginal symptoms. *Circulation* 1990; **82**: 1962–72.

11. Deanfield JE, Kensett M, Wilson RA, Shea M, Selwyn AP. Silent myocardial ischemia due to mental stress. *Lancet* 1984; **ii**: 1001–4.

12. Rozanski A, Bairey CN, Krantz DS et al. Mental stress and the induction of silent myocardial ischemia in patients with coronary artery disease. *N Engl J Med* 1988; **318**: 1005–12.

13. Yeung AC, Barry J, Orav J, Bonassin E, Raby KE, Selwyn AP. Effects of asymptomatic ischemia on long-term prognosis in chronic stable coronary disease. *Circulation* 1991; **83**: 1598–604.

14. Gordon JB, Ganz P, Nabel EG et al. Atherosclerosis and endothelial function influence the coronary vasomotor response to exercise. *J Clin Invest* 1989; **83**: 1946–52.

15. Nabel EG, Selwyn AP, Ganz P. Paradoxical narrowing of atherosclerotic coronary arteries induced by increases in heart rate. *Circulation* 1990; **81**: 850–9.

16. Deanfield JE, Shea MJ, Wilson RA, Horlock P, deLandsheere CM, Selwyn AP. Direct effects of smoking on the heart: silent ischemic disturbances of coronary flow. *Am J Cardiol* 1988; **57**: 1005–9.

17. Nabel EG, Ganz P, Gordon JB, Alexander RW, Selwyn AP. Dilation of normal and constriction of atherosclerotic coronary arteries caused by the cold pressor test. *Circulation* 1988; **77**: 43–52.

18. Vita JA, Treasure CB, Nabel EG et al. The coronary vasomotor response to acetylcholine relates to risk factors for coronary artery disease. *Circulation* 1990; **81**: 491–7.

19. Dyce MC, Anderson TJ, Yeung AC, Selwyn AP, Ganz P. Indices of LDL particle size closely relate to endothelial function. *Circulation* 1993; **88** **(suppl I)**: I-466–I-471.

20. Juul K, Nielsen LB, Munkholm K, Stender S, Nordestgaard BG. Oxidation of plasma low-density lipoprotein accelerates its accumulation and degradation in the arterial wall in vivo. *Circulation* 1996; **94**: 1698–704.

21. Williams JK, Adams MR, Herrington DM, Clarkson TB. Short-term administration of estrogen and vascular responses of atherosclerotic coronary arteries. *J Am Coll Cardiol* 1992; **20**: 452–7.

22. Rocco MB, Nabel EG, Campbell S et al. Prognostic importance of myocardial ischemia detected by ambulatory monitoring in patients with stable coronary disease. *Circulation* 1988; **78**: 877–84.

23. Tzivoni D, Gavish A, Zin D et al. Prognostic significance of ischemic episodes in patients with previous myocardial infarction. *Am J Cardiol* 1988; **62**: 661–4.

24. Hedblad B, Juul-Moller S, Svensson K et al. Increased mortality in men with ST segment depression during 24h ambulatory long-term ECG recording. Results from prospective population study 'Men born in 1914', from Malmo, Sweden. *Eur Heart J* 1989; **10**: 149–58.

25. Deedwania PC, Carbajal EV. Usefulness of ambulatory silent myocardial ischemia added to the prognostic value of exercise test parameters in predicting risk of cardiac death in patients with stable angina pectoris and exercise-induced myocardial ischemia. *Am J Cardiol* 1991; **68**: 1279–86.

26. von Arnim Th for the TIBBS (Total Ischemic Burden Bisoprolol Study) investigators. Prognostic significance of transient ischemic episodes; response to treatment shows improved

prognosis. Results of the TIBBS follow-up. *J Am Coll Cardiol* 1996; **28**: 20–4.

27. Raby KE, Goldman L, Cook EF et al. Long-term prognosis of myocardial ischemia detected by Holter monitoring in peripheral vascular disease. *Am J Cardiol* 1990; **66**: 1309–13.

28. deMarchena E, Asch J, Martinez J et al. Usefulness of persistent silent myocardial ischemia in predicting a high cardiac event rate in men with medically controlled stable angina pectoris. *Am J Cardiol* 1994; **73**: 390–2.

29. Stone PH, Chaitman BR, Forman S et al. Prognostic significance of myocardial ischemia detected by ambulatory ECG, exercise treadmill testing, and resting ECG to predict cardiac events by 1 year (the ACIP study). *Am J Cardiol* 1997 (in press).

30. Madjlessi-Simon T, Mary-Krause M, Fillette F, Lechat P, Jaillon P. Persistent transient myocardial ischemia despite beta-adrenergic blockade predicts a higher risk of adverse cardiac events in patients with coronary artery disease. *J Am Coll Cardiol* 1996; **27**: 1586–91.

31. Quyyumi AA, Panza JA, Diodati JG, Callahan TS, Bonow RO, Epstein SE. Prognostic implications of myocardial ischemia during daily life in low risk patients with coronary artery disease. *J Am Coll Cardiol* 1993; **21**: 700–8.

32. Moss AJ, Goldstein RE, Hall J et al. Detection and significance of myocardial ischemia in stable patients after recovery from an acute coronary event. *JAMA* 1993; **269**: 2379–85.

33. Pepine CJ, Cohn PF, Deedwania PC et al. for the ASIST Study Group. Effects of treatment on outcome in mildly symptomatic patients with ischemia during daily life. The Atenolol Silent Ischemia Study (ASIST). *Circulation* 1994; **90**: 762–8.

34. Dargie HJ, Ford I, Fox KM. Total Ischaemic Burden European Trial (TIBET). Effects of ischaemia and treatment with atenolol, nifedipine SR, or their combination on outcome in patients with chronic stable angina. The TIBET Study Group. *Eur Heart J* 1996; **17**: 104–12.

35. Knatterud GL, Bourassa MG, Pepine CJ et al. Effects of treatment strategies to suppress ischemia in patients with coronary artery disease: 12-week results of the Asymptomatic Cardiac Ischemia Pilot (ACIP) Study. *J Am Coll Cardiol* 1994; **24**: 11–20.

36. Rogers WJ, Bourassa MG, Andrews TC et al. The Asymptomatic Cardiac Ischemia Pilot (ACIP) Study: outcome at one year for patients with asymptomatic cardiac ischemia randomized to medical therapy or revascularization. *J Am Coll Cardiol* 1995; **26**: 594–605.

37. Shepherd J, Cobbe SM, Ford I et al. for the West of Scotland Coronary Prevention Study Group. Prevention of coronary artery disease with pravastatin in men with hypercholesterolemia. *N Engl J Med* 1995; **333**: 1301–7.

38. The Scandinavian Simvastatin Survival Study Group. Randomized trial of cholesterol lowering in 4444 patients with coronary heart disease: the Scandinavian Simvastatin Survival Study (4S). *Lancet* 1994; **344**: 1383–9.

39. Sacks FM, Pfeffer MA, Moye LA et al. for the Cholesterol and Recurrent Events Trial Investigators. The effect of pravastatin on coronary events after myocardial infarction in patients with average cholesterol levels. *N Engl J Med* 1996; **335**: 1001–9.

40. Brown BG, Lynn JT, Schefer SM, Kaplan CA, Dodge HT, Albers JJ. Niacin or lovastatin combined with cholesterol regress coronary atherosclerosis and prevent clinical events in men with elevated apolipoproteinlipoprotein B. *N Engl J Med* 1990; **323**: 1289–98.

41. Sacks FM, Pasternak RC, Gibson CM, Rosner B, Stone PH for the Harvard Atherosclerosis Reversibility Project Group. The effect on coronary atherosclerosis of improving plasma cholesterol levels in patients with normal plasma cholesterol levels. *Lancet* 1994; **344**: 1182–6.

42. Gould KL, Martucci JP, Goldberg DI et al. Short-term cholesterol lowering decreases size and severity of perfusion abnormalities by positron emission tomography after dipyridamole in patients with coronary artery disease. *Circulation* 1994; **89**: 1530–8.

43. van Boven AJ, Jukema JW, Zwinderman AH, Crijns HJGM, Lie KI, Bruschke AVG. Reduction of transient myocardial ischemia with pravastatin in addition to the conventional treatment in patients with angina pectoris. *Circulation* 1996; **94**: 1503–5.

44. Andrews TC, Raby K, Barry J et al. Effect of cholesterol reduction on myocardial ischemia in patients with coronary disease. *Circulation* 1997; **95**: 324–8.

45. Borzak S, Fenton T, Glasser SP et al. for the Angina and Silent Ischemia Study Group (ASIS). Discordance between effects of anti-ischemic therapy on ambulatory ischemia, exercise performance, and anginal symptoms in patients with stable angina pectoris. *J Am Coll Cardiol* 1993; **21**: 1605–11.

7

Sudden death and myocardial ischemia

Xavier Viñolas, Josep Guindo, Enrique Rodriguez and Antonio Bayés de Luna

INTRODUCTION

The explanation of the importance of the relationship between myocardial ischemia and sudden cardiac death is due to the significant epidemiological relevance of both and their socioeconomic implications. Although the incidence of sudden cardiac death is decreasing, in the United States alone between 350 000 and 400 000 people present sudden cardiac death annually.[1,2] Within the concept of 'total ischemic burden'[3] silent ischemia represents probably 70% of all ischemic crises and this percentage may be even greater if the silent ischemia of totally asymptomatic individuals is considered.[4] It has been estimated that silent myocardial ischemia is present in almost 5% of the asymptomatic population, in about 30% of uncomplicated myocardial infarction, and in many patients with unstable or stable angina.[4]

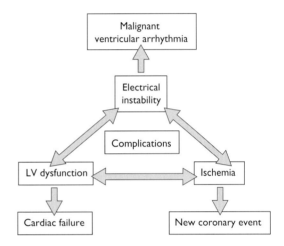

Figure 7.1 Triangle of risk of complications with heart disease, especially post-myocardial infarction patients.

SUDDEN DEATH AS A MULTIFACTORIAL PROBLEM

Nowadays it is absolutely clear that sudden cardiac death is a multifactorial problem. Risk factors for sudden cardiac death (center of triangle in Fig. 7.1) are related to three factors: ischemia, left ventricular dysfunction and electrical instability. The three factors are not independent and interact with each other. From a simplified point of view each parameter has bi-directional interactions with the other two. In Tables 7.1, 7.2 and 7.3 we summarize the most important relationships between them.

The relationship between myocardial ischemia and sudden cardiac death is currently not known in detail in spite of the great interest that the topics of ischemia[3–18] and sudden death[1,2,19–25] have awakened in recent years. The result from the CAST study appears to strengthen the idea of this relationship because it has been thought that silent ischemia could explain at least to some extent the appearance of late proarrhythmia and sudden death in this study.[26,27]

One important aspect when discussing ischemia and sudden death is the differentiation

Table 7.1   Interactions between ischemia and left ventricular function.

1) Left ventricular dysfunction ⟶ ischemia
   - Increase of telediastolic pressures and reduction of subendocardial blood flow
   - Reduction of cardiac output
   - Increase of ischemia during exercise

2) Ischemia ⟶ left ventricular dysfunction
   - Hibernated myocardium
   - Stunned myocardium
   - Ischemic cascade

Table 7.2   Interactions between ischemia and electrical instability.

1) Ischemia ⟶ electrical instability
   - Slowing of conduction
   - Prolongation of excitability recovery
   - Changes in refractoriness (shorter than in normal myocytes)
   - Refractoriness dispersion (allowing re-entrant circuits)

2) Electrical instability ⟶ ischemia
   - Decrease of coronary flow during arrhythmias with rapid heart rates
   - Increase of telediastolic pressures and reduction of subendocardial blood flow

Table 7.3   Interaction between left ventricular dysfunction and electrical instability.

1) Left ventricular dysfunction ⟶ electrical instability
   - Neurohumoral factors
   - Ionic disturbances
   - Renin–angiotensin–aldosterone axis activation
   - Proarrhythmic effect of drugs
   - Morphofunctional factors
     - Anatomical block allowing re-entry
     - Functional block
     - Automatic activity

2) Electrical instability ⟶ left ventricular dysfunction
   - Hemodynamic alterations during rapid heart rates
   - Loss of atrial contraction

IS SILENT ISCHEMIA TRUE ISCHEMIA?

It has been clearly demonstrated that angina is no more than a late manifestation of the ischemic cascade phenomenon[28] (Fig. 7.2). Both experimental and clinical evidence indicate the existence of a series of events which appear consecutively after occlusion of a coronary artery, [29–32] these being successively metabolic changes, alterations in relaxation and contractility of the myocardium, hemodynamic changes, electrocardiographic changes, and, finally, the appearance of angina.

It has been observed, since the pioneering work of Stern and Tzivoni[33] with Holter ECG, and using exercise testing,[34] that some coronary patients may present with painless electrocardiographic ST-segment changes. Using simultaneously Holter ECG and positron emission tomography, Deanfield et al.[35,36] demonstrated

between painful and painless ischemia. As most of the episodes of ST changes are silent it is very important to clarify first if silent ischemia (expressed with electrocardiological techniques as silent ST depression) corresponds to true ischemia, that is, decreased coronary blood flow.

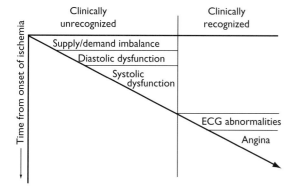

Figure 7.2 Ischemic cascade. (Adapted from Nesto et al.[28])

that ST-segment depression detected by Holter ambulatory electrocardiography corresponds to true ischemia detected by positron emission tomography. Lastly, in ambulatory patients wearing conventional ECG and nuclear Holter devices,[37] a decrease in the ejection fraction in the nuclear Holter may be detected before the appearance of the ST-segment depression as a manifestation of silent ischemia. These data confirm the phenomenon of the myocardial ischemic cascade in ambulatory patients, and verify the ischemic nature of electrocardiographic (Holter or exercise testing) ST-segment changes.

From this perspective it can be summarized that ST-segment deviations detected by exercise testing and Holter ECG in coronary patients without pain correspond to true ischemia, and at least for some patients they have a similar prognosis to ST deviations with angina. Whether the presence of silent ischemia implies a greater risk of cardiac events, and especially of sudden cardiac death, will be discussed later in this chapter.

PHYSIOPATHOLOGY OF ISCHEMIA AND ARRHYTHMIAS

It is well known that acute ischemia may induce ventricular fibrillation and, consequently, sudden death. Some factors that may favor myocardial vulnerability to ventricular fibrillation are the following: (1) slow conduction and blocks, (2) refractoriness dispersion, (3) total ventricular mass, and (4) increase in automaticity.

Harris demonstrated in 1950[38] that ventricular arrhythmias after acute occlusion showed a bimodal incidence. The peak was observed during the first 30 minutes with a second peak hours after occlusion. As we will see later, this has a quite acceptable clinical correlation. From a biochemical point of view an increase in extracellular potassium is observed soon after coronary occlusion.[39] It is important to note that extracellular $K+$ shows the same bimodal peaks as ventricular arrhythmias.

At the same time some other phenomena occur: as anaerobic metabolism begins, lactate acid is accumulated, intracellular pH decreases, intracellular sodium increases, and cytolitic $Ca++$ increases. All these phenomena produce a hyperpolarized cell and activity triggered by electrophysiological phenomena and early after-depolarizations is seen.[29,40] These phenomena are also accompanied by a slowing and fragmentation of conduction.[41]

Chronic ischemia represents different phenomena. In post-myocardial infarction patients two situations may be observed. In the first case a myocardial necrosis is established without residual ischemia. In this situation an anatomical scar is present, and ventricular arrhythmias (especially monomorphic ventricular tachycardia) may occur without ischemia being usually a triggering mechanism. In the second case a zone of ischemia surrounding a necrosis is observed (peri-infarction zone). The ischemia in this zone can be augmented during increased oxygen demands (exercise, etc.), or during decreased coronary blood flow (e.g. coronary spasm). In this latter situation the physiopathological phenomena are different from the experimental models of coronary occlusion in which the primary event is a decrease in coronary blood flow. Ischemia-related arrhythmia appears when an increase in ischemia triggers the final event.

It is not yet entirely clear why ischemia is sometimes silent and sometimes painful, but it is probably due to two main reasons.[42,43] In some patients the pain threshold is higher owing to several factors (e.g. alterations in the level of endogenous endorphins) and in these cases myocardial ischemia may be as severe as symptomatic ischemia. In the remaining cases, those with a normal pain threshold, crises of silent ischemia are probably less severe (e.g. crises of lesser intensity and/or duration) than crises with pain. Moreover, the pain threshold in the same individual may sometimes be variable[44] so that ischemic crises of the same intensity may appear either with or without pain.

THE IMPORTANCE OF GRADE AND TYPE OF ISCHEMIA

We have seen that several physiopathological links exist between myocardial ischemia and ventricular arrhythmias. Although from an experimental point of view these links are well known, the clinical correlations are less well defined. Probably it is due to the fact that laboratory-induced ischemia is usually different from that seen in the different clinical settings. In the laboratory we induce a decreased coronary flow; in clinical practice most ischemic episodes are due to an increased oxygen demand. Furthermore, the relationship between myocardial ischemia and sudden death is very different according to the severity and duration of ischemia.

Severe transmural and persistent ischemia

The observation that experimental coronary occlusion[45] or acute myocardial infarction[46] often results in a variety of ventricular arrhythmias that precede ventricular fibrillation demonstrates a casual relationship between myocardial ischemia and sudden death. Acute myocardial infarction is the clinical model of an acute, severe and long-lasting ischemia. It is well known that myocardial infarction causes a series of electrical, mechanical, and biochemical changes that facilitate the onset of ventricular arrhythmias. We have seen in the previous section some of the pathophysiological mechanisms that may cause these hyperactive arrhythmias, which are usually not due to re-entry phenomena. As the myocardium is more sensitive to ischemia than the specialized conduction system, hyperactive ventricular arrhythmias are more often seen than conduction disturbances or depressed automatism. The incidence of sudden death during acute myocardial infarction is similar whether painful or painless, as has been shown in the Framingham study (Table 7.4).[47]

Furthermore, ischemia may also cause supraventricular or bradyarrhythmias, although these are less frequent. Any of these three types

Table 7.4 Risk of sudden death in recognized versus unrecognized myocardial infarction: 30 year follow-up from the Framingham study.

Myocardial infarction	10-year survival age-adjusted mortality per 1000 at risk			
	Coronary heart disease deaths		Sudden deaths	
	Men	Women	Men	Women
Unrecognized	26	20	10	5
Recognized	27	22	12	5

of arrhythmia may potentially be the cause of sudden cardiac death.

Severe transmural but short-lasting ischemia

It is therefore evident that severe transmurual and persistent myocardial ischemia may trigger malignant ventricular arrhythmias and sudden cardiac death[46] as occurs in the acute phase of clinical or experimental myocardial infarction. However, severe transmural but short-lasting myocardial ischemia, as occurs in Prinzmetal's angina[48–51] or during percutaneous transluminal coronary angioplasty (PTCA),[32,52] frequently gives rise to ventricular arrhythmias, but these are only rarely malignant.[53] The present authors have studied 121 crises of coronary spasm recorded by Holter monitoring in patients with ambulatory Prinzmetal's angina in a stable clinical situation.[48] In this series, 35% of the crises were silent. The crises likely to develop ventricular arrhythmias were those presenting greater ST-segment elevation and longer duration. The same conclusion was reached in the experience of Meinertz et al.[54] during PTCA. In 98 PTCAs performed in 36 patients, 40% of the ischemic episodes were silent. An increase in the number of premature ventricular complexes of 100% or greater, or its appearance, were observed in 40% of either symptomatic or silent episodes. Nevertheless, complex ventricular arryhthmias were observed in only 10% of PTCA procedures, and no patient presented with malignant ventricular arrhythmias. Thus it can be concluded that malignant ventricular arrhythmias resulting in sudden death are very infrequent when the ischemia, although severe and transmural, is of short duration.

Ventricular arrhythmias during ischemic crises may appear not only during the acute phase of ischemia, but also during the reperfusion phase. Although arrhythmias due to reperfusion are a reality from an experimental point of view, they do not seem to represent a harmful clinical problem, as they are rarely malignant. Reperfusion arrhythmias probably appear more often in relation to transient transmural ischemia.[48–51]

Subendocardial ischemia

The clinical relationship between subendocardial ischemia and ventricular arrhythmias is not well defined. Ventricular arrhythmias appear occasionally during positive exercise testing, but are rarely malignant.[55,56] In reported Holter recording studies, when subendocardial ischemia ($\downarrow$ST) is mild to moderate, a clear relationship between ventricular arrhythmias and silent myocardial ischemia is slight or nil.[57–59] Stern et al.[59] and Carboni et al.[60] found that in some patients ventricular ectopic activity increased during ischemic episodes identified by Holter monitoring. On the contrary, no relationship was found between ventricular arrhythmias and silent myocardial ischemia detected by Holter ECG in the series of Graboys et al.[57] and Hausman et al.[58]

In the present authors' experience, there is no relationship between subendocardial ischemia and ventricular arrhythmias.[61,62] The Holter tapes of 70 post-myocardial infarction patients (65 men, 5 women; mean age 54.35 years) recorded 10–20 days after the acute phase were studied. The incidence was analysed of ventricular arrhythmias during evident silent ischemia (ST descent between 1 and 2 mm), probable silent ischemia (five minutes before and after ST descent), and the period without silent ischemia. Evidence was found of silent ischemia in 29 tapes with a total of 110 crises. Premature ventricular complexes were observed in 19 crises (17.2%). There was no significant difference between crises with and without ventricular arryhthmias regarding lengthening of crises and ST descent. The incidence of ventricular arrhythmias during silent ischemia (evident, probable and global), compared with periods without silent ischemia, was not significant (Table 7.5). Thus, at least in this population of post-myocardial infarction patients with mild ST descent, there was no positive relationship between silent myocardial ischemia and ventricular arrhythmias.

On the other hand, in a study of patients who died suddenly while wearing a Holter device,[63] a crisis of silent ischemia, expressed by a new

Table 7.5   Relationship between silent myocardial ischemia and ventricular arrhythmias in Holter ECG.

Period	Time	PVC	Couplets and runs
Without SI	601 h 20 s	6 400 = 10.64 x h	48 = 0.07 x h
With evident SI	24 h 18 s	176 = 7.33 x h	2 = 0.08 x h
With probable SI	18 h 10 s	339 = 18.8 x h	2 = 0.11 x h
Global SI	42 h 28 s	515 = 12.2 x h	4 = 0.10 x h

PVC: Premature ventricular contractions; SI: silent myocardial ischemia; xh = /hour

ST-segment descent, was observed in only 12.5% of patients in whom the final event was a classical ventricular fibrillation. On the contrary, ST-segment ascent is very frequent in ambulatory patients who suddenly die due to bradyarrhythmia (approximately 90%). We can therefore conclude that myocardial ischemia, as a triggering mechanism of sudden death, is globally present in about one-third of all cases.

A new ischemic episode of subendocardial ischemia before sudden death does not seem to be frequent. In the series of Gomes et al.,[64] no relationship was found between silent myocardial ischemia and triggering of ventricular arrhythmias. In the series of Pepine et al.[65] the incidence was greater. Of the 35 cases of patients who died while wearing a Holter ECG, the recording was not interpretable in approximately one-third, ischemic ST-segment changes were observed in another third, while no ischemic changes were observed in the remaining third. Therefore, in cases where the Holter ECG was interpretable, ST changes were observed in 50%. However, there was an important number of cases of bradyarrhythmia as a cause of sudden death in this study, which may explain the high incidence of ST-segment alterations. As we have already mentioned, the patients dying suddenly due to a bradyarrhythmia also showed a higher incidence of acute ST changes. These patients reflect the fact that in most of these patients the bradyarrhythmia was merely the final step of important myocardial damage (massive myocardial infarction, myocardial rupture, etc.).

PROGNOSTIC SIGNIFICANCE OF MYOCARDIAL ISCHEMIA

Some discrepancies exist regarding the role of silent ischemia in coronary patients, especially regarding the prognostic value for malignant ventricular arrhythmias and sudden cardiac death (Table 7.6). As we will see, its prognostic value depends on the groups of patients studied, and also on how close to the coronary event the ischemia is detected.

Different authors[34,66] have demonstrated that post-myocardial infarction patients with painless ST-segment depression during exercise testing have the same prognosis as patients with angina. Theroux et al.[34] performed exercise tests in 210 post-myocardial infarction patients and found ischemic ST changes in 64 (34%). In 37 (58%) ischemia was silent, whereas 27 (42%) had symptomatic ischemia. During 1-year follow-up the mortality rate was 27% (17/64) in patients with ST-segment depression and only 2.1% (3/146) in those without. Sudden cardiac death occurred in 16% (10/64) of patients with ST changes and in 0.7% (1/146) of those without, whether the ischemia was painful or painless. Weiner et al.[66] studied 424 patients with silent myocardial ischemia during the exercise test and

Table 7.6 Prognosis of silent ischemia.

Coronary event	Risk group	Result	Authors
Unstable angina	–	Poor prognosis	Gottlieb et at.[67]
			Nademanee et al.[68]
Stable angina	High-risk patients	Poor prognosis	Tzivoni et al.[69]
			Rocco et al.[71]
			Deedwania et al.[70]
	Low-risk patients	Low prognostic value	Quyyumi et al.[44]
			Mulcahy et al.[72]

found that the risk of sudden cardiac death at 7 years was 9%. This risk was similar to that of patients with symptomatic ST depression during the effort test (7% at 7 years), and significantly greater than that of patients without coronary artery disease (1% at 7 years; $P < 0.001$).

Among patients with silent ischemia, the risk of sudden death was related to the severity of coronary artery disease and the degree of left ventricular dysfunction. Patients with preserved left ventricular function and one-vessel disease had a risk of myocardial infarction or sudden death of 10% at 7 years, compared with 62% of risk in patients with three-vessel disease and abnormal left ventricular function ($P < 0.001$). Interestingly, among patients with three-vessel disease the risk of sudden death was significantly greater in patients with silent ischemia than in patients with angina (21% versus 7%; $P < 0.001$).

The poor prognostic implications of ST-segment depression detected by Holter are also established (Table 7.6), both in patients with unstable[67,68] and stable[69,70] angina (Figs 7.4 and 7.5). Tzivoni et al.[69] analysed the prognostic value of ischemia detected by Holter monitoring in 224 post-infarction patients. Transient episodes of ST depression were observed in 33%. The frequency of cardiac events (cardiac death, reinfarction, unstable angina, bypass surgery or coronary angioplasty) was 51% among patients with

silent ischemia compared with 12% among patients without ischemia ($P < 0.001$). Furthermore, in patients with a positive exercise test and with ischemia in Holter the number of cardiac events was significantly higher (51% versus 20%; $P < 0.001$). The event rate in patients with ischemic changes either on Holter or on exercise test was only 8.5%. It was observed that Holter adds information about the prognosis of ischemia after myocardial infarction and that the information given by exercise testing and Holter monitoring is not redundant.

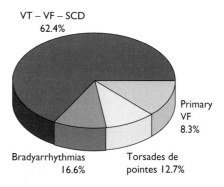

Figure 7.3 Final arrhythmia detected in patients dying while wearing a Holter device. VF: ventricular fibrillation; VT: ventricular tachycardia; SCD: sudden cardiac death. (Adapted from Bayés de Luna et al.[63])

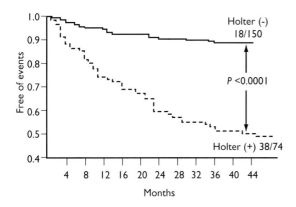

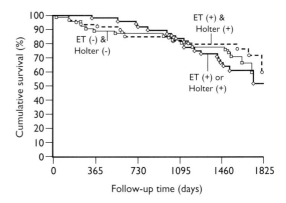

Figure 7.4 Prognostic significance of myocardial ischemia. (Adapted from Tzivoni et al.[69])

Figure 7.6 As we can observe no differences in survival were seen between the three groups of patients. ET (+): exercise test positive; Holter (+): Holter with ischemia. (Adapted from Mulcahy et al.[72])

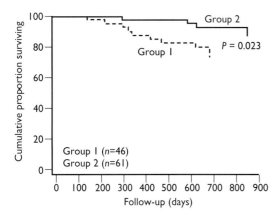

Figure 7.5 Prognostic significance of myocardial ischemia in patients with stable angina. (Adapted from Deedwania et al.[70])

Deedwania et al.[70] analysed the prognostic significance of silent ischemia detected by ambulatory monitoring in 107 patients. All the patients had long-term stable angina, controlled symptomatically with oral medications. Ischemia was observed in 46 patients. In those, 87% of the episodes were silent. In the remaining 61 patients no ischemia was observed. During the follow-up (mean 24 months) more cardiac events were observed in the 46 patients with Holter-detected

ischemia (five sudden cardiac deaths and six nonsudden cardiac deaths) when compared with patients without ischemia (five nonsudden cardiac deaths). Kaplan–Meier survival analysis between the two groups confirmed that patients with silent ischemia had a worse prognosis during the follow-up ($P = 0.023$). In this study the presence of ischemia in Holter ECG was the most powerful predictor of outcome.

It has also been shown by Rocco et al.[71] that coronary heart disease patients who present ST-segment changes during exercise testing had a worse prognosis if they had spontaneous ST-segment changes detected by Holter.

Some other studies in patients at low risk show that the presence of silent ischemia in Holter monoitoring has no prognostic implications. Mulcahy et al.[72] studied 174 patients with chronic stable angina. Sixty percent of these patients showed ischemia during an exercise test and 40% during daily life activity. Thirty percent showed alterations in both tests. As can be seen in Fig. 7.6, no differences in mortality were found during a long follow-up (median 50 months). Arrhythmic events and sudden cardiac death were similar in the different groups. Quyyumi et al.[73] found

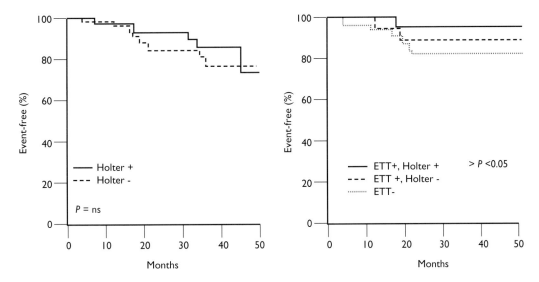

Figure 7.7 Prognostic value of Holter-detected ischemia. Quyyumi et al.[44]

similar results when evaluating 116 low-risk (selected by coronary angiography and left ventricular function) coronary artery disease patients as can be seen in Fig. 7.7. None of the clinical, treadmill exercise, radionuclide ventriculography or cardiac catheterization variables were predictive of outcome.

Recently, two major multicenter studies[74,75] have presented some discordant results regarding the prognostic value of ischemia in ischemic heart disease patients. The Multicenter Myocardial Ischemia Research Group[74] studied 936 patients who were clinically stable 1–6 months after hospitalization for an acute coronary event. Patients with unstable angina and myocardial infarction were included. Resting ECG, ambulatory ECG, exercise testing and stress thallium-201 scintigraphy were performed. It is important to stress that the study was designed to evaluate recurrent primary events (cardiac death, nonfatal infarction, or unstable angina), or restricted events (cardiac death or nonfatal infarction). The study was not specifically directed to evaluation of sudden cardiac death. ST-segment depression was detected by resting ECG in 11%, by Holter

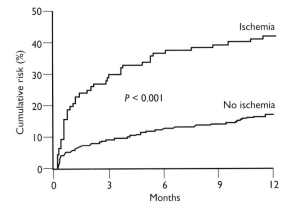

Figure 7.8 Prognostic significance of silent ischemia in 48-hour Holter ECG regarding total events (cardiac death + myocardial infarction + unstable angina).

in 8%, by exercise test in 29% and by stress thallium scintigraphy in 41%. In Fig. 7.8 and Table 7.7 we can see the summary of the results of the study. ST-segment depression in resting ECG was the only noninvasive marker of an increased risk for primary recurrent coronary

Table 7.7 Factors associated with recurrent restricted events (cardiac death or myocardial infarction).	Hazard ratio	P
Resting ECG	2.27	< 0.01
Holter ECG	1.24	0.60
Exercise electrocardiogram	0.74	0.30
Stress thallium scintigraphy	1.40	0.17

Source: Adapted from Moss et al.[74]

Table 7.8 Prognostic importance of different tests in post-myocardial infarction patients.	Positive	Negative	Not done
Holter	11.6*	3.9	–
Exercise testing	3.9	3.0	16.4*
EF < 35%	18.2*	3.5	14.7*

*Statistically significant.
Source: Adapted from Gill et al.[75]

events (hazard ratio 1.5, $P < 0.05$). The presence of ischemia in the thallium stress test indicated a slightly increased risk of coronary events ($P = 0.048$). The presence of ischemia in Holter ECG or in conventional exercise testing does not indicate an increased risk of death. No specific data regarding sudden cardiac death or ventricular arrhythmias were reported. It is important to stress that the risk of cardiac events was greater when exercise-induced ST depression was coherent with data of reduced left ventricular function (increased lung uptake during the thallium exercise test). This multicenter study confirms that the presence of ischemia is probably not of great prognostic value when we study 'low-risk' patients. One must bear in mind that all patients were enrolled at least 1 month after the coronary event and in a stable condition.

On the contrary, another multicenter study recently showed the value of detection of ambulatory ischemia by Holter ECG as a prognostic tool in post-myocardial infarction patients.[75] In this study 406 out of 952 patients were enrolled very soon after a myocardial infarction (5–7 days). In all patients, 48-hour Holter ECG, submaximal exercise testing and measurement of left ventricular function were performed. The end points of the study were death, nonfatal myocardial infarction and

unstable angina. It is also important to remember that ventricular tachycardias or sudden cardiac death are not reported specifically, so we must extrapolate the data from the total for cardiac death. Silent ischemia in Holter was present in 23% of patients, in exercise testing in 31% and in ejection fraction below 50% it was present in 40% of patients. As one can see by comparison with the study of Moss et al.,[74] the incidence of abnormal tests is much higher, thus indicating a higher-risk population. At 1-year follow-up the incidence of death was 5.7%, the incidence of death or myocardial infarction was 12.8%, and the incidence of death or myocardial infarction or unstable angina was 25%. Left ventricular dysfunction (detected by ejection fraction < 35%) was the stronger predictor of mortality. Table 7.8 summarizes the results of the prognostic value of each test. It can be seen that ejection fraction is the strongest predictor of total mortality and also, in confirmation of the results of previous studies, that the inability to perform an exercise test is predictive of bad outcome. The importance of silent ischemia as a risk factor was striking. The mortality rate at 1 year was 3.9% among patients without ambulatory ischemia and 11.6% among those with ischemia. It is important to note that only small differences were found regarding the outcome of patients with

Table 7.9   Joint prognostic value of Holter and ejection fraction.

		Death (%)	Death+MI (%)	Death+MI+UA (%)
EF > 50%	Holter(−)	3.4	6.7	17.4
	Holter(+)	4.3	19.6	34.8
EF 35–50%	Holter(−)	1.1	12.1	19.8
	Holter(+)	12.5	25.0	50.0
EF < 35%	Holter(−)	15.0	25.0	30.0
	Holter(+)	23.0	30.8	61.5

MI: myocardial infarction; UA: unstable angina; EF: ejection fraction.
Source: Adapted from Gill et al.[75]

conserved ejection fraction (>50%) and patients with only moderate reduction (35–50%), but mortality increases when a marked low ejection fraction is present (< 35%). Although the ejection fraction was the strongest predictor of mortality, ischemia on Holter ECG represented additional prognostic information (Table 8.9).

On the other hand, transient myocardial ischemia (subendocardial and subepicardial) does not induce late potentials in the signal-averaged ECG, thus supporting the idea that silent subendocardial ischemia does not change arrhythmogenic substrate. Turitto et al.[76] investigated 100 patients with known coronary artery disease who underwent serial recording of the signal-averaged ECG before, during and after dipyridamole. During the test, 47 patients developed transient myocardial ischemia (ST-segment ascent in 14 cases and ST-segment descent in 33). Baseline signal-averaged ECG was abnormal in 20 patients and there were no significant differences between them regarding inducible ischemia (26 versus 15% respectively). Absence of significant differences was also observed before, during and after the dipyridamole test. Normal signal-averaged ECG recordings became abnormal during dipyridamole infusion in only two patients. This suggests that the substrate for chronic re-entrant ventricular tachyarrhythmias is not influenced

by the electrophysiologic changes induced during transient myocardial ischemia.[76]

SILENT ISCHEMIA IN EXERCISE TEST VERSUS AMBULATORY MONITORING

Although there is evidence that ischemia can be detected both in ambulatory monitoring[33] and exercise test their relationship has not been fully reported. Very recently Stone et al.[77] studied whether the prognostic value from each risk-stratifying test is unique or redundant. The study demonstrated that: (1) angina was more frequent among patients with ambulatory ischemic episodes compared with patients free of them (P < 0.001); (2) patients with Holter ischemia presented more ischemia during exercise testing than patients without ischemia during ambulatory monitoring; (3) patients likely to have Holter ischemic episodes could be predicted on the basis of the exercise test performance characteristics. In spite of these results the relationship between silent ischemia in Holter monitoring and exercise testing is limited, indicating that the two tests are both of use in characterizing coronary patients. The magnitude of ischemia identified by one test does not appear to be a substitute for the magnitude of ischemia detected by the other test. These results suggest that the mechanisms responsible for ischemia identified by both tests may be different. Exercise testing looks more specifically to an increase in oxygen demand as a response to exercise. Holter looks not only at this aspect but also at the possibility of a decrease in oxygen supply (due for example to an increased coronary tone). A larger study with long follow-up for clinical events is required to investigate the relative prognostic importance of ST deviations detected by each modality and the value of both tests in the management of coronary patients.

DIRECT (TRIGGERING) AND INDIRECT (*MILIEU*) RELATIONSHIP BETWEEN SILENT MYOCARDIAL ISCHEMIA AND SUDDEN CARDIAC DEATH

The role of silent myocardial ischemia in sudden cardiac death must be differentiated with regard to its direct and indirect relationship. A direct relationship means we have certain evidence, at least according to our present knowledge, that acute myocardial ischemia triggers sudden death, as in the case of malignant ventricular arrhythmia preceded by ST-segment descent with or without pain (for example in Holter or exercise testing). An indirect relationship means that sudden death appears in the presence (*milieu*) of chronic ischemia. This difference is important, since a direct relationship indicates a cause and effect mechanism, while in the case of an indirect relationship, this would only be an associated phenomenon, although myocardial ischemia could interact in the mechanisms leading to sudden death. The phenomenon of sudden cardiac death in summarized in Fig. 7.9. Some trigger factors act on a vulnerable myocardium leading to the final step: sudden cardiac death.

A direct relationship between silent transient ischemia and sudden death exists. In favor of this:

1) Some isolated cases of ST alterations before sudden death have been published.[78]
2) In the authors' series[63] of patients dying suddenly while wearing a Holter device

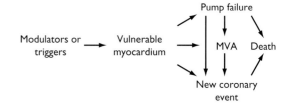

Figure 7.9   Sudden cardiac death. Some modulators or triggers act on a vulnerable myocardium and this leads to a new coronary event, a malignant ventricular arrhythmia or pump failure. Each of these three alterations can trigger the other and finally can degenerate to cardiac or sudden cardiac death. MVA: malignant ventricular arrhythmia.

only a small percentage presented ST alteration beforehand when the final event was a ventricular tachyarrhythmia. Almost the same incidence was reported by Gomes et al.[64] and Pepine et al.[65] The incidence of myocardial ischemia as a trigger of sudden death ranges between 30 and 50%, and depends on the number of patients in whom bradyarrhythmia was the final event, as many of these present ischemic ST alterations, especially due to myocardial infarction with electromechanical dissociation.

3) When silent ischemia is severe, transmural, and persistent, as occurs in some cases of silent myocardial infarction, the problem is different. In the Framingham study, the incidence of cardiac death and sudden death is similar in patients with silent or symptomatic myocardial infarctions. These results suggest a direct relationship between silent ischemia and sudden death, as silent myocardial ischemia must be the triggering mechanism in cases of sudden death in patients with painless myocardial infarction. This likely represents only a small percentage of myocardial infarction patients, as silent myocardial infarction represents only 20% of all infarctions, and sudden cardiac death, in turn, only appears

in 20% of these, representing about 5% of all myocardial infarction.

Some arguments against a direct relationship between transient silent ischemia and sudden cardiac death are:

1) the very low incidence of malignant ventricular arrhythmias during positive exercise testing, PTCA or Prinzmetal's angina;[54,79]
2) the low incidence of ventricular arrhythmias during subendocardial ischemia;[80,57]
3) the low incidence of cardiac symptoms before sudden death;[81-83]
4) the low incidence of myocardial infarction in out-of-hospital sudden death[84] (especially in patients with known coronary artery disease).

Regarding an indirect relationship it has been demonstrated by epidemiological, clinical and pathological studies that ischemia plays a very important role as a *milieu* in which sudden death appears.

1) From an epidemiological point of view, at least 80–90 cases of sudden death present ischemic heart disease. In the authors' series, 90% of patients who die presenting ventricular fibrillation as a final event are ischemic heart disease patients.
2) The papers of Sharma et al.[85] and Warnes and Roberts[86] demonstrated that sudden cardiac death occurs in patients with silent myocardial ischemia, but these findings are also a manifestation of an indirect relationship. Sharma et al.[85] studied 15 patients who survived out-of-hospital ventricular fibrillation (nine without history of angina or myocardial infarction). No patient had angina during exercise at catheterization, but 12 of 15 had ST-segment depression, and 11 presented abnormal wall motion, suggesting that silent myocardial ischemia is present in the majority of patients who survive an out-of-hospital cardiac arrest. Silent myocardial ischemia may therefore play a role in out-of-hospital cardiac arrest.

3) Warnes and Roberts[86] carried out necropsy studies in 70 victims of sudden cardiac death to determine the amount and distribution of cross-sectional area luminal narrowing in each five-interval segment of the four major coronary arteries, and compared the amount of narrowing both qualitatively and quantitively in those with ($n = 31$) and without ($n = 39$) previous evidence of myocardial ischemia. Comparison of the number of coronary arteries severely narrowed (>75%) (qualitative analysis) revealed no significant differences between previously asymptomatic and symptomatic patients. However, symptomatic victims had a significantly higher mean percentage of severely narrowed (>75%) 5 mm segments (30% versus 25%; $P < 0.005$) (quantitative analysis).

CONCLUSION

There are extensive data favoring an indirect relationship between silent myocardial ischemia and sudden cardiac death. However, a direct relationship detected by current methods is present in only a small percentage of cases when the cause of sudden cardiac death is ventricular fibrillation. The relationship between ischemia and sudden death is not uniform but depends on the duration and intensity of the ischemia, and the risk group of patients studied. The relation may be direct or indirect and future studies will reveal the therapeutic consequences of this association.

Table 7.10   Evolution of silent ischemia.

Authors	Year	Advances
Stern and Tzivoni[33]	1974	Concept
Deanfield et al.[36]	1984	Confirmation
Gill et al.[75]	1996	Prognosis
ACIP II	?	Treatment?

REFERENCES

1. Lown B. Sudden cardiac death: the major challenge confronting contemporary cardiology. *Am J Cardiol* 1979; **43**: 313–28.

2. Working Group on Arteriosclerosis of the National Heart, Lung, and Blood Institute. *Volume 2: Patient Oriented Research – Fundamental and Applied, Sudden Cardiac Death.* DHEW, NIH Publication no. 82-2035. (Washington, DC: US Government Printing Office, 1981): 114–22.

3. Cohn PF. Total ischemic burden: definition, mechanisms, and therapeutic implications. *Am J Med* 1986; **81 (suppl 4A)**: 2–6.

4. Cohn PF, ed. *Silent Myocardial Ischemia and Infarction* (New York: Marcel Dekker, 1989).

5. Rutishauser W, Roskman H eds. *Silent Myocardial Ischemia* (Berlin: Springer Verlag, 1984).

6. Parmley W. Silent myocardial ischemia. *Am J Med* 1985; **79 (suppl 3A)**: 1–34.

7. Singh B. Detection, quantification and clinical significance of silent myocardial ischemia in coronary artery disease. *Am J Cardiol* 1986; **58 (suppl B)**: 1–60.

8. Pepine C. Silent myocardial ischemia. *Cardiol Clin* 1986; **4**: 577–8.

9. Cohn P, Kannel W. Recognition, pathogenesis and management options in silent coronary artery disease. *Circulation* 1987; **75 (suppl II)**: 1–53.

10. Bayés de Luna A. Avances en electrocardiología: isquemia miocárdica silente. *Rev Latina Cardiol* 1987; **8 (suppl 1)**: 1–61.

11. Morris JJ. Medical management of silent ischemia and myocardial infarction. *Am J Cardiol* 1988; **61 (suppl B)**: 1–31.

12. Morganroth J, Moore EN, eds. *Silent Myocardial Ischemia* (Boston: Kluwer Academic, 1988).

13. Sing BN, Phil D, eds. *Silent Myocardial Ischemia and Angina* (New York: Pergamon Press, 1988).

14. Von Armin T, Maseri A, eds. *Silent Ischemia: Current Concepts and Management* (Darmstadt: Steinkopff, 1987).

15. Lauler DP. Silent myocardial ischemia and infarction. Past, present and future. *Am J Cardiol* 1988; **61 (suppl F)**: 1–49.

16. Roskman H, Rutishauser W. Silent myocardial ischemia. Treatment strategies of ischemia. *Eur Heart J* 1988; **9 (suppl N)**: 1–185.

17. Kellermann JJ, Braunwald E, eds. *Silent Myocardial Ischemia: A Critical Appraisal* (Basel: Karger, 1990).

18. Pepine CJ. Silent myocardial ischemia: definition, magnitude, and scope of the problem. *Cardiol Clin* 1986; **4**: 577–81.

19. Bayés de Luna A, Brugada J, Cosin J, Navarro Lopez F, eds. *Sudden Cardiac Death* (Dordrecht: Kluwer Academic, 1991).

20. Kulbertus HE, Wellens HJJ, eds. *Sudden Death* (The Hague: Martinus Nijhoff, 1980).

21. Morganroth J, Horowitz LN. *Sudden Cardiac Death* (Orlando, FL: Grune & Stratton, 1985).

22. Myerburg RJ, Castellanos A. Cardiovascular arrest and sudden cardiac death. In: Braunwald E, ed. *Heart Disease* (Philadelphia, PA: WB Saunders, 1988): 742–77.

23. Greenberg HM, Dwyer EM. Sudden coronary death. *Ann N Y Acad Sci* 1982; **382**: 1–484.

24. Kostis JB, Sanders M. *The Prevention of Sudden Cardiac Death* (New York: Wiley-Liss, 1990).

25. DiMarco JP, Haines DE. Sudden cardiac death. *Curr Probl Cardiol* 1990; **15**: 183–232.

26. The Cardiac Arrhythmia Suppression Trial (CAST) Investigators. Preliminary report: effect of encainide and flecainide on mortality in a randomized trial of arrhythmia suppression after myocardial infarction. *N Engl J Med* 1989; **321**: 406–12.

27. Kennedy HL. Late proarrhythmia and understanding the time of occurrence. *Am J Cardiol* 1990; **66**: 1139–43.

28. Nesto R, Kowalchuk G. The ischemic cascade: temporal sequence of hemodynamic, electrocardiographic and symptomatic expressions of ischemia. *Am J Cardiol* 1987; **57 (suppl C)**: 23–30.

29. Janse MJ, Kléber AG. Electrophysiological changes and ventricular arrhythmias in early phase of myocardial ischemia. *Circ Res* 1981; **49**: 1064–81.

30. Kléber AJ, Janse MJ. Impulse propagation in myocardial ischemia. In: Zipes DP, Jalife J, eds. *Cardiac Electrophysiology. From Cell to Bedside* (Philadelphia, PA: WB Saunders, 1990): 156–61.

31. Sigwart U, Grebic M, Payot M, Boy JJ, Essinger A, Fischer A. Ischemic events during coronary artery balloon obstruction. In: Rutishauser W, Roskman H, eds. *Silent Myocardial Ischemia* (Berlin: Springer Verlag, 1984): 29–36.

32. Hauser AM, Gangadharan V, Ramos RG, Gordon S, Timmis GC. Sequence of mechanical, electrocardiographic and clinical effects of repeated coronary artery occlusion in human

beings: echocardiographic observations during coronary angioplasty. *J Am Coll Cardiol* 1985; **5**: 193–7.

33. Stern S, Tzivoni D. Early detection of silent ischemic heart disease by 24-hour ECG monitoring during daily activity. *Br Heart J* 1974; **36**: 481–6.

34. Theroux P, Waters D, Halphen C, Debaisieux JC, Mizgala H. Prognostic value of exercise testing soon after myocardial infarction. *N Engl J Med* 1979; **301**: 341–5.

35. Deanfield J, Shea M, Ribiero P et al. Transient ST-segment depression as a marker of myocardial ischemia during daily life. *Am J Cardiol* 1984; **54**: 1195–200.

36. Deanfield J, Ribeiro P, Oakley C, Kliker S, Selwyn AP. Critical analysis of ST segment changes in normal subjects: implications for ambulatory monitoring of myocardial ischemia in patients with angina. *Am J Cardiol* 1984; **54**: 1321–5.

37. Taki J, Yasuda T, Gold HK et al. Characteristics of transient left ventricular dysfunction detected by ambulatory left ventricular function monitoring device in patients with coronary artery disease. *Circulation* 1987; **76 (suppl IV)**: 336.

38. Harris HS. Delayed development of ventricular ectopic rhythms following experimental coronary occlusion. *Circulation* 1950; **I**: 1318–28.

39. Harris HS, Bisteni A, Russell RA et al. Excitatory factors in ventricular tachycardia resulting from myocardial ischemia: potassium a major excitant. *Science* 1954; **199**: 200–3.

40. Katzing BG. Effects of extracellular calcium and sodium on depolarization induced automaticity in guinea pigs' papillary muscle. *Circ Res* 1975; **37**: 118–27.

41. Kleber AG, Riegger CB, Janse MJ. Electrical uncoupling and increased extracellular resistance after induction of ischemia in isolated, arterially perfused rabbit papillary muscle. *Circ Res* 1987; **61**: 271–9.

42. Falcone C, Specchia G, Rondanelli R et al. Correlation between beta-endorphin plasma levels and anginal symptoms in patients with coronary artery disease. *J Am Coll Cardiol* 1988; **11**: 719–23.

43. Falcone C, Sconocchia R, Guasti L, Codega S, Montemartine C, Specchia G. Dental pain threshold and angina pectoris in patients with coronary artery disease. *J Am Coll Cardiol* 1988; **12**: 348–52.

44. Quyyumi AA, Panza JA, Lakatos E, Epstein SE. Circadian variation in ischemic events: causal role of variation in ischemic threshold due to changes in vascular resistance. *Circulation* 1988; **78 (suppl II)**: 331.

45. Kléber AJ, Janse MJ. Impulse propagation in myocardial ischemia. In: Zipes DP, Jalife J, eds. *Cardiac Electrophysiology. From Cell to Bedside* (Philadelphia, PA: WB Saunders, 1990): 156–61.

46. Rosen M, Palti Y. *Lethal Arrhythmias Resulting from Myocardial Ischemia and Infarction* (Boston, MA: Kluwer Academic, 1989).

47. Kannel WB, Cupples LA, D'Agostino RB. Sudden death risk in overt coronary heart disease: the Framingham study. *Am Heart J* 1987; **113**: 799.

48. Bayés de Luna A, Carreras F, Cladellas M, Oca F, Sagués F, Garcia Moll M. Holter ECG study of the electrocardiographic phenomenon in Prinzmetal angina attacks with emphasis on the study of ventricular arrhythmias. *J Electrocardiol* 1985; **18**: 267–76.

49. Previtali M, Klersy C, Salerno J. Ventricular arrhythmias in Prinzmetal's variant angina. Clinical significance and relation to the degree and time course of ST segment elevation. *Am J Cardiol* 1983; **52**: 19–25.

50. Puddu PE, Bourassa M, Waters DD, Lesperance J. Sudden death in two patients with variant angina and apparently minimal fixed coronary stenoses. *J Electrocardiol* 1983; **16**: 213–20.

51. Tzivoni D, Keren A, Granot H, Gottlieb S, Benhorin J, Stern S. Ventricular fibrillation caused by myocardial reperfusion in Prinzmetal's angina. *Am Heart J* 1983; **105**: 323–5.

52. Sigwart U, Grebic M, Payot M, Boy JJ, Essinger A, Fischer A. Ischemic events during coronary artery balloon obstruction. In: Rutishauser W, Roskman H, eds. *Silent Myocardial Ischemia* (Berlin: Springer Verlag, 1984): 29–36.

53. Nakamura M, Takeshita A, Nose Y. Clinical characteristics associated with myocardial infarction, arrhythmias, and sudden death in patients with vasospastic angina. *Circulation* 1987; **75**: 1110–16.

54. Meinertz T, Zeheder M, Hohnloser S, Just H. Prevalence of ventricular arrhythmias during silent myocardial ischemia. *Cardiovasc Rev & Rep* 1988; **(suppl A)**: 34–8.

55. Fintel DJ, Platia EV. Exercise testing and cardiac arrhythmias. In: Platia EV, ed. *Cardiac Arrhythmias: Nonpharmacological Approach* (Philadelphia, PA: JB Lippincott, 1987): 28–35.

56. Hong R, Bhandari A, McKay C, Au P, Rahimtoola S. Lifethreatening ventricular tachycardia and fibrillation induced by painless myocardial ischemia during exercise test. *JAMA* 1987; **257**: 1937–40.

57. Graboys TB, Stein IM, Cueni L, Lampert S, Lown B. Is the presence of silent ischemia associated with the provocation of ventricular arrhythmias? *Circulation* 1987; **76 (suppl IV)**: 365.

58. Hausmann D, Nikutta P, Trappe HJ, Daniel WG, Wenzlaff P, Lichtlen PR. Incidence of ventricular arrhythmias during transient myocardial ischemia in patients with stable coronary artery disease. *J Am Coll Cardiol* 1990; **16**: 49–54.

59. Stern S, Banai S, Keren A, Tzivoni D. Ventricular ectopic activity during myocardial ischemia episodes in ambulatory patients. *Am J Cardiol* 1990; **65**: 412–15.

60. Carboni GP, Lahiri A, Cashman PMM, Raftery EB. Mechanisms of arrhythmias accompanying ST-segment depression on ambulatory monitoring in stable angina pectoris. *Am J Cardiol* 1987; **60**: 1246–51.

61. Bayés de Luna A, Camacho AM, Guindo J et al. Is there a relationship between crises of silent ischemia and appearance of ventricular arrhythmias? *Eur Heart J* 1989; **10 (suppl A)**: 29.

62. Camacho AM, Guindo J, Bayés de Luna A. Usefulness of silent myocardial ischemia detected by ST segment depression in postmyocardial infarction as a predictor of ventricular arrhythmias. *Am J Cardiol*, 1992; **69**: 1243–45.

63. Bayés de Luna A, Coumel Ph, Leclercq JF. Ambulatory sudden death: mechanisms of production of fatal arrhythmias on the basis of data from 157 cases. *Am Heart J* 1989; **117**: 151–54.

64. Gomes JA, Alexopoulos D, Winters SL, Deshmukh P, Fuster V, Suh K. The role of silent ischemia, the arrhythmic substrate and the short–long sequence in the genesis of sudden cardiac death. *J Am Coll Cardiol* 1989; **14**: 1618–22.

65. Pepine CJ, Gottlieb SO, Morganroth J. Ambulatory ischemia and sudden death: analysis of 35 cases of sudden death during ambulatory ECG monitoring. *J Am Coll Cardiol* 1991; **17**: 63–5.

66. Weiner DA, Ryan TJ, McCabe CH et al. Significance of silent myocardial ischemia during exercise testing in patients with coronary artery disease. *Am J Cardiol* 1987; **59**: 725–9.

67. Gottlieb LS, Weisfeldt M, Ouyang P, Mellits D, Gertenblinth G. Silent ischemia as a marker for

68. Nademanee K, Intrarachot V, Josephson MA, Rieders D, Mody FV, Singh PN. Prognostic significance of silent myocardial ischemia in patients with unstable angina. *J Am Coll Cardiol* 1987; **10**: 1–9.

early unfavorable outcomes in patients with unstable angina. *N Engl J Med* 1986; **314**: 1214–19.

69. Tzivoni D, Gavish A, Gottlieb S et al. Prognostic significance of ischemic episodes in patients. *Am J Cardiol* 1988; **62**: 661–4.

70. Deedwania P, Carbajai E, Nelson J. Silent ischemia during Holter monitoring: a marker of mortality and adverse clinical outcome in stable angina. *Circulation* 1988; **78 (suppl II)**: 43.

71. Rocco MB, Nabel EG, Campbell S et al. Prognostic importance of myocardial ischemia detected by ambulatory monitoring in patients with stable coronary artery disease. *Circulation* 1988; **78**: 877–84.

72. Mulcahy D, Knight D, Patel D et al. Detection of ambulatory ischemia is not of practical clinical value in the routine management of patients with stable angina. A long-term follow-up study. *Eur Heart J* 1995; **16**: 317–24.

73. Quyyumi A, Panza J, Diodati J et al. Prognostic implications of myocardial ischemia during daily life in low risk patients with coronary artery disease. *J Am Coll Cardiol* 1993: **21**: 700–8.

74. Moss AJ, Goldstein R, Hall J et al. Detection and significance of myocardial ischemia after recovery from an acute coronary event. *JAMA* 1993; **269**: 2379–85.

75. Gill JB, Cairns J, Roberts R et al. Prognostic importance of myocardial ischemia detected by ambulatory monitoring early after acute myocardial infarction. *N Engl J Med* 1996; **334**: 65–70.

76. Turitto G, Zanchi E, Risa AL et al. Lack of correlation between transient myocardial ischemia and late potentials on the signal-averaged electrocardiogram. *Am J Cardiol* 1990; **65**: 290–6.

77. Stone PH, Chaitman BR, McMahon RP et al. Asymptomatic Cardiac Ischemia Pilot (ACIP) Study. Relationship between exercise-induced and ambulatory ischemia in patients with stable coronary disease. *Circulation* 1996; **94**: 1537–44.

78. Gradman AH, Bell PA, DeBusj RF. Sudden death during ambulatory monitoring: clinical and electrocardiographic correlations. Report of a case. *Circulation* 1977; **55**: 210–11.

79. McHenry PL. Clinical role of exercise testing for detection, evaluation and treatment of ventricular arrhythmias. In: Zipes P, Jalife J, eds. *Cardiac Electrophysiology. From Cell to Bedside* (Philadelphia, PA: WB Saunders, 1990): 832–7.

80. Farré J, Brugada P. Extrasystoles ventriculares postinfarto y el uso de fármacos antiarrítmicos: un peligro anticipado por los electrofisiólogos. *Rev Esp Cardiol* 1989; **42**: 498–500.

81. Goldstein S, Landis JR, Leighton R et al. Characteristics of the resuscitated out-of-hospital cardiac arrest victim with coronary heart disease. *Circulation* 1981; **64**: 977–82.

82. Goldstein S, Landis JR, Leighton R et al. Predictive survival models for resuscitated victims of out-of-hospital cardiac arrest with coronary heart disease. *Circulation* 1985; **71**: 873–78.

83. Goldstein S, Medendrop SV, Landis RJ et al. Analysis of cardiac symptoms preceding cardiac arrest. *Am J Cardiol* 1986; **58**: 1195–98.

84. Cobb LA, Baum RS, Alvarez H, Shaffer WA. Resuscitation from out of hospital ventricular fibrillation: 4 years' follow-up. *Circulation* 1975; **52 (suppl III)**: 223–27.

85. Sharma B, Asinger R, Francis G, Hodges M, Wyeth R. Demonstration of exercise-induced painless myocardial ischemia in survivors of out-of-hospital ventricular fibrillation. *Am J Cardiol* 1987; **59**: 740–45.

86. Warnes C, Roberts W. Sudden coronary death: relation of amount and distribution of coronary narrowing at necropsy to previous symptoms of myocardial ischemia, left ventricular scarring and heart weight. *Am J Cardiol* 1984; **54**: 65–8.

8

The importance of ambulatory (silent) ischemia in 'low-risk' stable angina patients: observations from the Total Ischemic Burden European Trial (TIBET)

David Mulcahy

INTRODUCTION

Asymptomatic (silent) ischemia in patients with coronary artery disease is today fully characterized in terms of presence, frequency, relationship to the findings of exercise testing, and relationship to ischemic change accompanied by angina.[1–5] 'Silent' ischemia has been confirmed as representing true ischemia in patients with coronary syndromes,[2,6,7] and its characteristics of heart rate at onset, heart rate increase prior to onset of ischemia, in addition to duration of transient ischemic episodes have been shown to be the same as those episodes accompanied by pain.[8,9] Silent ischemia during daily life is now known to occur predominantly in patients with a positive exercise test for ischemia,[10,11] usually at low workload. Silent ischemia is more likely to occur in patients with three-vessel disease than in those with single-vessel disease[5,12] and in those with good rather than poor left ventricular function (greater ischemic burden).[5,13] Approximately 50% of patients with documented coronary artery disease and stable symptoms have transient ischemia during daily activities when off antianginal therapy,[5] and approximately 33% will continue to have silent ischemia despite medical therapy.[14]

An analysis of all the published characteristics data reflects the fact that silent ischemia is very common in patients with coronary artery disease, and is frequent in patients with severe coronary disease and a positive exercise test at low workloads. Most of such patients will also experience anginal symptoms during their daily lives.

By the late 1980s the stage had been reached when it was clear that silent ischemia was common in stable coronary syndromes, and the question to be answered was 'What does it all mean?' If silent ischemia is silent then the patient is not symptomatically affected by it, and thus treatment is unlikely to improve quality of life. If silent ischemia is of prognostic importance then perhaps we should be looking for and aggressively treating it in the hope of improving prognosis, even if the patient is not aware of any improvement. The first published papers assessing the prognosis of silent ischemia confirmed what was expected in patients with stable angina: that patients with silent ischemia during daily life had a significantly worse short- and medium-term prognosis compared with similar patients without silent ischemia.[15–17] It is probably fair to say that all those who commenced prognostic studies at the time expected this to be the case. Many of the early prognostic reports, however, were single-institution affairs with small numbers of subjects, and without a proper 'trial' format. Furthermore, many patients included in these reports were 'high-risk' patients who might, under present circumstances, be more likely candidates for intervention rather than inclusion in natural history studies by virtue of our increased knowledge of those subgroups of stable coronary patients who benefit prognostically from such intervention (left main stem disease; three-vessel disease with reduced left ventricular function; three-vessel disease with proximal left anterior descending involvement, etc.).[18–20] What was not clear from an early stage was what to do with the asymptomatic or mildly symptomatic stable angina patient who had silent ischemia, and whether they were indeed at greater risk of an adverse short- and medium-term outcome compared with similarly characterized patients without silent ischemia. This question was of added clinical importance as such patients represent 'low-risk' patients, in whom intervention had, and has, not been shown to be of prognostic benefit, and thus where management is less straightforward. Furthermore, while it was known that standard antianginal therapies were effective in reducing (but in many cases not abolishing) silent ischemia in stable angina,[21,22] there was no information on whether patients who had a reduction or abolition of their transient ischemic activity had a better outcome than those on the same medications who did not respond similarly in terms of ischemia reduction or abolition.

With these issues in mind a large international European multicentre study (Total Ischemic Burden European Trial—TIBET) was planned with the following objectives:

1) to assess the frequency of transient (silent) ischemia in patients with mild chronic stable angina who were not being considered for intervention;
2) to assess the effects of standard antianginal therapies (atenolol and nifedipine SR) both

individually and in combination, administered in a parallel group format, on the total ischemic burden;
3) to assess the medium-term (2-year) prognosis of such patients with particular reference to whether patients with transient ischemia at the outset had an adverse prognosis compared with those without;
4) to assess whether reduction or abolition of the total ischemic burden by different forms of standard therapy resulted in an improved outlook compared with patients who did not have such a response to therapy;
5) to assess whether any one type of standard medical therapy (or the combination) resulted in an improved prognosis compared with other therapy options.

The trial commenced in the early 1990s and was reported on in 1996.[23–25] The following paragraphs will detail the demographics of the TIBET study population and the results. The discussion will center on the results of the TIBET study but also incorporate all the other studies assessing the medium- and long-term prognostic significance of transient (silent) ischemia in stable coronary syndromes reported in the intervening time from commencement to publication of the TIBET study. The issue of (silent) ischemia in unstable coronary syndromes, either in the setting of unstable angina or in the early postinfarction phase, will not be addressed in detail as the pathophysiological mechanisms underlying the ischemic response in such circumstances (acute plaque rupture, thrombus formation, etc.) will differ considerably from those in stable but significantly obstructive coronary artery disease.

Patient selection for TIBET

Patients of both sexes between the ages of 40 and 79 years with stable angina (of at least 3 months' duration) who had an ischemic response to treadmill or bicycle exercise testing (>1.5 mm ST-segment depression) after a two-week washout period, and who were not being

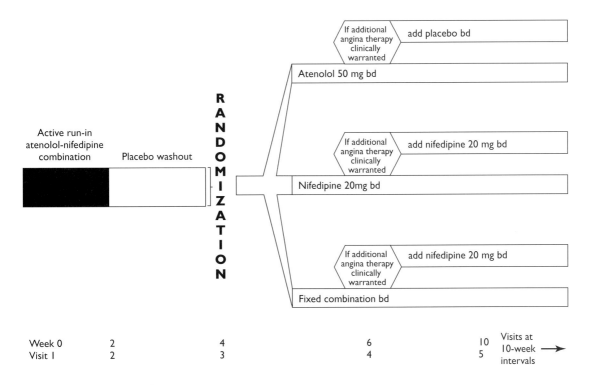

Figure 8.1 TIBET study design.

considered for further investigation or intervention, were considered suitable for inclusion. Over the period of patient recruitment, 682 such patients were enrolled in 69 centers from nine different countries; however, only 608 were considered to have fulfilled properly the (exercise ischemia) inclusion criteria. Standard exclusion criteria had applied, including a history of recent cardiac events, intolerance of any of the study drugs, the taking of medications likely to affect interpretation of the ST-segment, and the presence of significant conduction disturbances on the electrocardiogram.

Study design

Figure 8.1 graphically displays the study design. In short, the TIBET study was a double-blind parallel group comparison of twice daily randomized treatment with atenolol (50 mg bd), nifedipine slow-release (20 mg bd), or their combination, following a one-month run-in period consisting of two weeks of combination therapy (to ensure tolerance of the medications) and then two weeks of single-blind placebo treatment. Baseline measurements (exercise testing and 48 hours of ambulatory ST-segment monitoring) were performed at the end of the two-week placebo phase and prior to randomization. Both investigations were repeated 6 weeks following randomization to allow for assessment of the effects of the various chosen therapies on the total ischemic burden when comparing the findings with baseline. All patients were then followed for an average 2-year period for the purposes of assessing overall medium-term prognosis in a low-risk

Table 8.1 Baseline characteristics of the TIBET subjects (n = 608): age, gender, and clinical history.

	Patients on atenolol	Patients on nifedipine	Patients on combination
Number of patients	205	202	201
Age; years (mean SD)	59.6 (7.7)	60.2 (7.7)	59.7 (7.9)
Males	178	165	180
Previous MI	70	59	69
Previous heart failure	2	3	0
Hypertension	43	45	42
Diabetic	9	5	16
Current smokers	36	27	38
Previous angiogram	58	50	59
Previous angioplasty	4	4	5
Previous CABG	12	10	8

MI: myocardial infarction; CABG: coronary artery bypass grafting.

population, and to investigate the relationship between transient ischemia, therapeutic intervention, and outcome.

Results

Table 8.1 details the demographic data of the 608 subjects in the study population considered to have accurately fulfilled the exercise inclusion criteria. Data are presented according to randomized treatment received. The large majority were males. The mean age was 60 years. One-third had suffered a previous myocardial infarction, one-quarter had angiographically documented coronary disease, and one-fifth were hypertensive.

As required for inclusion in the study, all patients had a positive exercise test for ischemia at baseline (70% had an associated anginal response). Of the 537 patients with interpretable ambulatory monitoring recordings at baseline 50% had evidence of transient ischemia, the majority of episodes being silent. Exercise testing after 6 weeks of randomized therapy resulted in highly significant changes from baseline for all

standard variables (time to onset of ischemia, angina and total exercise time) in all treatment groups, and there were no differences between any of the treatment groups with respect to these changes. Table 8.2 details the effects of 6 weeks of treatment on the frequency of transient ischemia during daily life. The effect of each treatment can be assessed by the asymmetry in the 2×2 tables. The abolition of ischemia was highly significant for all three treatment groups; however, no individual treatment group was more effective in abolishing transient ischemic activity than any other. Considering only those patients who had transient ischemia at baseline, the frequency of patients free from ischemia after 6 weeks of therapy (atenolol 44/89; nifedipine SR 40/87; combination 35/80) revealed no intertreatment differences. Thus, in terms of influencing the total ischemic burden, atenolol, nifedipine SR, and their combination were all equally effective in significantly reducing the ischemic burden, and improving exercise parameters in a large number of 'low-risk' stable angina patients. Of particular interest was the lack of any apparent further benefit from using a combination of treatments in

Table 8.2 Distribution of subjects by presence or absence of episodes of transient ischemia on ambulatory ST-segment monitoring before and after treatment (n = 504).

			After Absent	After Present
Patients on atenolol	Before	Absent	71	19
		Present	44	45
Patients on nifedipine	Before	Absent	66	11
		Present	40	47
Patients on combination	Before	Absent	76	5
		Present	35	45

attempting to modify the total ischemic burden in mildly symptomatic patients. This observation has been previously made and questions the (routine) clinical practice of adding a second anti-ischemic agent when ischemic activity persists despite baseline therapy in the setting of stable coronary artery disease.

Prognostic assessment

The end-points chosen as cardiac events during the average 2-year follow-up period following inclusion in the trial were cardiac death, nonfatal myocardial infarction, unstable angina, the requirement for revascularization, and the necessity for withdrawal from prescribed treatment (treatment failure was defined as symptoms persisting despite high-dose trial therapy and prophylactic GTN). Cardiac death, nonfatal myocardial infarction, and unstable angina (chest pain of increasing frequency or severity requiring admission to hospital) were classified as 'hard' end-points, and revascularization/treatment failure as 'soft' endpoints. For the purposes of analysis of frequency of events, the total number originally randomized to the TIBET study (n = 682) were considered, as follow-up data were available on them.

One hundred and twenty-four patients had a total of 163 trial end-points (13 cardiac death; 38 nonfatal myocardial infarction; 26 unstable angina; 34 interventions (coronary artery bypass grafting/percutaneous transluminal coronary angioplasty (CABG/PTCA)); 52 treatment failures). Table 8.3 shows the distribution of the

Table 8.3 Distribution of the 682 subjects by treatment group and most serious end-point.

Severest end-point	Atenolol	Nifedipine	Combination	Total
Cardiac death	3	6	4	13
Nonfatal MI	14	15	7	36
Unstable angina	12	4	8	24
CABG	7	6	4	17
PTCA	1	0	0	1
Treatment failure	10	15	8	33
No end-point	179	186	193	558
Total	226	232	224	682

MI: myocardial infarction; CABG: coronary artery bypass graft; PTCA: percutaneous transluminal coronary angioplasty.

Table 8.4 Cross-tabulations of subjects by the presence or absence of an end-point and the presence or absence of one or more ischemic episodes on ambulatory ST-segment monitoring off-treatment and on-treatment, for each of the combinations of 'hard' and 'hard + soft' end-points with ST-segment monitoring outcome. Results are for subjects with at least 23 hours of analyzable tapes at the visits considered in each subtable.

		Off-treatment event on Holter		On-treatment event on Holter	
		Yes	No	Yes	No
Hard	Yes	33	30	23	40
End-point	No	265	299	183	383
			(P=0.42)		(P=0.50)
		Yes	No	Yes	No
Hard + soft	Yes	58	51	41	71
End-point	No	240	278	165	352
			(P=0.19)		(P=0.34)

most severe end-point in the 682 subjects by treatment group. Of note is that in a preselected low-risk population of stable angina patients, the majority of whom had a significantly ischemic response to exercise (70% having angina), the mean 2-year follow-up (most severe) event rate for both hard events and for 'elective revascularization' was 91/682 or 13.3%, thus reflecting the good medium-term prognosis associated with such a condition.

Transient ischemia and outcome

Table 8.4 details the cross-tabulation of both 'hard' and 'hard/soft' end-points in subjects with and without transient ischemia during ambulatory ST-segment monitoring both at baseline (off-treatment) and while on-treatment. In those patients with transient ischemia at baseline, 11% suffered a subsequent hard end-point, compared with 9% of those without transient ischemia at baseline. For hard/soft

end-points this frequency was 20% versus 16%. For the on-treatment data, 11% of those with transient ischemia suffered hard events compared with 9% of those without ischemia. The figures for hard/soft events were 20% versus 17%. None of these comparisons achieved statistical significance. There was, furthermore, no evidence of any association between the frequency or duration of ischemic events either at baseline or following 6 weeks of treatment and the risk of any end-point. In assessing the relationship between treatments and outcome, there was a nonsignificant trend toward fewer events on combination therapy when combined with the two individual therapy groups; however, no statistically significant differences could be found (Fig. 8.2). When considering only patients who had five or more episodes of transient ischemia during monitoring, no prognostic impact could be detected either in the total group or in the individual therapy groups.

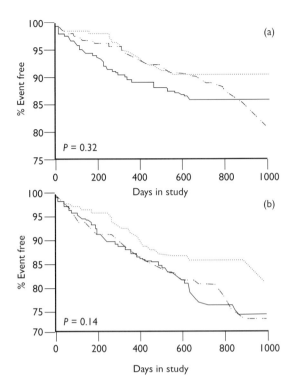

Figure 8.2 Kaplan–Meier survival curves showing percentage of subjects event-free by days in study for the three treatment arms, for (a) hard end-points, and (b) hard + soft end-points. ————: atenolol; ··········: nifedipine; ----------: combination treatment.

CONSIDERATION OF TIBET (AND OTHER) RESULTS AND THEIR IMPLICATIONS

In analyzing the results of the TIBET study one must ensure that the characteristics of the population chosen for study are reflected in the results. This was the case, 50% of patients having transient ischemia off-therapy, and 13.3% suffering some cardiac event over a mean 2-year follow-up period on a range of standard medical therapies (annual mortality 1%). Despite this the term 'low-risk' must be used a little cautiously, as the mean ST-segment depression on exercise testing was 2 mm, and total mean exercise time was approximately 7 minutes. There was a significant reduction in the total ischemic burden in all subgroups studied; however this did not translate into an improved outlook in any group, and, moreover, the patients without transient ischemia at baseline did not have a better outlook than either those with transient ischemia at baseline or those with persisting ischemia after introduction of therapy. Thus, in a large number of previously or currently symptomatic but stable coronary patients on treatment, the results of the TIBET study strongly suggest that the presence of ambulatory ischemia does not predict outcome. It is thus of no surprise that modification of such ischemic activity did not significantly influence outcome either, although the finding of a trend for reduction in hard events on combination therapy compared with individual therapy should be borne in mind when planning further studies. When considering only cardiac death and nonfatal myocardial infarction as end-points, 21 such events occurred on nifedipine, 17 on atenolol, and 11 on the combination, representing a reduction of 48% on the combination compared with nifedipine, and 35% compared with atenolol. This trend cannot be linked to reduction in ischemia per se, as all treatment groups had an equally significant impact on the total ischemic burden. An interesting finding of the study was a significant reduction in resting blood pressure on combination treatment compared with either therapy alone. It is interesting to speculate that more effective modification of the systolic pressure (and perhaps shear stresses at the sites of coronary stenoses) by the use of the combination might lead to a greater reduction in the incidence and frequency of acute plaque rupture, the likely pathophysiological mechanism underlying most acute cardiovascular events.[26]

An important clinical message from the TIBET study is that there appears little indication to intervene surgically on stable angina patients with mild symptoms but with evidence of significant reversible myocardial ischemia for prognostic reasons. In almost 700 patients followed for 1300 patient-years on medical therapy, these patients had an annual mortality which is probably less than the accepted risk of

CABG. Thus revascularization should remain the treatment of choice for patients restricted by anginal symptoms *despite* optimal medical therapy, and for occasional patients with angiographically documented left main stem and subsets of patients with three-vessel disease. These findings only confirm those of others who have shown that surgery does not carry prognostic benefit in low-risk subgroups.

The delay between initiation of the TIBET study and its publication allowed for a stream of other prognostic studies commenced in the late 1980s and early 1990s to be completed and published. These data should be compared with those of the TIBET study to try more clearly to assess the prognostic implications of transient ischemia, and then to formulate a policy of identifying the likely place of ambulatory ST-segment monitoring in our investigative bag for patients with stable angina, and the place for treating predominantly silent ischemia, having detected it. While the TIBET study suggests that there is no practical value to identifying transient (silent) ischemia in predominantly 'low-risk' stable angina patients, what have the other published studies found?

Following the publication in 1990 of a study of 107 patients suggesting that the presence of silent ischemia during daily life was an independent predictor of cardiac death in the short and medium term in patients with stable angina,[17] a series of larger studies on patients with stable coronary syndromes have been reported which have not been able to substantiate this observation. Kennedy et al.[27] noted that over 200 patients with persisting ambulatory ischemia in the stable phase following CABG had the same outlook as those without such ischemia at up to 4 years of follow-up. Patel et al. have confirmed this finding at up to 10 years following surgery.[28] While Rocco et al. in 1988 had reported an adverse short-term prognosis in patients with stable angina who had silent ischemia during daily life,[15] a 2-year follow-up report on the original cohort of patients and further subjects showed that the link between silent ischemia and an adverse prognosis in terms of death and nonfatal myocardial infarction was lost.[29] Mulcahy et al. subsequently reported that in 172 stable angina patients on medical therapy who were followed for 2[30] and then 5 years,[31] there was no link between the presence or absence of transient (silent) ischemia, and outcome. Quyyumi et al. reported no link between ambulatory ischemia and an adverse prognosis in 116 'low-risk' patients with documented coronary artery disease who were monitored off-therapy.[13] Moss et al., in a study of almost 900 patients who underwent ambulatory ST-segment monitoring in the stable phase (1–5 months) following admission with acute coronary syndromes, reported no link between the presence or absence of transient ischemia and outcome.[32] All studies reported a relatively low overall annual mortality, similar to that reported by Brunelli et al., who had previously assessed long-term survival in over 1000 medically treated patients with ischemic heart disease.[33] Interestingly, the original paper which suggested that silent ischemia was an independent predictor of sudden death in stable coronary disease[17] reported a 25% 2-year actual mortality rate in those with silent ischemia. Most of the 'negative' studies quoted above, and others which have not been specifically referred to, and which in total incorporate well over 2000 patients, report an annual mortality in the region of that reported by Brunelli et al.,[33] about 1.6%.

In 1995 an interesting study, the Atenolol Silent Ischemia Study (ASIST), was published which looked at the effects of atenolol versus placebo on transient ischemia during daily life, and 1-year follow-up information was gleaned.[34] The study format was randomization of patients with documented episodes of transient (silent) ischemia to either atenolol or placebo, and repeat ambulatory monitoring at various stages throughout the 1-year follow-up period. The authors found that there was a significantly greater reduction in transient ischemic activity on atenolol than on placebo (although 46% of placebo-treated patients had abolition of transient ischemia at 6-month follow-up!), and that there was a nonsignificant trend toward fewer overall cardiac events on atenolol when compared with placebo after 1-year follow-up. While it would be tempting to assume that the reduction in transient ischemia by atenolol was responsible for the trend toward an improved outcome, it is much more likely that this is not the case; otherwise, one might have expected those 46% of placebo-treated patients whose transient ischemia was 'abolished' on follow-up monitoring to have had a better outcome than the 54% who continued to have transient ischemia on placebo.[35] It is likely that atenolol is of potential benefit compared with placebo for reasons such as blood pressure reduction, and membrane stabilization. As with ASIST, the TIBET study (and many others) showed that atenolol does indeed significantly reduce transient ischemic activity, as does nifedipine SR; however this is not translated into a significantly improved prognosis compared with those who had continued ischemic activity. In addition, ASIST only included patients who had transient ischemia. TIBET showed that patients who did not have transient ischemia during daily life had a similar prognosis to those who did.

One can at the present time conclude that the findings of the TIBET study are generally reflective of the majority of publications assessing the prognostic significance of transient ischemia and the total ischemic burden in patients with *stable* coronary syndromes. While many would not have expected such an outcome when prognostic studies commenced in the late 1980s, it is an interesting lesson on how much there is still to learn about the relationship between plaque and its stability, imbalance of myocardial oxygen supply and demand, and what triggers plaque rupture and acute coronary events. On reflection it seems reasonable to accept that transient ischemia reflects the imbalance between myocardial oxygen demand and supply across at least one 'fixed' coronary stenosis, but that such an ischemic response per se is unlikely to precipitate plaque rupture which we know to be the pathophysiological mechanism underlying the majority of acute coronary syndromes. Thus

transient ischemia is a marker of significant coronary artery disease rather than the cause of acute coronary events. The findings of the TIBET study support this assertion: despite a significant reduction in the total ischemic burden as assessed electrocardiographically, there was no difference in outcome between those with or without transient ischemia, or between those with abolition of, or with persisting transient ischemia on various therapies. Thus modification of the ischemic burden may be achievable, but reduction of acute cardiovascular events will require a treatment or treatments which will stabilize the atherosclerotic plaque. It is interesting to note that while this has not to date been achieved with any antianginal agent, it has to a certain extent been achieved with the latest generation of cholesterol-reducing agents, the HMG CoA reductase inhibitors.[36–38] It is likely that, by either direct or indirect means, these agents stabilize the atherosclerotic plaque and reduce the tendency to rupture for whatever reason. While such plaques may still be sufficiently significant to result in ischemia due to imbalance in the myocardial oxygen supply–demand ratio, the ischemia in itself is simply an effect, rather than a cause, of the significant lesion. If the plaque remains stable the ischemic response will remain consistent, as evidenced by many patients in the author's research bases who have documented coronary artery disease which does not significantly progress over years, and where ambulatory ischemia can be demonstrated to occur at similar demand levels for many years, reflecting this 'static atherosclerotic state'. To influence prognosis, treatment may have to be directed at the plaque (the cause), rather than the ischemia (the effect).

This issue of the relationship between the stable plaque and transient ischemia reflects the importance of not considering together patients with unstable and stable coronary syndromes with associated transient ischemia. While transient ischemia during daily life in stable coronary syndromes reflects the presence of at least one significant 'stable' lesion, transient ischemia in the setting of an unstable coronary syndrome (unstable angina or in the peri-infarction state) reflects the acute (significant) hemodynamic effects of the lesion generated by the acute plaque rupture. Transient ischemia is thus much more likely to be of prognostic importance in the setting of the unstable plaque, by virtue of directly reflecting the instability of such an acutely ruptured plaque.[39–41] Whether the eradication of the ischemia, rather than the stabilization of the plaque, would improve matters is not so clear however. In the final analysis the question of the prognostic importance of transient (silent) ischemia in stable angina will depend on whether the cart follows the horse or vice versa. If ischemia (the horse) causes a significant excess of acute cardiac events (the cart) in stable coronary syndromes, then it will be of prognostic importance and should be eradicated if possible. If ischemia results from the development of significant stenoses, or from acute plaque rupture, then it will remain a marker of underlying coronary disease, its eradication being unlikely to improve outlook significantly when compared with coronary patients without ischemia. At the present time there is little evidence that the cart follows the horse, that transient ischemia causes acute plaque rupture, and the findings of the TIBET study do not detract from this conclusion.

REFERENCES

1. Stern S, Tzivoni D. Early detection of silent ischemic heart disease by 24-hour electrocardiographic monitoring in active subjects. *Br Heart J* 1974; **35**: 481.

2. Deanfield JE, Maseri A, Selwyn AP et al. Myocardial ischaemia during daily life in patients with stable angina: its relation to symptoms and heart rate changes. *Lancet* 1983; **ii**: 753–8.

3. Cecchi AC, Dovellini EV, Marchi F et al. Silent myocardial ischaemia during ambulatory electrocardiographic monitoring in patients with effort angina. *J Am Coll Cardiol* 1983; **1**: 934–9.

4. Quyyumi AA, Efthimiou J, Quyyumi A, Mockus LJ, Spiro SG, Fox KM. Nocturnal angina: precipitating factors in patients with coronary artery disease and those with variant angina. *Br Heart J* 1986; **56**: 346.

5. Mulcahy D, Keegan J, Crean P et al. Silent myocardial ischaemia in chronic stable angina: a study of its frequency and characteristics in 150 patients. *Br Heart J* 1988; **60**: 417–23.

6. Levy RD, Shapiro LM, Wright C et al. The haemodynamic significance of asymptomatic ST-segment depression assessed by ambulatory pulmonary artery pressure monitoring. *Br Heart J* 1986; **56**: 526.

7. Rozanski A, Bairey CN, Krantz DS et al. Mental stress and the induction of silent myocardial ischaemia in patients with coronary artery disease. *N Engl J Med* 1988; **318**: 1005.

8. Stern S, Gavish A, Weisz G et al. Characteristics of silent and symptomatic myocardial ischaemia during daily activities. *Am J Cardiol* 1988; **61**: 1223.

9. Mulcahy D, Keegan J, Fox KM. Comparative characteristics of silent and painful ischaemia during ambulatory ST-segment monitoring in patients with coronary artery disease. *Int J Cardiol* 1990; **28**: 377.

10. Campbell S, Barry J, Rocco MB et al. Features of the exercise test that reflect the activity of ischemic heart disease out of hospital. *Circulation* 1986; **74**: 72–80.

11. Mulcahy D, Keegan J, Sparrow J et al. Ischaemia in the ambulatory setting—the total ischemic burden: relation to exercise testing and investigative and therapeutic implications. *J Am Coll Cardiol* 1989; **14**: 1166.

12. Kunkes SH, Pichard AD, Smith H et al. Silent ST-segment deviations and the extent of coronary artery disease. *Am Heart J* 1980; **100**: 813.

13. Quyyumi AA, Panza JA, Diodati JG, Callahan TS, Bonow RO, Epstein SE. Prognostic implications of myocardial ischaemia during daily life in low risk patients with coronary artery disease. *J Am Coll Cardiol* 1993; **21**: 700–8.

14. Mulcahy D, Keegan J, Lindsay D et al. Silent myocardial ischaemia in patients referred for coronary artery bypass surgery because of angina: a comparison with patients whose

symptoms were well controlled on medical treatment. *Br Heart J* 1989; **61**: 496.

15. Rocco MB, Nabel EG, Campbell S et al. Prognostic importance of myocardial ischaemia detected by ambulatory monitoring in patients with stable coronary artery disease. *Circulation* 1988; **78**: 877–84.

16. Tzivoni D, Weisz G, Gavish A, Zin D, Keren A, Stern S. Comparison of mortality and myocardial infarction rates in stable angina pectoris with and without ischemic episodes during daily activities. *Am J Cardiol* 1989; **63**: 273.

17. Deedwania PC, Carbajal EV. Silent ischaemia during daily life is an independent predictor of mortality in stable angina. *Circulation* 1990; **81**: 748–56.

18. The Veterans Administration Coronary Artery Bypass Surgery Cooperative Study Group. Eleven-year survival in the Veteran Administration randomized trial of coronary bypass surgery for stable angina. *N Engl J Med* 1984; **311**: 1333.

19. Varnauskas E and the European Coronary Study Group. Twelve-year follow-up of survival in the randomized European Coronary Surgery Study. *N Engl J Med* 1988; **319**: 332.

20. Aldermen EL, Bourassa MG, Cohen LS et al. Ten-year follow-up of survival and myocardial infarction in the Randomized Coronary Artery Surgery Study. *Circulation* 1990; **82**: 1629.

21. Quyyumi AA, Crake T, Wright CM et al. Medical treatment of patients with severe exertional and rest angina: double-blind comparison of beta-blocker, calcium antagonist, and nitrate. *Br Heart J* 1987; **8**: 124.

22. Frishman WH, Teicher M. Antianginal drug therapy for silent myocardial ischaemia. *Am Heart J* 1987; **114**: 140.

23. The TIBET Study Group. The Total Ischemic Burden European Trial (TIBET): design, methodology, and management. *Cardiovasc Drug Ther* 1992; **6**: 379–86.

24. Fox KM, Mulcahy D, Findlay I, Ford I, Dargie HJ. The Total Ischaemic Burden European Trial (TIBET). Effects of atenolol, nifedipine SR and their combination on the exercise test and the total ischaemic burden in 608 patients with stable angina. *Eur Heart J* 1996; **17**: 96–103.

25. Dargie HJ, Ford I, Fox KM. Total Ischaemic Burden European Trial (TIBET). Effects of ischaemia and treatment with atenolol, nifedipine SR and their combination on outcome in patients with chronic stable angina. *Eur Heart J* 1996; **17**: 104–12.

26. Davies MJ, Thomas AC. Plaque fissuring—the cause of acute myocardial infarction, sudden ischaemic death, and crescendo angina. *Br Heart J* 1985; **53**: 363.

27. Kennedy HL, Seiler SM, Sprague MK et al. Relation of silent myocardial ischaemia after coronary artery bypass grafting to angiographic completeness of revascularisation and long-term prognosis. *Am J Cardiol* 1990; **65**: 14–22.

28. Patel D, Mulcahy D, Curzen N et al. Prognostic significance of transient ST-segment changes following coronary artery bypass surgery: a long-term (4–10-year) follow-up study. *Br Heart J* 1993; **70**: 337.

29. Yeung AC, Barry J, Orav J et al. Effects of asymptomatic ischaemia on long-term prognosis in chronic stable coronary disease. *Circulation* 1991; **83**: 1598.

30. Mulcahy D, Parameshwar J, Holdright D et al. Value of ambulatory ST-segment monitoring in chronic stable angina: does measurement of the 'total ischaemic burden' assist with management? *Br Heart J* 1992; **67**: 47.

31. Mulcahy D, Knight C, Patel D et al. Detection of ambulatory ischaemia is not of practical clinical value in the routine management of patients with stable angina. A long-term follow-up study. *Eur Heart J* 1995; **16**: 317–24.

32. Moss LJ, Goldstein RE, Hall J et al. Detection and significance of myocardial ischaemia in stable patients after recovery from an acute coronary event. *JAMA* 1993; **269**: 2379–85.

33. Brunelli C, Cristofani R, L'Abbate A. Long-term survival in medically treated patients with ischemic heart disease and prognostic importance of clinical and electrocardiographic data. *Eur Heart J* 1989; **10**: 292.

34. Pepine CJ, Cohn PF, Deedwania PC et al. Effects of treatment on outcome in mildly symptomatic patients with ischaemia during daily life. The Atenolol Silent Ischaemia Study (ASIST). *Circulation* 1994; **90**: 762.

35. Mulcahy D. Pointers from recent multicentre trials using ambulatory monitoring—placing placebo in perspective. *Eur Heart J* 1995; **16**: 1754.

36. Scandinavian Simvistatin Survival Study Group. Randomized trial of cholesterol lowering in 4444 patients with coronary heart disease: the Scandinavian Simvistatin Survival Study (4S). *Lancet* 1994; **344**: 1383.

37. Shepherd J, Cobbe SM, Ford I et al. Prevention of coronary heart disease with pravastatin in men with hypercholesterolemia. *N Engl J Med* 1995; **333**: 1301.

38. Sacks FM, Pfeffer MA, Moye LA et al. The effect of pravastatin on coronary events after myocardial infarction in patients with average cholesterol levels. *N Engl J Med* 1966; **335**: 1001.

39. Gottlieb SO, Weisfeldt ML, Ouyang P et al. Silent ischaemia as a marker of early unfavorable outcomes in patients with unstable angina. *N Engl J Med* 1986; **314**: 1214.

40. Gottlieb SO, Gottlieb SH, Achuff SC et al. Silent ischaemia on Holter monitoring predicts mortality in high-risk post-infarction patients. *JAMA* 1988; **259**: 1030.

41. Patel DJ, Holdright DR, Knight CJ et al. Early continuous ST-segment monitoring in unstable angina: prognostic value additional to the clinical characteristics and the admission electrocardiogram. *Heart* 1996; **75**: 222.

9

Asymptomatic cardiac ischemia: insights from the NHLBI-sponsored Asymptomatic Cardiac Ischemia Pilot (ACIP) study

Barry D Bertolet, Christopher S Brown, Carl J Pepine and C Richard Conti

Asymptomatic cardiac ischemia can be defined as objective evidence of reversible myocardial cellular hypoxia in the absence of symptoms.[1] Presently, millions of patients with all forms of coronary artery disease experience frequent episodes of transient asymptomatic cardiac ischemia.[2] Approximately 30–50% of patients with stable as well as unstable coronary syndromes will demonstrate evidence of asymptomatic cardiac ischemia despite medical therapy.[1] Studies have suggested that the presence of such asymptomatic cardiac ischemia yields a similar significance and prognosis to that of symptomatic ischemia.[1] In fact, in patients with symptomatic cardiac ischemia, the asymptomatic ischemic episodes outnumber the symptomatic episodes by at least three to one. In the next two decades, as the baby-boom generation reaches retirement age, it is predicted that the number of patients with coronary disease and asymptomatic ischemia will double. Therefore, understanding and defining the proper management of this condition becomes increasingly paramount. Studies have shown that therapy with beta-blockers, calcium antagonists, and long-acting nitrates as well as myocardial revascularization will suppress asymptomatic cardiac ischemia.[1] However, the optimal treatment to suppress transient cardiac ischemia, and more importantly its effects on long-term prognosis, has not

been determined. Some information is available from a prospective randomized trial initiated by the National Heart, Lung and Blood Institute called the Asymptomatic Cardiac Ischemia Pilot (ACIP) study. This chapter will review the design and results of the ACIP study.

DESIGN

The purpose of ACIP was to determine the feasibility of conducting a full-scale trial of therapies to prevent adverse outcomes in patients with chronic stable coronary artery disease and asymptomatic cardiac ischemia. In order to qualify for the study, patients were required to have:

1) angiographic evidence of coronary artery diameter stenosis greater than 50% (by electronic calipers) in one or more vessels suitable for mechanical revascularization;

2) at least one episode of asymptomatic cardiac ischemia on 48-hour ambulatory electrocardiographic (ECG) monitoring; and,

3) evidence of exercise-induced myocardial ischemia on treadmill testing.[3]

The qualifying angiography had to be performed within 3 years of the qualifying ambulatory ECG recording. If the patient was

Table 9.1 ACIP exercise protocol.			
Stage	Speed/grade (mph/%)	Time (min)	METs
I	2.0/0.0	1	2.5
II	2.5/2.0	2	3.5
III	3.0/3.0	4	4.5
IV	3.0/7.0	6	6.2
V	3.0/10.5	8	7.6
VI	3.0/14.0	10	9.1
VII	3.0/17.5	12	10.5
VIII	3.0/21.0	14	12.0
IX	3.1/24.0	16	13.4
X	3.4/24.0	18	15.1

METs: metabolic equivalents.

gradual linear increase in oxygen consumption with 1.5 metabolic equivalent increments between stages (Table 9.1). This protocol was modified for elderly or short patients so that they had a walking speed of 2 miles per hour versus 3 miles per hour in the standard protocol. When compared with the Bruce protocol, the ACIP protocol produced similar peak aerobic capacities and peak rate–pressure products yet allowed a more linear increase in VO_2, and better correlation of VO_2 to work rate.[4] The sensitivity for detection of ischemic ST-segment changes using the ACIP protocol was similar to the Bruce (94% versus 100%). These exercise ECG signals were recorded continually and also read centrally at an ECG core laboratory. Ischemic-type ST-segment shifts were defined as 1 mm of horizontal or downsloping ST depression or greater than 1.5 mm of upsloping ST-segment depression noted 80 ms after the J-point.[3]

Notable exclusions from ACIP included recent myocardial infarction, coronary angioplasty, or coronary artery bypass surgery; unstable angina; significant noncardiac illnesses that may result in death within five years; New York Heart Association Class III or IV congestive heart failure; contraindications to either beta-blockers or calcium-channel antagonists; coronary artery disease not amenable to revascularization; left main coronary artery disease greater than 50% in diameter; ECG abnormalities that interfere with analysis of ischemia; and/or need for digitalis.[3]

Eligible patients were randomized to receive one of three initial treatment strategies—angina-guided medical therapy, ischemia-guided medical therapy after suppression of angina, or mechanical revascularization (Fig. 9.1). The pharmacological agents chosen for the medical regimens were atenolol and nifedipine XL or diltiazem SR and isosorbide dinitrate. These agents were chosen to reflect current clinical practice and maximize potential anti-ischemic benefits by using drugs with different pharmacological properties. The initial component of each medical treatment arm was an agent that decreased heart rate. The second

unable to perform treadmill exercise, they must have had a reversible stress-related radionuclide myocardial perfusion defect or an abnormal arm ergometry exercise ECG in order to qualify.

Prior to the ambulatory ECG recording period, patients were withdrawn from cardiac active medications for at least five half-lives. Low-dose beta-blocker or diltiazem therapy was permitted for those who were postinfarction. Two leads, usually II and V5, with isoelectric ST-segments at baseline were monitored for 48 hours. These tapes were read centrally by an ambulatory ECG core laboratory. Asymptomatic cardiac ischemia was defined as the presence of at least 1 mm of ST-segment depression lasting for at least 1 minute in the absence of symptoms recorded by pressing the event button.[3]

The treadmill exercise tests were performed according to the ACIP protocol, a modification of the Naughton and Balke protocols.[4] This protocol starts with two 1-minute warm-up stages followed by 2-minute stages providing a

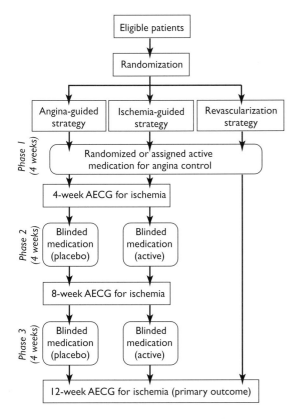

Figure 9.1 The Asymptomatic Cardiac Ischemia Pilot (ACIP) study design outlining the three treatment strategies and the initial 12-week evaluation schema. (Reproduced with permission from Knatterud et al.[6])

The goal of the ischemia-guided treatment strategy was to eliminate ambulatory ECG evidence of ischemia which persisted after control of angina. The titration of the ischemia medications was based on the ambulatory ECG recording performed at 4 and 8 weeks. Patients with ischemia received atenolol 50 mg/day or diltiazem SR 60 mg bid. If tolerated, the dose was increased one week later to atenolol 100 mg/day or diltiazem SR 90 mg bid. If ischemia was present on subsequent monitoring, nifedipine XL 30 mg/day or isosorbide dinitrate 20 mg bid was started. This was titrated to nifedipine XL 60 mg/day or isosorbide dinitrate 40 mg bid the following week.

The third treatment strategy was the mechanical revascularization strategy. The goal of this arm was to achieve as complete a revascularization as possible using either coronary angioplasty or bypass surgery. The choice of revascularization procedure was determined by the site study physician using the following guidelines. Bypass surgery was preferred for patients with diffuse coronary artery disease greater than 20 mm in length, excessive tortuosity or angulation of the stenosed vessel, completely occluded vessels, coronary lesions involving major side-branches, and for lesions which would result in cardiogenic shock if abrupt vessel closure should occur. Angioplasty was preferred if the American College of Cardiology/American Heart Association guidelines for angioplasty were met. Angioplasty was deemed successful if the final residual stenosis was less than 50% diameter. The mechanical revascularization of the reference vessel was to be performed within 4 weeks of randomization. All angiograms were read centrally at an angiographic core laboratory.

The primary outcome of this pilot study was the absence of any ischemia-related event and cardiac ischemia on ambulatory ECG recording at 12 weeks after entry (Fig. 9.1). By this time, the drug titration should have been completed and patients assigned to mechanical revascularization stable. Secondary outcome variables included determination of the number and duration of ischemic episodes and maximal ST-segment depression on the ambulatory ECG

agent in each arm provided a coronary vasodilatory effect.[3]

Active medication to control angina was available at any time during the study in all three treatment strategies. The goal of the angina-guided treatment strategy was to have adequate angina control, defined as fewer than three episodes of angina per week which were easily controlled with sublingual nitroglycerin and did not interfere with the patient's daily activities. The study medicines were increased on a weekly basis until anginal control was obtained. If angina persisted despite maximal medications, mechanical revascularization was then considered.

Table 9.2   Baseline demographics.

	Symptom strategy	Ischemia strategy	Revascularization
Mean age (years)	61 ± 8	62 ± 8	61 ± 8
Male	165 (90%)	155 (85%)	159 (83%)
Diabetes	11 (6%)	19 (10%)	18 (9%)
Hypertension	32 (17%)	41 (22%)	39 (20%)
Current smoker	19 (10%)	17 (9%)	13 (7%)
Previous MI	38 (21%)	40 (22%)	43 (22%)
Previous CABG	5 (3%)	7 (4%)	5 (3%)
Previous PTCA	20 (11%)	18 (10%)	16 (8%)
LV function			
EF < 35%	0	4 (2%)	4 (2%)
EF 35–49%	18 (10%)	18 (10%)	17 (9%)
EF > 50%	165 (90%)	161 (88%)	171 (89%)
Coronary anatomy			
One-vessel disease	40 (22%)	46 (25%)	50 (26%)
Two-vessel disease	66 (36%)	64 (35%)	81 (42%)
Three-vessel disease	77 (42%)	73 (40%)	61 (32%)

recording. Other secondary analyses were based on the follow-up exercise treadmill test. Variables evaluated were the presence or absence of ST-segment depression, time to onset of angina, time to onset and maximum depth of ST depression, total number of abnormal ECG leads, rate–pressure product achieved, and reasons for termination. Even though this study was not powered to examine clinical events, these were also recorded.[3]

In addition, the patients' responses to ischemia testing at 6 and 12 months, as well as adverse clinical outcomes such as death, myocardial infarction (MI), or need for non-protocol revascularization occurring at 6, 12, and 24 months, were recorded. All variables were analyzed according to the patient's assigned initial treatment strategy.

RESULTS

A total of 1959 patients with known or suspected coronary artery disease (CAD) and exercise-induced ischemia were recruited. Nine hundred and fifty-two of these patients (48.6%) had evidence of asymptomatic daily-life cardiac ischemia. Of these, 618 patients, or 65%, met all the prerandomization entry criteria. The main reason many patients were excluded was due to the coronary angiographic findings. Patients were randomized to one of the three treatment strategies: 204 to the angina-guided therapy, 202 to the ischemia-guided therapy, and 212 patients to the revascularization arm. Of the patients assigned to the revascularization arm, 49% had an angioplasty and 41% underwent bypass surgery.[3] At the time of final data editing, the clinical coordinating center determined that there was evidence of unacceptable performance in the conduct of the trial at one clinical site.[5] These 60 patients were removed from the cohort and not used in any analysis. The numbers of patients used for subsequent analysis were 183 in the angina-guided arm, 183 in the ischemia-guided arm, and 192 patients in the revascularization arm, for a total of 558 acceptable patients enrolled. After removal of these patients from the final analysis, no change in any parameter tested could be observed. The baseline characteristics of these patients are shown in Table 9.2.

Short-term outcomes

After 12 weeks, 24% of the patients assigned to the angina-guided treatment strategy did not require any medication, 51% were taking only one drug, and 25% were taking both drugs.[6] In the ischemia-guided treatment strategy group, 22% did not require any therapy, 54% required only one drug, and 24% required both agents. Among the patients assigned to initial revascularization, 65% of the patients did not require any drugs, 28% required one drug, and 7% required both drugs (Fig. 9.2). Additionally, few patients were advanced to the higher-dose drug therapy in any of the three treatment strategies.

According to the 12-week follow-up ambulatory ECG study, the angina-guided treatment strategy abolished all daily-life cardiac ischemia in 38.6% of patients, ischemia-guided treatment strategy abolished 41.4%, and the revascularization treatment strategy abolished 53.6% (P = 0.01 compared with both medical therapy arms) (Fig. 9.3). Examining the patients assigned to the revascularization, 71% of the patients who underwent coronary bypass were ischemia-free, whereas only 53% of the angioplasty patients had no evidence of daily-life cardiac ischemia ($P < 0.05$).

At 12 weeks, all patients demonstrated an improvement in exercise tolerance and a reduction in exercise-induced angina and ECG evidence of ischemia. Of the three treatment strategies, patients assigned to revascularization showed the most improvement; however, more than 70% of all cohorts still had exercise-induced ischemia (Fig. 9.4).

Long-term outcomes

After 1 year, these patients were re-evaluated with regard to clinical events and the presence of cardiac ischemia on ambulatory ECG and

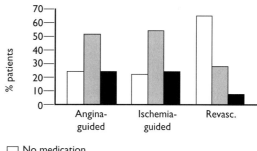

No medication
One drug
Two drugs

Figure 9.2 Anti-ischemia drug use for each of the three treatment strategies at 12 weeks. Note the similarities between the angina-guided and ischemia-guided groups. Most patients who underwent revascularization did not require anti-ischemia medical therapy. (Adapted from Knatterud et al.[6])

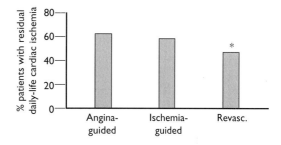

Figure 9.3 Residual daily-life cardiac ischemia noted on 48-hour ambulatory ECG monitoring. The percentage of patients from each treatment group with residual daily-life cardiac ischemia at 12 weeks is shown. Coronary revascularization was the therapy most likely to abolish the daily-life cardiac ischemia (denoted by *). (Adapted from Knatterud et al.[6])

exercise treadmill tests.[7] Total elimination of daily-life cardiac ischemia was achieved in 31% of the patients assigned to the angina-guided treatment strategy, 36% in the ischemia-guided treatment strategy, and 57% of patients randomized to initial revascularization. These results demonstrate that suppression of cardiac ischemia is relatively stable over a 1-year period

(Fig. 9.5). Additionally, over the course of a year, patients randomized to revascularization could exercise to a higher rate–pressure product, achieve a higher percentage of age-predicted maximal heart rate, and demonstrated less exercise-induced angina depression than their counterparts randomized to the medical treatment strategies. Of particular interest, the benefit seen for initial revascularization therapy over medical therapy regarding the reduction of exercise-induced ischemia at the 12-week and 6-month testing was not evident at the 1-year testing (Fig. 9.6).

Over the two years of follow-up, patients randomized to initial revascularization had a significantly lower total mortality than patients assigned to either medical treatment strategy (Fig. 7).[8] Cardiac outcomes of death or nonfatal myocardial infarction occurred in 12.1% of the patients in the angina-guided treatment strategy, 8.8% of those in the ischemia-guided treatment strategy, and 4.7% of those assigned to initial revascularization. Moreover, the likelihood for ischemia-related hospitalization was greater in the two medical treatment strategies. These hospitalizations were mainly for non-protocol revascularization procedures. Hospitalizations for a cardiac event occurred in 29.5% of those patients assigned to the medical treatment strategies versus 18.2% of those assigned to revascularization ($P < 0.05$).

Overall, the initial revascularization strategy was the most successful therapy in suppressing asymptomatic cardiac ischemia on ambulatory ECG and exercise test, giving patients freedom from medications and improving clinical outcomes. These pilot data suggest that suppression of asymptomatic cardiac ischemia, particularly when using mechanical revascularization, may improve clinical outcomes in these patients; however, a larger trial is needed.[8]

Critical commentary

One of the important criticisms of this study involves the drug titration protocol in the medical treatment strategies. It was expected that patients assigned to the ischemia-guided

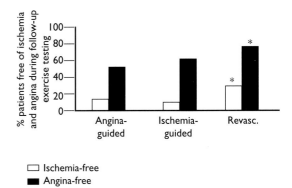

Figure 9.4 Percentage of patients free of cardiac ischemia and/or angina at the time of follow-up exercise testing. Note that patients who underwent successful coronary revascularization were more likely to be angina- and ischemia-free (denoted by*). (Adapted from Knatterud et al.[6])

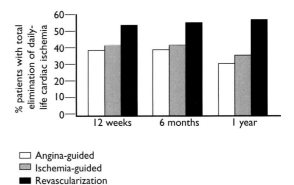

Figure 9.5 Suppression of ambulant daily-life ischemia by treatment group over time. The extent of ischemia suppression provided by each treatment strategy was relatively stable over the course of a year. (Adapted from Rogers et al.[7])

strategy would be more likely to receive a combination drug regimen or at least a higher dosage of medications when compared with the angina-guided strategy. As this was not the case, patients assigned to the ischemia-guided treatment strategy probably had less than optimal

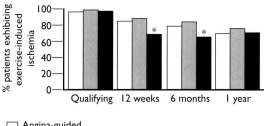

☐ Angina-guided
▨ Ischemia-guided
■ Revascularization

Figure 9.6 Percentage of patients exhibiting exercise-induced ischemia by treatment group over time. At 12 weeks and 6 months, patients randomized to revascularization therapy had significantly less exercised-induced ischemia than those assigned to the medical groups (denoted by *). This advantage seems to be lost at 1 year of follow-up. It is surprising at the degree of residual cardiac ischemia present across all the treatment groups. (Adapted from Rogers et al.[7])

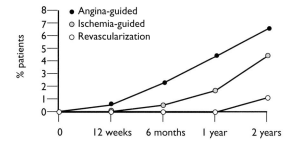

Figure 9.7 Mortality according to treatment strategy over 2 years of follow-up. Even though the number of events was small, the survival benefit for those patients assigned to mechanical revascularization is striking. (Adapted from Davies et al.[8])

drug titration, which limits the ability to test the utility of an angina-guided versus ischemia-guided treatment protocol. The trend toward fewer clinical events in the ischemia-guided group suggests a benefit of this approach. This observation would support the hypothesis that

abolition of all cardiac ischemia results in an improved long-term clinical outcome.

Another concern was the strikingly large number of patients with ischemia still present following 'successful' revascularization. The explanation may be that over 10% of patients randomized to initial revascularization did not undergo revascularization. Many patients had angioplasty of a single lesion in the presence of multiple lesions.[8] Moreover, some ischemia might be a likely result of restenosis at angioplasty sites. It is also possible that 'complete revascularization' in a diffuse disease like CAD is more hypothetical than practical.

Other study observations

Several ACIP substudies warrant comment. One study reported results of the ambulatory ECG tapes obtained on all the 1820 patients with known or suspected CAD and myocardial ischemia who were screened for the ACIP study.[9] The overall prevalence of asymptomatic cardiac ischemia was 49%. Ischemia seemed to be more prevalent in those patients with larger increases in heart rate above their daily mean values. This prevalence ranged from 33% in patients with heart rate increases less than 38 beats per minute over the daily mean to 64% of those with heart rate increases greater than 74 beats per minute (Fig. 9.8). Two other independent predictors of asymptomatic cardiac ischemia were increased age and recent history of angina (Table 9.3). No differences in prevalence of ischemic episodes with respect to season, temperature, or day of week could be

Table 9.3   Predictors of asymptomatic daily-life cardiac ischemia.
Large increases in heart rate over the 24-hour mean heart rate
Increasing age
Recent history of angina

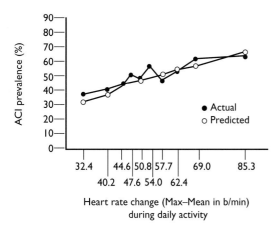

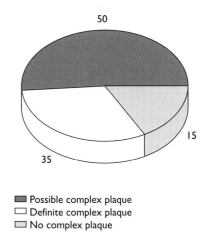

Possible complex plaque
Definite complex plaque
No complex plaque

Figure 9.8 The prevalence of asymptomatic cardiac ischemia related to the change in heart rate. The heart rate change was calculated as the maximum (Max) minus the mean value for 48 hours of monitoring. With larger heart rate increases over the mean level, the prevalence of ischemia also increases in a predictable fashion. (Reproduced with permission from Pratt et al.[13])

Figure 9.9 Coronary artery lesion morphology in those patients with asymptomatic cardiac ischemia. Complex lesions were seen in a majority of these patients. Asymptomatic myocardial ischemia seemed to serve as a 'marker' for these complex lesions. (Adapted from Sharaf et al.[11])

identified. A higher prevalence of asymptomatic ischemia was noted among northern as opposed to southern USA residents; however, this difference could have resulted from a difference in screening practices between clinical sites. There was a tendency for the northern sites (northern USA, Canada, and London) to screen a higher proportion of patients with early ST-segment depression during exercise testing. There was also a higher prevalence of cardiac ischemia in Caucasian patients; however, one of the limitations of the study was that the population screened contained limited numbers of women and African Americans.[9] The percentage of women with ischemia enrolled was lower than the prevalence of ischemia in the general population because, at the participating centers, women were found to have ischemia less often than men in the course of routine clinical care, and screening tests for ischemia were less predictive of protocol-defined coronary disease in women.[10]

The features of coronary angiographic pathology were particularly interesting and may relate to the mechanism for ambulatory ischemia and ischemia-related adverse outcomes. The 558 patients enrolled in the ACIP study with asymptomatic cardiac ischemia were compared with 43 patients who did not qualify because they lacked evidence for asymptomatic cardiac ischemia.[11] Patients with asymptomatic cardiac ischemia were more likely to have proximal coronary stenosis (64% versus 42%) as well as coronary stenosis greater than 70% (40% versus 21%) than those patients without daily-life cardiac ischemia. Additionally, the presence of ambulatory ischemia seemed to serve as a marker of complex plaque or thrombus on the angiogram (Fig. 9.9). This unstable coronary pathology was found almost twice as frequently in patients with ambulatory ischemia compared with those without ambulatory ischemia. Presence of complex plaque may account for the higher cardiac event rate in

Table 9.4 Determinants of ischemia-related adverse outcomes.

Presence of asymptomatic daily-life cardiac ischemia

Increasing number of asymptomatic daily-life cardiac ischemic episodes

Assignment to medical therapy as opposed to revascularization therapy

those patients with demonstrable asymptomatic cardiac ischemia as compared with those without ambulant cardiac ischemia.[11]

Patient characteristics at study entry that predict ischemia-related adverse outcomes at 1 year were evaluated in detail.[12] The ACIP population of patients were primarily elderly white men with multivessel coronary disease, a proximal coronary stenosis greater than 50%, and angiographic evidence of complex plaque formation. Given this population, the only baseline characteristic to predict independently a poor outcome was the number of ischemic episodes noted on ambulatory ECG monitoring at entry. Surprisingly, age, symptom status, and exercise stress variables as well as coronary angiography variables did not yield additional independent prognostic information. Assignment to an initial medical strategy, as opposed to initial revascularization, was also independently associated with adverse outcome (Table 9.4). These data confirm that the presence of daily-life cardiac ischemia, much of which is asymptomatic, denotes patients who are at high risk for future adverse events. Complete myocardial revascularization appears to modify this risk significantly.

Some of ACIP substudies have examined the effectiveness of the medical treatment regimens for asymptomatic cardiac ischemia. The effectiveness of the two assigned medical regimens (atenolol/nifedipine versus diltiazem/isosorbide dinitrate) was analyzed in the patients who had these regimens randomly assigned.[13] At the

time of the 12-week ambulatory ECG, 47% of the patients randomized to the atenolol/nifedipine regimen had total suppression of ischemia as compared with 31% of the patients who were assigned to diltiazem/ isosorbide dinitrate regimen. This greater ischemia suppression with the atenolol/ nifedipine regimen correlated with a greater reduction in the heart rate. However, after adjusting for imbalances in ischemia at entry (randomization was not stratified for ischemia), only a trend favoring the atenolol/nifedipine combination in suppressing ischemia could be recognized.[13] When examining the exercise treadmill tests, both drug combination regimens improved all subjective and objective measurements of ischemia. This improvement included increases in exercise time, reductions in ST-segment depression, and increases in time to ischemia onset and inducible angina. In both drug combination regimens, patients with the greatest heart rate reductions had the greatest suppression of daily-life cardiac ischemia. After 12 weeks of therapy, patients whose heart rate was greater than 80 beats per minute had twice as many ischemic episodes as those with heart rates less than 70 beats per minute (Fig. 9.10). A criticism in the evaluation of these two different medical combination therapies is that, due to the study design, a large portion of the patients (approximately 50%) were not taking 'optimal (two drugs) or maximal (manufacturer recommended peak doses)' therapy by the 12-week testing period.[13] Nevertheless, these medication dosages were maintained for the remainder of the first year of follow-up[7] and were very similar to those used in clinical practice.

The efficacy of the two treatment options in the revascularization group was also analyzed.[14,15] At baseline, patients assigned to bypass surgery had more ischemia (both ischemic and asymptomatic) than those assigned to angioplasty.[14] Five or more ischemic episodes were noted in 56% of the bypass-surgery-assigned patients compared with only 32% of the angioplasty-assigned patients. Exercise-induced angina was frequent in the bypass group (80% versus 49%). Despite this

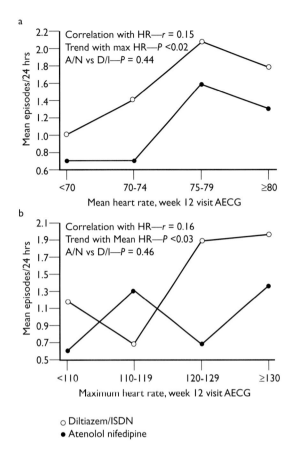

Figure 9.10 Relation of mean (a) and maximal (b) heart rate to the mean number of ischemic episodes on ambulatory ECG monitoring at 12 weeks by medical regimen. In essence, the faster the heart rate, the more likely the patient was to have asymptomatic ischemia. (Reproduced with permission from Pepine et al.[12])

average of 3.7 minutes longer for patients assigned to coronary bypass surgery compared with only 1.7 minutes longer for those assigned to angioplasty. At the 12-week follow-up, only 10% of the bypass-surgery-assigned patients had exercise-induced angina compared with 30% of the angioplasty-assigned patients (P < 0.01); however, this advantage for bypass disappeared by 12 months, probably related to repeat angioplasty in those assigned initial angioplasty. These data suggest that the patients assigned coronary artery bypass had less residual cardiac ischemia (by both ambulatory ECG monitoring and exercise testing) following revascularization than patients assigned to angioplasty. Even with these striking results of ischemia suppression, there does seem to be considerable residual ischemia that persists even after 'apparently successful' coronary bypass surgery.[15]

In addition to less cardiac ischemia on testing, patients assigned bypass had fewer ischemia-related clinical events such as death, nonfatal MI, or repeat revascularization procedure compared with those assigned angioplasty. At 1 year, there were no deaths. One patient in the bypass surgery and three in the angioplasty-assigned group had a nonfatal MI. There were 16 non-protocol revascularizations in the angioplasty-assigned group and only one in the bypass-surgery-assigned group. Although these data suggest that bypass may be a better choice for initial therapy of ischemia, the number of events is too small to draw definitive conclusions as to which therapy reduces overall risk.[15] It should be noted that ACIP was carried out prior to the widespread use of intracoronary stenting, and it is possible that this adjunctive procedure to balloon angioplasty would have reduced the need for repeat revascularization in those assigned angioplasty and thereby lessened ischemia-related clinical events.

A preliminary assessment of the cost implications of these treatment strategies for cardiac ischemia was performed.[16] As expected, initial revascularization consumed more resources ($13 030/patient) than the angina-guided ($4265/patient) or the ischemia-guided ($4692/

bias against bypass surgery, at the 12-week follow-up visit, daily-life cardiac ischemia was suppressed in 70% of the bypass-assigned patients compared with only 46% of the angioplasty-assigned patients. Moreover, exercise-induced ischemia was no longer present in 46% of the coronary artery bypass grafting surgery patients compared with only 23% of patients randomized to angioplasty. After revascularization, patients were able to exercise longer—an

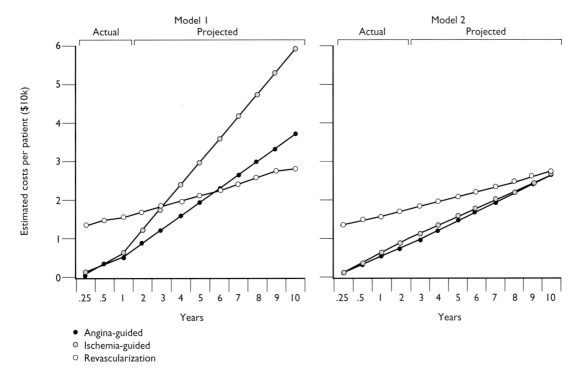

Figure 9.11 Cost implications of each treatment strategy over time. As expected, the cost of revascularization was higher in the first year; however, in subsequent years the cost of medical therapy exceeded that of the revascularization group. It is extrapolated that the costs of the medical group will meet or exceed those of the mechanical revascularization group in 4–5 years. (Adapted from Pepine et al.[16])

patient) strategies early in the first year of care. However, due to the higher number of clinical events and the need for non-protocol coronary revascularization procedures, the subsequent follow-up costs of the medically treated patients were higher than those of the revascularization group ($1694 versus $504/patient). When extrapolated over the expected lifetime of these patients with chronic stable coronary artery disease, the costs of the medical therapy groups would equal or exceed those of the initial revascularization group in 4–9 years depending on the economic model used (Fig. 9.11). Initial revascularization may, therefore, provide the best treatment to control ischemia as well as prove to be the most cost-effective therapy over the lifetime of these patients.

An ACIP ancillary substudy performed at five of the ACIP study centers compared the ischemia detected by ambulatory ECG monitoring with that found by single photon emission computed tomography (SPECT) in 106 patients screened for the ACIP study.[17] Only 50 of these patients were enrolled in the ACIP trial, mainly due to lack of ambulatory ECG ischemia. Seventy-four percent of patients with significant coronary stenosis by angiography had SPECT abnormalities, whereas 61% had ischemia by ambulatory ECG monitoring. Only a 50% concordance between normal or abnormal was noted between the ambulatory ECG and SPECT imaging. These data suggest that ischemia detected from ambulatory ECG monitoring may be related more to altered coronary vasomotion (i.e., endothelial dysfunction) rather than an anatomic abnormality.

SUMMARY AND CONCLUSIONS

The ACIP study demonstrated that among clinically stable patients with coronary artery disease a cohort can be identified using relatively simple, inexpensive noninvasive monitoring for cardiac ischemia. This cohort represents a subgroup at relatively high risk for adverse outcomes. At 1 year in the entire cohort this risk exceeded 50% for composite ischemia-related adverse outcomes (clinical events and recurrent ambulatory ECG ischemia despite treatment), 22% for any clinical event (including non-protocol revascularization) and exceeded 13% for only death, nonfatal MI, or hospitalization for an ischemia-related event. These adverse outcomes were all significantly more frequent in those randomized to initial medical strategy. Furthermore, this cohort of patients can be randomized to different treatment strategies using a complex and demanding protocol. It also revealed that cardiac ischemia can be suppressed in approximately 40–50% of patients with low to moderate doses of medications titrated over a period of 2–3 months. Revascularization therapy proved to be the most effective of these treatment strategies in reducing ischemia (ambulatory ECG and exercise treadmill) as well as ischemia-related clinical events. More importantly, this pilot study has confirmed the need for a large prognosis trial with a similar design. It is estimated that such a study will need to consist of approximately 5300 patients followed for 5 years. Until these data become available, it would be prudent for the physician caring for patients with coronary artery disease or those at high risk for coronary disease to be concerned about the prognostic implications associated with myocardial ischemia. If ischemia is identified, such patients deserve very aggressive treatments with either medication or revascularization because they are at high risk for adverse events. If initial revascularization was not employed, ischemia despite medical therapy demands strong consideration for revascularization.

REFERENCES

1. Bertolet BD, Pepine CJ. Daily life cardiac ischemia: should it be treated? *Drugs* 1995; **49**: 176–95.
2. Cohn PF. Silent myocardial ischemia. *Ann Intern Med* 1988; **108**: 312–17.
3. Pepine CJ, Geller NL, Knatterud GL et al. The Asymptomatic Cardiac Ischemia Pilot (ACIP) study: design of a randomized clinical trial, baseline data, and implications for a long-term outcome trial. *J Am Coll Cardiol* 1994; **24**: 1–10.
4. Tamesis B, Stelken A, Byers S et al. Comparison of the asymptomatic cardiac pilot and modified asymptomatic cardiac ischemia pilot versus Bruce and Cornell exercise protocols. *Am J Cardiol* 1993; **72**: 715–20.
5. Conti RC, Knatterud GL, Sopko G. Correction. *J Am Coll Cardiol* 1995; **842**: 842.
6. Knatterud GL, Bourassa MG, Pepine CJ et al. Effects of treatment strategies to suppress ischemia in patients with coronary artery disease: 12-week results of the Asymptomatic Cardiac Ischemia Pilot (ACIP) study. *J Am Coll Cardiol* 1994; **24**: 11–20.
7. Rogers WJ, Bourassa MG, Andrews TC et al. Asymptomatic Cardiac Ischemia Pilot (ACIP) study: outcome at one year for patients with asymptomatic cardiac ischemia randomized to medical therapy or revascularization. *J Am Coll Cardiol* 1995; **26**: 594–605.
8. Davies RF, Goldberg AD, Pepine CJ et al. Asymptomatic Cardiac Ischemia Pilot (ACIP) study two-year follow-up: outcomes of patients randomized to initial strategies of medical therapy versus revascularization. *Circulation* 1997 (in press).
9. Pepine CJ, Andrews T, Deanfield JE et al. Relation of patient characteristics to cardiac ischemia during daily life activity (an Asymptomatic Cardiac Ischemia Pilot data bank study). *Am J Cardiol* 1996; **77**: 1267–72.

10. Steingart RM, Forman S, Coglianese M et al. Factors limiting the enrollment of women in a randomized coronary artery disease trial. *Clin Cardiol* 1996; **19**: 614–18.

11. Sharaf BL, Williams DO, McMahan RP et al. A detailed angiographic analysis of patients with ambulatory electrocardiographic ischemia: a database study from the Asymptomatic Cardiac Ischemia Pilot (ACIP). *J Am Coll Cardiol* 1997; **29**: 78–84.

12. Pepine CJ, Sharaf B, Andrews T et al. Relationship between clinical, angiographic and ischemia findings at baseline and ischemia-related adverse outcomes at one year in the Asymptomatic Cardiac Ischemia Pilot trial. 1997 (in press).

13. Pratt CM, McMahan RP, Goldstein S et al. The Asymptomatic Cardiac Ischemia Pilot (ACIP) study: comparison of subgroups assigned to medical regimens used to suppress cardiac ischemia. *Am J Cardiol* 1996; **77**: 1302–9.

14. Bourassa MG, Pepine CJ, Forman SA et al. Asymptomatic Cardiac Ischemia Pilot (ACIP) study: effects of coronary angioplasty and coronary artery bypass graft surgery on recurrent angina and ischemia. *J Am Coll Cardiol* 1995; **26**: 606–14.

15. Bourassa MG, Knatterud GL, Pepine CJ, Sopko G. Asymptomatic Cardiac Ischemia Pilot (ACIP) study: improvement of cardiac ischemia at one year after PTCA and CABG. *Circulation* 1995; **92** (suppl II): 1–7.

16. Pepine CJ, Mark D, Bourassa M et al. Cost implications for treatment of cardiac ischemia: ancillary Asymptomatic Cardiac Ischemia Pilot (ACIP) study. *J Am Coll Cardiol* 1996; 186A.

17. Mahmarian JJ, Steingart RM, Forman S et al. Relation between ambulatory electrocardiographic monitoring and myocardial perfusion imaging to detect coronary artery disease and myocardial ischemia: an ACIP ancillary study. *J Am Coll Cardiol* 1997; **29**: 764–69.

10

Beta-blocking therapy for silent myocardial ischemia

Enrique V Carbajal and Prakash C Deedwania

Recent studies have demonstrated frequent episodes of silent myocardial ischemia in coronary artery disease (CAD) patients who were considered to be under adequate control of symptoms while receiving conventional antianginal drugs.[1] Although asymptomatic, such transient episodes of ischemia detected during daily life have been found to be associated with adverse clinical outcome and increased risk of coronary events and cardiac death.[2] Similar findings have been noted in patients suffering from acute coronary syndromes such as unstable angina[3] and acute myocardial infarction.[4]

Although minimally symptomatic myocardial ischemia is associated with adverse prognosis, at the present time there is no defined treatment approach for optimal therapy for patients with silent ischemia. It is, however, well established that rational therapy should be based on pathophysiologic consideration and therefore the pathophysiologic features of silent ischemia will first be summarized.

PATHOPHYSIOLOGIC EVENTS LEADING TO MYOCARDIAL ISCHEMIA AND THE ROLE OF BETA-BLOCKERS

Episodes of myocardial ischemia generally occur in association with obstructive atheromatous involvement of the coronary arteries. Myocardial ischemia occurs at the point where there is an imbalance between (increased) myocardial oxygen demand and (decreased) coronary blood flow. The onset of ischemia triggers several events including profound metabolic abnormalities and development of other clinically significant events such as diastolic and systolic dysfunction of the myocardium.[5]

The occurrence of ischemia in patients with stable CAD can become an unpredictable recurrent event. When this happens, it suggests the presence of variability in the coronary vasomotor tone that produces a more significant reduction in the cross-sectional lumen in the area of the coronary artery affected by an atheromatous lesion. The alteration of coronary vasomotor tone occurs due to varying degrees of endothelial dysfunction at the site of the atheroma and luminal stenosis. Although an atherosclerotic lesion may be fairly stable, the perfusion to a particular area of the myocardium can be reduced due to dynamic changes in the luminal diameter associated with altered endothelial activity overlying the area with stenosis. Vasoconstriction of the vessel can occur through several mechanisms such as loss of normal dilator responses and development of abnormal (paradoxical) constrictor activity in response to exercise, acetylcholine, and several other vasodilating substances.[6–12]

Other potential mechanisms for reduction in regional or global myocardial blood flow could involve an increased resistance to blood flow in the coronary arterioles,[13] constriction of distal coronary arteries, collateral vessels, or both,[14] and a decrease in subendocardial flow due to increased intracavitary pressures, for example congestive heart failure.[15] Although more work is required to determine the clinical significance of endothelial dysfunction in patients with CAD, it is evident that abnormalities of endothelial function, abnormalities of the distal coronary artery tone, as well as abnormal hemodynamic status can affect blood supply to the myocardium, resulting in the development of ischemia in patients with stable CAD.

In the vast majority of patients with obstructive CAD, the predominant cause of myocardial ischemia appears to be an increase in myocardial oxygen demand in the presence of a fixed coronary artery reserve. The increase in myocardial oxygen demand occurs largely due to increased heart rate, increased blood pressure or enhanced myocardial contractility. In most patients this is characterized by development of ischemia during periods of exertional activities or mental stress.

Some studies have suggested that most episodes of myocardial ischemia during daily activities occur with minimal or no physical activity.[16,17] Findings from recent studies, however, indicate that most silent ischemic episodes detected during electrocardiographic (ECG) monitoring are associated with an increase in hemodynamic parameters.[17,18] In one study, simultaneous evaluation of heart rate and blood pressure monitoring on a continuous basis in silent patients with stable CAD revealed that most silent ischemic episodes were preceded by an increase in the heart rate and systolic blood pressure.[17] Similar findings were noted in another study[18] in which evaluation of ischemic activity during electrocardiographic monitoring was performed while patients initiated physical activities at different times of the day. In this study it was noted that the most ischemic episodes were preceded by initiation of physical activity of sufficient magnitude to result in an increase in the heart rate. The increased myocardial O_2 demand preceding silent ischemia was seen in patients who started daily activities in the early morning

and in those patients who started activities at a later time in the day. Although the majority of silent ischemic episodes noted in these studies were preceded by increases in heart rate and blood pressure, some 20–30% of ischemic episodes did occur without any preceding increases in hemodynamic parameters. For the minority of ischemic episodes that were not preceded by hemodynamic changes, it is likely that abnormalities of coronary blood flow might have played a more significant role.

The findings from these studies evaluating the pathophysiologic mechanism of silent myocardial ischemia suggest a significant role of increased myocardial oxygen demand in the exercise laboratory and during ambulatory monitoring. This is an important issue to consider when evaluating management strategies for patients with established CAD. In most of these patients, a therapeutic strategy aimed at preventing or minimizing increases in heart rate or blood pressure will result in significant reduction or suppression of myocardial ischemia and relief of angina, and such treatment may provide the most therapeutic benefit. Limited evidence that helps support this concept comes from a study in patients with mixed angina (exertional and at rest) and CAD who were randomized to receive treatment with metoprolol (beta-blocker) or nifedipine (calcium-channel blocker). The patients underwent evaluation by exercise testing and Holter monitoring.[19] In this study, compared with long-acting nifedipine, therapy with long-acting metoprolol was found to be more effective. Metoprolol significantly reduced the number and duration of the ischemic events during ambulatory monitoring regardless of the clinical angina pattern and exercise tolerance.[19] The results from this study suggest an important role of beta-blockade in such patients.

CARDIOPROTECTIVE EFFECTS OF BETA-BLOCKERS

For several years the relationship between treatment with beta-blockers and clinical outcome has been extensively evaluated in

Table 10.1   General actions of antianginal drugs by class.

	Beta-blockers	Nitrates	Ca++-blockers[a]
Parameters of myocardial oxygen demand			
Inotropic activity	↓	↑	↑↔↓
Systolic pressure	↓↓	↓	↓↓
LV cavity volume	↑	↓↓	↑↓
Heart rate response	↓	↑	↑↓
Coronary flow			
Epicardial coronary blood flow	↓	↑	↑↑
Vasodilatation at site of atheroma	↓	↑	↑
Distal coronary flow	↑	↓	↑↑
Aortic pressure	↓	↓	↓
Antiplatelet effect	+	+	?

[a]Calcium-channel blockers.

↓: decreased; ↑: increased; ?: not known; ↔: no predominance of effect; LV: left ventricular; +: present.

patients who have suffered acute myocardial infarction.[20–36] In such patients, early and late treatment with beta-blockers has resulted in statistically significant modest reductions in the relative risk of total early (13–32%) and late (10–45%) mortality,[20,22,24,25,28,30] nonfatal reinfarction (19–47%),[20,21,23,28,32,33,39] sudden cardiac death (16–52%),[20,21,22–24,28,30,33,34] mortality in higher-risk patients with congestive heart failure (CHF) (47% versus 13% reduction in patients without CHF),[26] and in older patients (33% versus 19% reduction in younger patients).[27] Also, treatment with beta-blockers during the acute phase of myocardial infarction has been associated with a reduction in cardiac arrhythmias,[29,37] particularly in patients with enzymatic evidence of larger-size myocardial infarction (reduction in early and late ventricular fibrillation, primary and secondary ventricular fibrillation).[37] The beneficial effect of beta-blockers on mortality in acute myocardial infarction has been noted during extended follow-up of up to 6 years (18.2%).[31] In addition, treatment with beta-blockers has been associated with a reduc-

tion in the circadian variation of sudden death in the postacute myocardial infarction phase.[35] The results from these studies indicate a beneficial cardioprotective effect of beta-blockers in acute myocardial infarction. As yet, no other type of antianginal drug has demonstrated such beneficial effect in patients suffering from acute myocardial infarction or in other subsets of patients with CAD.

The cardioprotective effects of beta-blockers in acute myocardial infarction may be explained through several mechanisms such as ability to reduce the parameters of myocardial oxygen demand, antiarrhythmic activity, and potential antithrombotic properties (Table 10.1). In patients with stable CAD, beta-blockers may provide relief of symptoms primarily by affecting the determinants of myocardial oxygen demand, and perhaps by helping to avoid sudden hemodynamic stresses on the atheromatous coronary stenosis, thereby reducing the risk of plaque fissuring and potential associated thrombosis. These beneficial effects of beta-blockers on clinical outcome in patients with acute myocardial infarction might well be quite relevant when considering treatment of patients with stable CAD who are at risk of silent myocardial ischemia. Before discussing the specific role of beta-blockers in silent ischemia it would be useful to review the important pharmacologic features of beta-blockers.

PHARMACOLOGIC PROPERTIES OF BETA-ADRENERGIC BLOCKERS

Beta-blockers have achieved an important role in the management of patients with CAD. In the cardiac tissue, beta-blockers exert several actions aimed primarily at helping to decrease the myocardial oxygen demand (Table 10.1). These actions include a reduction in heart rate at rest, attenuation of the heart rate response to exertional activities, lowering of blood pressure, and reduction in force of myocardial contraction. Through other mechanisms such as prolongation of the diastolic phase of the cardiac cycle it has been suggested that beta-blockers might also help improve myocardial oxygen supply, particularly to the ischemic regions. Beta-blockers also appear to exert a beneficial influence on endothelial function, particularly at the level of coronary atheromas, and they may have some antiplatelet action as well.

Beta-blockers exert their actions through bindings to specific receptors in cardiac muscle (particularly β_1 receptors) and by doing so they competitively inhibit the binding of catecholamines. This action results in attenuated cardiac response to sympathetic stimulation. Through a negative inotropic effect, beta-blockers may increase left ventricular (LV) volume, LV end-diastolic pressure, and increase pulmonary capillary pressure. These actions could cause a patient to experience dyspnea and perhaps limit functional capacity. In patients with evidence of left ventricular dysfunction there is a risk that these agents may precipitate development of congestive heart failure.

The effects of beta-blocker therapy on regional myocardial flow and coronary vasomotion have been studied on a limited basis in the animal model[38] and in patients with CAD.[39,40] Compared with findings during exercise without beta-blocker therapy, treatment with a cardioselective beta-blocker (atenolol) in chronic CAD in the animal model was associated with improved myocardial blood flow per beat, increase in the endocardial-to-epicardial blood flow ratio, and improved regional wall motion during exercise.[38] In a study of patients with CAD, the vasomotion of normal and stenosed coronary arteries was evaluated during exercise testing before and after treatment with propranolol. Compared with the angiographic findings during exercise testing before therapy, treatment with propranolol was associated with prevention of exercise-induced narrowing of stenotic areas.[39] Furthermore, in this study, the use of propranolol was not associated with potentiation of coronary vasoconstriction. In another study, patients with CAD underwent angiographic evaluation before and after exercise testing, prior to and after administration of propranolol. In this study, exercise testing was associated with vasodilatation of normal coronaries and vasoconstriction of stenosed segments. After administration of propranolol there was decreased luminal diameter in normal and stenosed segments of coronary arteries at rest. However, during subsequent dynamic exercise there was vasodilatation of both normal and stenosed segments in patients receiving propranolol.[40] These results suggest that, although nonselective beta-blockade might potentiate vasoconstriction, the use of beta-blockers attenuates the vasoconstrictory response to catecholamines during exercise.

Several beta-blockers have been found to affect platelet aggregability. Studies in healthy persons and in patients with CAD have provided evidence of the ability of beta-blockers to prevent or reduce platelet aggregability during exposure to aggregating agents and during exercise stress testing.[41–45] Although this potential beneficial action of beta-blockers may be more relevant to patients suffering from acute coronary syndromes (unstable angina, acute myocardial infarction), it might indeed

Table 10.2   Suggested antianginal drugs in the presence of other medical conditions.

	1st drug	2nd drug	3rd drug
History of prior MI	Beta-blocker	Nitrate	Ca^{++}-blocker (?!)
Chronic exercise or effort angina	Beta-blocker	Nitrate	Ca^{++}-blocker
Angina at rest or nocturnal	Ca^{++}-blocker	Nitrate	Beta-blocker (cardioselective)
Supraventricular tachyarrhythmias	Beta-blocker	Ca^{++}-blocker (D,V)	Nitrate
Bradyarrhythmias or AV blocks	Nitrate	Ca^{++}-blocker (N,A)	
Peripheral vascular disease	Ca^{++}-blocker	Nitrate	Beta-blocker (cardioselective)
Congestive heart failure	Nitrate	Ca^{++}-blocker (A,N)	Beta-blocker (cardioselective)
COPD	Nitrate	Ca^{++}-blocker	Beta-blocker (cardioselective)
IDDM	Nitrate	Ca^{++}-blocker	Beta-blocker (cardioselective)
Renal failure	Nitrate	Ca^{++}-blocker (D)*	Beta-blocker *, (cardioselective)
IHSS	Beta-blocker	Ca^{++}-blocker (D,V)	

MI: myocardial infarction; Ca^{++}: calcium channel; ?!: caution; D: diltiazem; V: verapamil; AV: atrioventricular; N: nifedipine; A: amlodipine; COPD: chronic obstructive pulmonary disease; IDDM: insulin-dependent diabetes mellitus; *: hepatic metabolism; IHSS: idiopathic hypertrophic subaortic stenosis.

also play a therapeutic role in patients with stable CAD and episodes of silent myocardial ischemia.

In patients with stable CAD, beta-blockers have proved to be important therapeutic agents as monotherapy as well as adjunctive therapy to other antianginal drugs in the treatment of angina pectoris.[46] Beta-blockers are especially useful in the management of angina during exercise. In the treatment of patients with stable CAD the so-called cardioselective beta-blockers (β_1-receptor blockers) are preferred over agents that also possess β_2-receptor blocking activity. Stimulation of β_2-receptors is associated with arterial vasodilatation. This property may be of clinical significance in patients with CAD since blockade of β_2 vasodilator activity may be associated with risk of developing generalized, and particularly focal, coronary vasoconstriction due to unopposed alpha-vasoconstrictor activity in the areas of coronary atheroma.[47] Some evidence indicates that this is a relatively frequent problem during treatment with noncardioselective beta-blockers.[48] In contrast to this notion, there is available evidence to suggest that in the presence of increased sympathetic activity beta-blockers do not adversely affect coronary vasodilatation associated with exertion, and may even help attenuate or reverse coronary vasoconstriction in areas of coronary atheroma during exertional activity.[38–40]

The addition of a nitrate or a calcium-channel antagonist appears to counteract the potential vasoconstrictive influence of nonselective beta-blockers. Stimulation of β_2-receptors is associated with relaxation of bronchial smooth muscle, and if inhibited there is a risk of triggering various degrees of bronchospasm and wheezing. It should, however, be noted that at progressively higher doses the cardioselective beta-blockers also begin to lose β_1-selective action because of a greater degree of binding to β_2-receptors.

Treatment with beta-blockers can produce various side-effects that may limit their clinical usefulness (Table 10.2). For example, one should exert caution using beta-blockers in patients

Table 10.3 Comparative doses and actions of commonly used beta-blockers.

	Dose/day (mg)	Cardio-selective	Lipid-soluble	Plasma half-life, h	Elimination route	CNS effects	ISA	DM safety	PVD safety
Metoprolol	100–200	+	++	3–4	Hepatic	+	–	+	+
Atenolol	50–200	+	+	6–9	Renal	+,–	–	+	+
Betaxolol	10–20	+	+	14–22	Renal	+	–	+	+
Propranolol	160–480	–	++++	3–6	Hepatic	+++	–	–	–
Nadolol	40–320	–	+	12–24	Renal	–,+	–	–	–
Timolol	20–40	–	+,++	3–5	Hepatic	++	–,+	–	–
Pindolol	20–40	–	++	8	Renal	++	+++	–	–
Labetalol	200–800	–, also α_1	+	6–8	Hepatic	–,+	+	–	–

CNS: central nervous system; ISA: intrinsic sympathomimetic activity; DM: diabetes mellitus; PVD: peripheral vascular disease; (+): present; (–): not present; α_1: alpha$_1$ adrenergic receptor blocker.

with persistent bradyarrhythmias, atrioventricular conduction abnormalities, or the presence of clinical congestive heart failure. Other relative contraindications to the use of beta-blockers are the presence of reactive airway disease, peripheral arterial insufficiency, and diabetes mellitus in patients who have had problems with previous clinically significant hypoglycemic episodes.

Beta-blockers have different properties such as water- or lipid-solubility and mild intrinsic ability to stimulate the β-receptors (partial intrinsic sympathomimetic activity (ISA)) (Table 10.3). The water-soluble beta-blockers such as nadolol and atenolol appear to be less likely to diffuse across the blood–brain barrier. This translates into a lower incidence of central nervous system (CNS) side-effects such as depression and generalized fatigue. These are fairly uncommon side-effects (especially in the elderly) but any beta-blocker has the potential for these side-effects. Beta-blockers with alpha-adrenergic blocking activity may be useful in CAD patients with angina who suffer from intermittent claudication in the extremities.

It is appropriate to initiate treatment with a low dose and progressively increase the dose while monitoring for adverse reactions. The maintenance dosage of beta-blockers should be titrated to achieve the desired therapeutic effects. Evaluation of adequate dosage can be made during exercise stress testing while monitoring for the occurrence of symptoms and the heart rate and blood pressure responses. Although the use of continuous Holter monitoring for ischemia is not fully established in clinical practice, it should be considered to help evaluate the anti-ischemic effects of beta-blockers in high-risk patients. After initiating treatment with a beta-blocker, ideal therapeutic goals should include a significant reduction in frequency or abolition of anginal attacks, a relative attenuation of the heart rate response during exercise (to approximately 50% increment above the resting heart rate), a heart rate at rest of 50–60 beats/min, attenuation of blood pressure response during exercise, and absence of adverse reactions.[49]

A significant potential problem in patients with CAD who are receiving treatment with a beta-blocker is the risk of developing withdrawal symptoms after abrupt discontinuation of the drug.[50] A few of the manifestations of acute beta-blocker withdrawal in patients with

CAD include exacerbation of angina, frequent ventricular ectopy, and risk for developing acute myocardial infarction and sudden death.[51,52] Any condition or situation associated with enhanced sympathetic activity carries the potential for triggering the occurrence of beta-blocker withdrawal.

COMBINATION THERAPY WITH A BETA-BLOCKER AND OTHER ANTIANGINAL DRUGS

In patients with CAD the use of two or more antianginal agents in combination may allow for management with lower doses of each drug which can help reduce the rate of adverse effects and improve patient compliance with the prescribed treatment (Table 10.2). Such combination therapy can be more effective in suppressing anginal episodes when compared with either agent given alone. There is a rather limited amount of data from studies in patients with CAD which have evaluated the anti-ischemic efficacy of treatment with beta-blockers as monotherapy or in combination for suppression of silent ischemic episodes during continuous monitoring.

COMPARISON OF VARIOUS ANTI-ISCHEMIC DRUGS

Various classes of antianginal drugs (beta-blockers, nitrates, calcium-channel blockers) produce a wide range of cardiovascular effects (Table 10.1). These drugs have been extensively evaluated for the treatment of angina and myocardial ischemia. These drugs have undergone careful evaluation for their ability to reduce or suppress ischemia detected during exercise testing in patients with stable CAD. Because of the recent information concerning the clinical significance of ischemia detected during electrocardiographic monitoring in patients with CAD, conventional antianginal drugs have been evaluated in a more objective manner for their anti-ischemic effects outside the exercise laboratory. Specifically, recent studies have evaluated the anti-ischemic properties of antianginal drugs

during continuous Holter monitoring.[53–75] Although most of the antianginal drugs are effective in reducing the frequency and severity of anginal attacks, several recent studies in patients with acute coronary syndromes as well as in patients with stable angina have revealed that drug therapy aimed at control of symptoms does not eliminate or sufficiently suppress episodes of silent ischemia detected during Holter monitoring.[3,19] These findings may have important future clinical implications. The following sections will describe treatment with beta-blockers in patients with angina and stable CAD, their ability to reduce or suppress ischemia, and their role as anti-ischemic agents in the treatment of patients with stable CAD and silent episodes of ischemia.

COMPARISON OF BETA-BLOCKERS WITH OTHER DRUGS IN SILENT ISCHEMIA

Several recent studies have evaluated the anti-ischemic effects of various antianginal drugs given as monotherapy or as combination therapy during prolonged ambulatory Holter monitoring in patients with stable CAD.[18,53–75] Most of these studies have reported positive results characterized by significant reductions in the frequency and duration of silent myocardial ischemia during active treatment. However, despite control of angina and variable degrees in reduction of ischemic activity, in none of these studies was complete suppression of ischemia achieved in all patients who underwent active treatment. In each of these studies there were several patients (Fig. 10.1) who continued to demonstrate ischemic episodes during the monitoring period while receiving treatment.

In general, the findings from these studies indicate that treatment regimens which include a beta-blocker have a more prominent anti-ischemic effect compared with those without a beta-blocking agent.[57,58,62] The anti-ischemic effect seen during treatment with a beta-blocker may be explained in part by the ability of these drugs to attenuate the heart rate (hemodynamic) response to catecholamines.

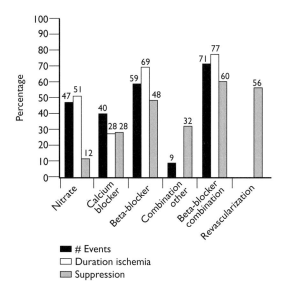

Figure 10.1 Effect of treatment with various classes of antianginal drug therapy and myocardial revascularization on the frequency, duration and total suppression of transient ischemic episodes.

EFFECTS OF BETA-BLOCKERS VERSUS OTHER DRUGS ON HEART RATE AND SILENT ISCHEMIA

As discussed under the section on pathophysiology, heart rate plays an important role in the pathogenesis of silent ischemic episodes recorded during continuous Holter monitoring.[17,18,56–58] Based on the available data from a few studies that have evaluated the effect of antianginal therapy on heart rate and silent myocardial ischemia, it appears that treatment with beta-blockers as monotherapy or in combination results in the greatest reduction in heart rate during the monitoring period and before the onset of silent ischemic episodes.

In the Atenolol Silent Ischemia Study (ASIST) in patients with chronic CAD and asymptomatic ischemia who were evaluated by Holter monitoring, patients were randomized to receive atenolol or placebo.[58] Compared with placebo, treatment with atenolol was associated with a significant decrease in mean heart rate (from 75 to 63 beats per minute (bpm) versus 75

to 75 bpm with placebo, $P < 0.0001$) during Holter monitoring. In the Total Ischemic Burden Bisoprolol Study (TIBBS), a greater anti-ischemic effect was seen during treatment with bisoprolol.[62] In the Asymptomatic Cardiac Ischemia Pilot (ACIP) study there was a consistent relationship between heart rate reduction and abolition of silent ischemia. Silent ischemia was detected on a more frequent basis when the mean heart rate was > 80 bpm and less likely ($P < 0.001$) to occur if the mean heart rate during monitoring was < 70 bpm.[65] This finding was seen in each medical treatment group regardless of the combination regimen (atenolol–nifedipine or diltiazem– nitrate) used during monitoring. There was a significant ($P = 0.03$) trend toward lower heart rate in favor of the group receiving the combination atenolol–nifedipine. In the ACIP study, however, several patients receiving the combination with the beta-blocker experienced heart rates greater than 100 bpm during the monitoring period. This finding suggests that insufficient dosage of beta-blocker might have been used in the study and a greater degree of beta-blockade manifested by a slower heart rate could have been associated with a greater proportion of patients showing complete abolition of transient silent ischemia during Holter monitoring.

BETA-BLOCKERS AS MONOTHERAPY FOR SILENT ISCHEMIA

Recent studies in patients with documented CAD and stable angina have evaluated the effect of treatment with beta-blockers on silent myocardial ischemia detected during continuous ambulatory electrocardiographic monitoring. Overall, compared with other antianginal agents, beta-blockers appear to be the significantly more effective anti-ischemic drugs when given as monotherapy (Fig. 10.1). Review of the available data indicates that compared with other antianginal drugs such as nitrates and calcium-channel blockers, treatment with beta-blockers in patients with stable CAD is associated with a greater relative reduction in the frequency (59%) and duration (69%) of transient

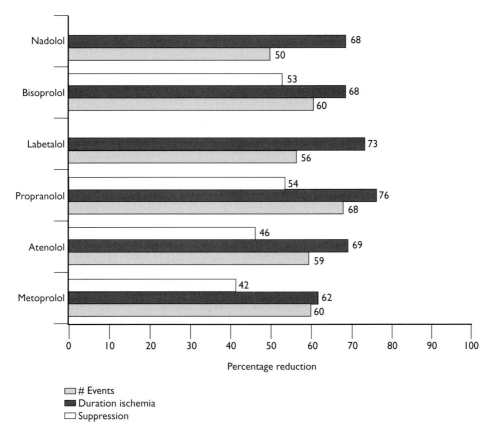

Figure 10.2 Effect of treatment with beta-blockers on the frequency, duration and total suppression of transient ischemic episodes.

myocardial ischemia detected during Holter monitoring (Fig. 10.1).[18,19,53,55,58,59,62,64,70,73–75] Although several different beta-blockers have been evaluated for their anti-ischemic efficacy on frequency and duration of silent ischemic episodes (Fig. 10.2), only a few studies provide data about total suppression of ischemia. Based on the available data it seems that therapy with a beta-blocker results in a relative total suppression of silent ischemia in approximately 48% of patients (Figs 10.1 and 10.2).[55,58,62,75] When beta-blockers are used in combination with other agents such as calcium-channel blockers there appears to be a further beneficial anti-ischemic effect characterized by greater reduction in the frequency and duration (71% and 77%, respec-

tively) of ischemic episodes detected during Holter monitoring and by an increase in the proportion (60%) of patients without evidence of silent ischemia during the monitoring period (Fig. 10.1). The rate of complete suppression of ischemic activity achieved during treatment with combination therapy that includes a beta-blocker compares favorably with the suppression rate (56%) achieved after myocardial revascularization with percutaneous transluminal coronary angioplasty and coronary artery bypass graft surgery (CABG) (Fig. 10.1).[57,60] In the ASIST trial the effect of atenolol on silent ischemia was evaluated in a double-blind, prospective, randomized manner in patients with documented stable CAD.[58] In this study, when compared with placebo, treatment with atenolol was associated with a significant decrease in the frequency (53% versus 30%), duration (45% versus 18%), and total suppression (60% versus 39%) of silent ischemic events at the 4-week evaluation ($P \leq 0.02$ for all comparisons).[58] In TIBBS, a randomized double-blind study with two parallel groups, the anti-ischemic effects of treatment with a long-acting beta-blocker (bisoprolol or nifedipine) were compared during Holter monitoring in patients with stable CAD.[62] In this study, therapy with bisoprolol, when compared with nifedipine, was far more effective in producing a greater reduction in the frequency (60% versus 29%, respectively, $P = 0.0001$) and duration (68% versus 28%, $P = 0.0001$) of ischemic events. Treatment with bisoprolol was also associated with a significantly greater rate (52.5% versus 15.6%, $P < 0.0001$) of suppression of ischemic activity.

COMBINATION THERAPY WITH BETA-BLOCKERS FOR SILENT ISCHEMIA

Limited data are available from a few studies evaluating the effects of combination anti-ischemic therapy on silent ischemia.[55,57,60,70,73,75] The combination of a beta-blocker, propranolol, metoprolol, or atenolol, and a calcium-channel antagonist, nifedipine or amlodipine, has been found to have greater anti-ischemic effect than treatment with any single agent.[55,73,75] The anti-ischemic effects of combination therapy in these studies were characterized by a lesser frequency and duration of ischemic episodes during Holter monitoring and greater rate of suppression of ischemia during ECG monitoring (Fig. 10.1).[55,57,73,75] Few data, however, are available on the effect of combination antianginal therapy on total suppression of silent ischemia. In one study, the use of combination therapy with propranolol and nifedipine resulted in total suppression of ischemia in 85% of the patients studied.[55] In the ACIP study, two drug combination schedules were used for patients randomized to receive angina-guided or ischemia-guided treatments. The combina-

tion of atenolol and nifedipine or the combination of diltiazem and isosorbide dinitrate resulted in more modest total suppression rates of 48% and 33%, respectively.[57] The modest effects on total ischemia suppression seen in the ACIP study could be partly explained by the fact that there was a limitation to upward adjustment of dosage for each drug used. It is possible that higher dosages could have resulted in even higher suppression rates of ambulatory silent ischemia during subsequent evaluation with Holter monitoring.

EFFECTS OF BETA-BLOCKERS AND OTHER DRUGS ON CLINICAL OUTCOME IN PATIENTS WITH SILENT ISCHEMIA

It is now well established that it is the presence of myocardial ischemia rather than the associated symptoms that predicts the adverse clinical outcome in patients with acute as well as chronic stable CAD. It would therefore seem logical to think that total suppression of ischemia might be associated with a much better clinical outcome. Based on the available prognostic data it has been suggested that the goal of antianginal therapy should be suppression of all ischemic episodes, whether they are associated with angina or are silent. Although this is an appealing concept there is, as yet, no definitive evidence to indicate that complete suppression of silent ischemia with aggressive anti-ischemic drug therapy will result in better clinical outcomes in patients with CAD and transient silent ischemia.

A few recent, well controlled, randomized, and large-scale studies have evaluated the impact of Holter-guided anti-ischemic therapy on the frequency and duration of silent ischemia during daily life. Some of these studies have also attempted to evaluate the effects of ischemia-guided therapy on clinical outcome in patients with stable CAD.[57,58,62] The evaluation of clinical outcome in some of these studies also revealed that, compared with control groups, the patients randomized to active therapy experienced a lower rate of adverse events which correlated with reduction or suppression of ischemia. In the

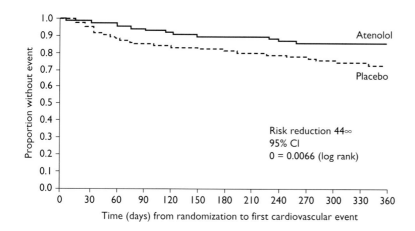

Figure 10.3 Event-free survival. Kaplan-Meier curves comparing the cumulative probabilities of not experiencing an adverse event during follow-up for patients with ambulatory electrocardiogram-monitored silent ischemia randomized to atenolol (upper curve) and placebo (lower curve). (With permission from the American Heart Association. *Circulation* 1994;**90**:762–8).

ASIST trial, patients with CAD and minimally symptomatic were randomized to receive atenolol 100 mg daily or placebo.[58] The patients randomized to atenolol therapy, compared with placebo, experienced a significantly lower frequency and duration of ischemic episodes during 48-hour Holter monitoring. Evaluation of clinical outcome during the 1-year follow-up (Fig. 10.3) revealed that, compared with placebo, patients treated with atenolol experienced fewer unfavorable events (11% versus 25%, respectively, $P <0.001$) and a longer event-free survival (120 versus 79 days, respectively), with a relative risk reduction of 56% ($P = 0.001$). Evaluation of specific events such as death, nonfatal myocardial infarction, resuscitation from ventricular tachycardia/ventricular fibrillation, or hospitalization for unstable angina, showed a nonsignificant trend in favor of treatment with atenolol compared with placebo.[58] In the TIBBS trial, compared with patients without total suppression of ischemia, patients with complete suppression of ischemic activity achieved a significantly lower incidence of clinical events (21.6% versus 38%, $P = 0.01$) during follow-up evaluation.[62]

So far only one large-scale study, the ACIP study, has evaluated the effect of combined anti-ischemic drug therapy compared with coronary revascularization on complete suppression of silent ischemia (primary end-point) and secondary end-points that included clinical events (death, myocardial infarction, cardiac arrest, unstable angina, sustained ventricular tachycardia, congestive heart failure), ambulatory ECG and exercise test findings.[57,60,61] The results of the ACIP study have revealed that although ischemia-guided therapy was effective in reducing the magnitude of ischemia, it failed to suppress ischemic episodes in all patients at the 12-week evaluation (primary end-point); myocardial revascularization (especially surgical revascularization) appeared to be a more effective anti-ischemic therapy compared with either combination drug therapy (atenolol–nifedipine or diltiazem–isosorbide dinitrate).

Although only partial data are available from the TIBBS trial regarding the relationship of suppression versus reduction in ischemic activity and clinical outcome, and the findings from that study indicate superiority of beta-blockade, these results do not provide definitive evidence that total suppression of ischemic activity is associated with better clinical outcome. Although suppression of ischemia was not achieved in all patients with conventional (symptoms-guided or ischemia-guided) therapy in these studies, the findings do indicate that anti-ischemic therapy should be designed to provide optimal reduction or even total suppression of ischemia. In order to determine whether complete suppression of ischemia is associated with better clinical outcome, long-term, large-scale studies need to be conducted utilizing various therapeutic strategies to achieve the desired anti-ischemic effects. Another important point to consider in the management of patients with silent ischemia and stable CAD is the fact that treatment with beta-blockers has been found to attenuate the morning increase (circadian variation) in ischemic activity in patients with CAD, which might be relevant for reducing the risk of acute myocardial infarction and sudden cardiac death rates.[18,56,62,74]

CONCLUSION

There are several antianginal drugs and therapeutic strategies available for the treatment of patients with CAD and silent ischemia. However, of the available antianginal drugs, beta-blockers appear to be most effective in suppressing myocardial ischemia and have become the most useful antianginal drugs. The unique beneficial anti-ischemic efficacy of beta-blockers can be explained by their actions on hemodynamic parameters, vasomotion, and platelet functions. Based on the available data it can be concluded that beta-blockers, when tolerated, are highly effective for the treatment of silent ischemia. Compared with other available anti-ischemic drugs, beta-blockers show a greater ability to attenuate the magnitude of myocardial ischemia (mostly silent) detected during routine daily activities. Although more data are needed the findings from recent studies suggest that treatment with beta-blockers is also beneficial in reducing the risk of adverse clinical outcome associated with silent ischemia.

REFERENCES

1. Cohn P, Vetrovec G, Nesto R, Gerber F. The nifedipine-total ischemia awareness program: a national survey of painful and painless myocardial ischemia including results of antiischemic therapy. *Am J Cardiol* 1989; **63**: 534–39.
2. Yeung A, Barry J, Orav J, Bonassin E, Raby K, Selwyn A. Effect of asymptomatic ischemia on long-term prognosis in chronic stable coronary disease. *Circulation* 1991; **83**: 1598–604.
3. Gottlieb S, Weisfeldt M, Ouyang P, Mellits E, Gerstenblith G. Silent ischemia as a marker for early unfavorable outcomes in patients with unstable angina. *N Engl J Med* 1986; **314**: 1214–19.
4. Gill J, Cairns J, Roberts R et al. Prognostic importance of myocardial ischemia detected by ambulatory monitoring early after acute myocardial infarction. *N Engl J Med* 1996; **334**: 65–70.
5. Braunwald E, Sobel B. Coronary blood flow and myocardial ischemia. In: Braunwald E, ed. *Heart Disease: A Textbook of Cardiovascular Medicine* (Philadelphia, PA: WB Saunders, 1988): 1191–221.
6. Gage J, Hess D, Murakami T, Ritter M, Grimm J, Krayenbueh H. Vasoconstriction of stenotic coronary arteries during dynamic exercise in patients with classic angina pectoris: reversibility by nitroglycerin. *Circulation* 1986; **73**: 865–76.
7. Gordon J, Ganz P, Nabel E et al. Atherosclerosis and endothelial function influence the coronary response to exercise. *J Clin Invest* 1989; **83**: 1946–52.
8. Nabel E, Ganz P, Gordon J, Alexander R, Selwyn A. Dilation of normal and constriction of atherosclerotic coronary arteries caused by the cold pressor test. *Circulation* 1988; **77**: 43–52.
9. Zeiher A, Drexler H, Wollschlager H, Just H. Modulation of coronary vasomotor tone in humans. Progressive endothelial dysfunction with different early stages of coronary atherosclerosis. *Circulation* 1991; **83**: 391–401.
10. Zeiher A, Drexler H, Wollschlager H, Saurbier B, Just H. Coronary vasomotion in response to sympathetic simulation in humans: importance of the functional integrity of the endothelium. *J Am Coll Cardiol* 1989; **14**: 1181–90.
11. Nabel E, Selwyn A, Ganz P. Large coronary arteries in humans are responsive to changing blood flow: an endothelium-dependent mechanism that fails in patients with atherosclerosis. *J Am Coll Cardiol* 1990; **16**: 349–56.
12. Crea F, Davies G, Romeo F et al. Myocardial ischemia during ergonovine testing: different

susceptibility to coronary vasoconstriction in patients with exertional and variant angina. *Circulation* 1984; **69**: 690–5.

13. Cannon R, Watson R, Rosing, Epestine S. Angina caused by reduced vasodilator reserve of the small coronary arteries. *J Am Coll Cardiol* 1983; **1**: 1359–73.

14. Pupita G, Maseri A, Kaski J et al. Myocardial ischemia caused by distal coronary artery constriction in stable angina pectoris. *N Engl J Med* 1990; **323**: 514–20.

15. Ellis A, Klocke F. Effect of preload of the transmural distribution of perfusion and pressure flow relationship in the canine coronary vascular bed. *Circ Res* 1980; **46**: 68–77.

16. Imperi GA, Lambert CR, Coy K, Lopez L, Pepine C. Effects of titrated beta blockade (metoprolol) on silent myocardial ischemia in ambulatory patients with coronary artery disease. *Am J Cardiol* 1987; **60**: 519–24.

17. Deedwania P, Nelson J. Pathophysiology of silent myocardial ischemia during daily life: hemodynamic evaluation by simultaneous electrocardiographic and blood pressure monitoring. *Circulation* 1990; **82**: 1296–304.

18. Parker J, Testa M, Jimenez A et al. Morning increase in ambulatory ischemia in patients with stable coronary artery disease. Importance of physical activity and increased cardiac demand. *Circulation* 1994; **89**: 604–14.

19. Ardissino D, Savonitto S, Egstrup K et al. Transient myocardial ischemia during daily life in rest and exertional angina and comparison of effectiveness of metoprolol versus nifedipine. *Am J Cardiol* 1991; **67**: 946–52.

20. Yusuf S, Sleight P, Hels P, McMahon S. Routine medical management of acute myocardial infarction. Lessons from overviews of recent randomized controlled trials. *Circulation* 1990; **82** (suppl II): 117–34.

21. Yusuf S. The use of beta-adrenergic blocking agents, i.v. nitrates and calcium channel blocking agents following acute myocardial infarction. *Chest* 1988; **93**: 25S–28S.

22. Friedman L. A randomized trial of propranolol in patients with acute myocardial infarction. Mortality results. *JAMA* 1982; **247**: 1707–14.

23. Curb J. A randomized trial of propranolol in patients with acute myocardial infarction. Morbidity results. *JAMA* 1983; **250**: 2814–19.

24. Golstein S. Propranolol therapy in patients with acute myocardial infarction: the beta-blocker heart attack trial. *Circulation* 1983; **67**(suppl I): 53–6.

25. Herlitz J, Hjalmarson A, Sweberg K et al. The influence of early intervention in acute MI on long-term mortality and morbidity as assessed in the Goteborg metoprolol trial. *Intern J Cardiol* 1986; **10**: 291–301.

26. Chadda K, Goldstein S, Byington R, Curb J. Effect of propranolol after acute myocardial infarction in patients with congestive heart failure. *Circulation* 1986; **73**: 503–10.

27. Hawkins C, Richardson D, Vokonas P. Effect of propranolol in reducing mortality in older myocardial infarction patients. *Circulation* 1983; **67**(suppl I): 94–7.

28. ISIS-1. Randomized trial of intravenous atenolol among 16 027 cases of suspected acute myocardial infarction. *Lancet* 1986; **i**: 57–66.

29. Norris R, Brown M, Clarke E, Barnaby P, Geary G, Logan R. Prevention of ventricular fibrillation during acute myocardial infarction by intravenous propranolol. *Lancet* 1986; **i**: 883–6.

30. The Norwegian multicenter study group. Timolol-induced reduction in mortality and reinfarction in patients surviving acute myocardial infarction. *N Engl J Med* 1981; **304**: 801–7.

31. Pedersen T. Six-year follow up of the Norwegian multicenter study on timolol after acute myocardial infarction. *N Engl J Med* 1985; **313**: 1044–58.

32. The TIMI study group. Comparison of invasive and conservative strategies after treatment with intravenous tissue plasminogen activator in acute myocardial infarction. *N Engl J Med* 1989; **320**: 618–27.

33. Roberts R, Rogers W, Mueller H et al. Immediate versus deferred beta-blockade following thrombolytic therapy in patients with acute myocardial infarction. *Circulation* 1991; **83**: 4422–37.

34. Hansteen V. Beta blockade after myocardial infarction: the Norwegian propranolol study in high-risk patients. *Circulation* 1983: **67** (suppl I): 57–60.

35. Peters R, Muller J, Golstein S, Byington R, Friedman L. Propranolol and the morning increase in the frequency of sudden cardiac death (BHAT study). *Am J Cardiol* 1989; **63**: 1518–20.

36. Frishman W, Lazar E. Reduction of mortality, sudden death and non-fatal reinfarction with beta-adrenergic blockers in survivors of acute MI: a new hypothesis regarding the cardiopro-

tective action of beta-adrenergic blockade. *Am J Cardiol* 1990; **66**: 66g–70g.

37. Herlitz J, Hjalmarson A, Swedberg K, Waagstein F, Holmberg S, Waldenstrom J. Relationship between infarct size and incidence of severe ventricular arrhythmias in a double-blind trial with metoprolol in acute MI. *Int J Cardiol* 1984; **6**: 47–60.

38. Matsuzake M, Patritti J, Tajimi T, Miller M, Kemper W, Ross J. Effects of beta-blockade on regional myocardial flow and function during exercise. *Am J Physiol* 1984; **247**: H52–H60.

39. Gaglione A, Hess O, Corin W, Ritter M, Grimm J, Krayenbuehl H. Is there coronary vasoconstriction after intracoronary beta-adrenergic blockade in patients with coronary artery disease? *J Am Coll Cardiol* 1987; **10**: 299–310.

40. Bortone A, Hess O, Gaglione A et al. Effect of intravenous propranolol on coronary vasomotion at rest and during dynamic exercise in patients with coronary artery disease. *Circulation* 1990; **81**: 1225–35.

41. Kerry R, Scrutton M, Wallis R. Beta-adrenoceptor antagonists and human platelets: relationship of effects to lipid solubility. *Biochem Pharmacol* 1984; **33**: 2615–22.

42. King M, Corrigan J, Fenster P. Antiplatelet effects of oral diltiazem, propranolol, and their combination. *Br J Clin Pharmacol* 1987; **24**: 615–20.

43. Frishman W, Weksler B, Christodoulou J, Smithen C, Killip T. Reversal of abnormal platelet aggregability and change in exercise tolerance in patients with angina pectoris following oral propranolol. *Circulation* 1974; **50**: 887–96.

44. Winther K, Willich S. Beta1-blockade and acute coronary ischemia. Possible role of platelets. *Circulation* 1991; **84** (suppl VI): 68–71.

45. Mehta J, Mehta P, Pepine C. Platelet aggregation in aortic and coronary venous blood in patients with and without coronary disease. *Circulation* 1978; **58**: 881–6.

46. Prichard B. Beta-adrenoreceptor blocking drugs in angina pectoris. In: Avery GX, ed. *Cardiovascular Drugs, Vol. 2: Beta-Adrenoreceptor Blocking Drugs.* (Baltimore, MD: University Park Press, 1978): 85–118.

47. Kern J, Ganz P, Horowitz J et al. Potentiation of coronary vasoconstriction by beta-adrenergic blockade in patients with coronary artery disease. *Circulation* 1983; **67**: 1178–85.

48. Prida X, Feldman R, Hill J, Pepine C. Comparison of selective (beta 1) and nonselec-

tive (beta 1 and beta 2) beta-adrenergic blockade on systemic and coronary hemodynamic findings in angina pectoris. *Am J Cardiol* 1987; **60**: 244–8.

49. Aellig W. Beta-adrenoceptor blocking activity and duration of action of pindolol and propranolol in healthy volunteers. *Br J Clin Pharm* 1976; **3**: 251–7.

50. Nattel S, Rangno R, Loon G. Mechanism of propranolol withdrawal phenomena. *Circulation* 1979; **59**: 1158–64.

51. Miller R, Olson H, Amsterdam E, Mason D. Propranolol withdrawal rebound phenomenon: exacerbation of coronary events after abrupt cessation of antianginal therapy. *N Engl J Med* 1975; **293**: 416–18.

52. Alderman E, Coltart K, Wettach G, Harrison D. Coronary artery syndromes after sudden propranolol withdrawal. *Ann Intern Med* 1974; **81**: 625–7.

53. Hassan E, Davies G. Optimal control of myocardial ischemia: the benefit of a fixed combination of atenolol and nifedipine in patients with chronic stable angina. *Br Heart J* 1992; **68**: 291–5.

54. Glasser S, Friedman R, Talibi T, Smith L, Weir E. Safety and compatibility of betaxolol hydrochloride combined with diltiazem or nifedipine therapy in stable angina pectoris. *Am J Cardiol* 1994; **73**: 213–18.

55. Kawanishi D, Reid C, Morrison E, Rahimtoola S. Response of angina and ischemia to long-term treatment in patients with stable angina: double blind randomized dosing trial of nifedipine, propranolol and their combination. *J Am Coll Cardiol* 1992; **19**: 409–17.

56. Stone P, Gibson R, Glasser S et al. Comparison of propranolol, diltiazem and nifedipine in the treatment of ambulatory ischemia in patients with stable angina. *Circulation* 1990; **82**: 1962–72.

57. Knatterud G, Bourassa M, Pepine C et al. Effects of treatment strategies to suppress ischemia in patients with CAD: 12-week results of the asymptomatic cardiac ischemia (ACIP) study. *J Am Coll Cardiol* 1994; **24**: 11–20.

58. Pepine C, Cohn P, Deedwania P et al. Effects of treatment on outcome in mildly symptomatic patients with ischemia during daily life. The atenolol silent ischemia study. *Circulation* 1994; **90**: 762–8.

59. Deanfield J, Detry J, Lichtlen P et al. Amlodipine reduces transient myocardial ischemia in patients with CAD: double blind circadian anti-

ischemia program in Europe (CAPE trial). *J Am Coll Cardiol* 1994; **24**: 1460–7.

60. Rogers W, Bourassa M, Andrews T et al. Asymptomatic cardiac ischemia pilot study: outcome at 1 year for patients with ischemia randomized to medical therapy or revascularization. *J Am Coll Cardiol* 1995; **26**: 594–605.

61. Chaitman B, Stone P, Knatterud G et al. Asymptomatic cardiac ischemia pilot (ACIP) study: impact of anti-ischemia therapy on 12-week rest electrocardiogram and exercise test outcomes. *J Am Coll Cardiol* 1995; **26**: 585–93.

62. von Arnim T for the TIBBS investigators. Medical treatment to reduce total ischemia burden: total ischemic burden bisoprolol study (TIBBS), a multicenter trial comparing bisoprolol and nifedipine. *J Am Coll Cardiol* 1995; **25**: 231–8.

63. von Arnim T. Prognostic significance of transient ischemic episodes: response to treatment shows improved prognosis. *J Am Coll Cardiol* 1996; **28**: 20–4.

64. Madjjlessi-Simon T, Mary-Kause M, Fillet F, Lechat P, Jaillon P. Persistent transient myocardial ischemia despite beta-adrenergic blockade predicts a higher risk of adverse cardiac events in patients with CAD. *J Am Coll Cardiol* 1996; **27**: 1586–91.

65. Pratt C, McMahon R, Golstein S et al. Comparison of subgroups assigned to medical regimens used to suppress cardiac ischemia (the asymptomatic cardiac ischemia pilot (ACIP) study). *Am J Cardiol* 1996; **77**: 1302–9.

66. Knuuti M, Wahl M, Wiklund I et al. Acute and long-term effects on myocardial ischemia of intermittent and continuous transdermal nitrate therapy in stable angina. *Am J Cardiol* 1992; **69**: 1525–32.

67. Dubiel J, Moczurad K, Bryniarski L. Efficacy of a single dose of slow release isosorbide dinitrate in the treatment of silent or painful myocardial ischemia in stable angina pectoris. *Am J Cardiol* 1992; **69**; 1156–60.

68. Rossetti E, Luca C, Bonetti F, Chierchia S. Transdermal nitroglycerin reduces the frequency of anginal attacks but fails to prevent silent ischemia. *J Am Coll Cardiol* 1993; **21**: 337–42.

69. Hamer A. Placebo effect of nitrate monotherapy for myocardial ischemia. *Am J Cardiol* 1992; **70**: 1238–42.

70. El-Tamini H, Davies G. Optimal control of myocardial ischemia: the benefit of a fixed combination of atenolol and nifedipine in patients with chronic stable angina. *Br Heart J* 1992; **68**: 291–5.

71. Donaldson K, Dawkins K, Waller D. A comparison of nisoldipine and nifedipine, in combination with atenolol, in the management of myocardial ischemia. *Eur Heart J* 1993; **14**: 534–9.

72. Siu S, Jacoby R, Phillips R, Nesto R. Comparative efficacy of nifedipine gastrointestinal therapeutic system versus diltiazem when added to beta blockers in stable angina pectoris. *Am J Cardiol* 1993; **71**: 887–92.

73. Davies R, Habibi H, Klinke P et al. Effect of amlodipine, atenolol and their combination on myocardial ischemia during treadmill exercise and ambulatory monitoring. *J Am Coll Cardiol* 1995; **25**: 619–25.

74. Deedwania PC, Carbajal EV, Nelson JR, Hait H. Anti-ischemic effects of atenolol versus nifedipine in patients with coronary artery disease and ambulatory silent ischemia. *J Am Coll Cardiol* 1991; **17**: 963–9.

75. Egstrup K. Randomized double-blind comparison of metoprolol, nifedipine, and their combination in chronic stable angina: effects on total ischemic activity and heart rate at onset of ischemia. *Am Heart J* 1988; **116**: 971–8.

11

A European multicenter study for comparing the effect of a beta-blocker with a calcium antagonist on transient ischemic episodes

Thomas von Arnim

INTRODUCTION

The 'total ischemic burden' is a term coined to comprise all detectable ischemia in patients with silent and/or symptomatic ischemia. Patients come to the attention of their physicians mostly driven by symptomatic disease. Patients with stable angina pectoris often show transient silent ischemic episodes together with symptomatic episodes of typical angina. Many studies which centered on the prognostic implication of transient ischemia have shown that it is more the ischemia than the angina which defines the prognostic impact for a given patient.[1–16] Thus several European studies focused on patients with angina pectoris and the total ischemic burden.[17–20] The APSIS study in Stockholm studied patients with stable angina pectoris and compared metoprolol with verapamil.[17] The TIBET study recruited patients mainly in England on the basis of stable angina pectoris and objective signs of ischemia on Holter monitoring and exercise testing.[18] The Total Ischemic Burden Bisoprolol Study (TIBBS)[19] recruited patients on the basis of several transient ischemic episodes documented in patients who had stable angina pectoris and a positive exercise electrocardiogram (ECG). The patient selection was somewhat different from the two studies mentioned above and so the results have to be compared with this difference in mind. The TIBBS study comprised 25 European centers and was a randomized controlled double-blind study with an open 1-year follow-up study[20] on the prognostic implications of transient ischemia and its medical treatment. Bisoprolol was chosen as a beta-blocker with the attractive features of single daily dosing and a balanced excretion combined with high beta-1-receptor selectivity. Nifedipine was the calcium antagonist that was most widely used for the indication of angina pectoris in Europe at the time when the study was planned.[19]

METHODS

Study design

TIBBS was a randomized multicenter double-blind controlled study with two parallel groups. A placebo prephase of 10 days was followed by two treatment phases of 4 weeks each. Treatment during phase 1 was either with 10 mg bisoprolol daily or 20 mg nifedipine slow-release twice a day. Treatment during phase 2 was double the dosage of phase 1 for each group, that is, 20 mg bisoprolol daily or 40 of nifedipine slow-release twice a day.

Sample size determination

A power of 90% for detection of a difference between the groups of at least 0.45 sd (alpha 5% two-tailed) was aimed for. This means that a difference of three episodes per 48 hours should have been detectable. Therefore, the sample size determination was 100 patients per treatment group who should have been evaluable with respect to number and duration of transient ischemic episodes.

Patient selection

In 30 European centers (see ref. 23 for participating institutions and personnel), ambulatory patients were recruited for the placebo prephase if they fulfilled the following inclusion criteria: history of typical stable angina pectoris and positive exercise tolerance test with ST-segment depression using a modified Bruce protocol on a treadmill or incremental workload of 25 W every 2 minutes on a bicycle. For women the presence of coronary artery disease had to be further documented by a definite history of myocardial infarction, positive findings on the coronary angiogram with >70% stenosis in a major vessel or positive findings on exercise thallium scintigraphy. For men these additional diagnostic criteria were desirable but not mandatory. During the placebo prephase, the patients underwent 48-hour ambulatory monitoring and were enrolled for randomized active treatment when they had had at least two episodes of transient myocardial ischemia, whether silent or symptomatic.

Patients were excluded if they met one or more of the following exclusion criteria: unstable angina pectoris; myocardial infarction within the past 3 months; bradycardia with < 50 beats/min during the day; significant first-degree atrioventricular (AV) block (PQ > 0.24 s); second- or third-degree AV block; hypertension with systolic blood pressure < 100 mmHg; or suspected poor compliance.

The following drugs were not given during the study: long-acting nitrates; beta-blockers (except the study medication); afterload-reducing agents, including calcium-channel blockers

and angiotensin converting enzyme (ACE) inhibitors (except the study medication); alpha1-adrenoceptor blockers and beta 2-stimulants; tricyclic antidepressants or drugs known to influence ST-segments (such as digitalis and antiarrhythmic agents).

Study protocol

If a patient met the inclusion criteria, he or she entered the 10-day placebo prephase and performed the qualifying exercise tolerance test on day 10. At the same time a physical examination and chemical laboratory tests were performed. From day 6 to day 4, the 48-hour ambulatory ECG monitoring was carried out. Express delivery of the tapes to the central laboratory, immediate evaluation and communication of the result by telephone or fax ensured the inclusion of suitable patients into the randomized treatment phase by day 0. At the end of treatment phase 1, after 4 weeks, and at the end of treatment phase 2, after 8 weeks, 48-hour Holter recordings were repeated, together with a check on anginal attacks, adverse events and a tablet count.

Follow-up

After the initial double-blind study, the patients were treated for their symptoms at the discretion of their physicians, to whom the results of the ambulatory monitoring during treatment were not disclosed.

At 6 months and 1 year from the randomization, screened patients underwent follow-up examinations. Patients who were screened on the basis of history of stable angina and a positive exercise ECG but who did not show two or more transient ischemic episodes were followed up as well as those who showed transient ischemia and had been randomized to controlled treatment in TIBBS.

Patients were excluded from follow-up if they had not technically acceptable 48-hour Holter tapes during the placebo prephase of TIBBS. In all 30 participating centers, the patients were followed up by repeated visits, telephone contacts, and/or interviews with their treating physicians. Information was obtained as to whether the patients had suffered any of the following events: (a) cardiac death, (b) non-cardiac death, (c) nonfatal myocardial infarction, (d) admission to hospital due to unstable angina, (e) need for percutaneous transluminal coronary angioplasty (PTCA) or (f) bypass grafting. Events (a–d) were evaluated together with the other events and separately as 'hard events', because they do not have the bias problem of an elective treatment decision. The definition of nonfatal acute myocardial infarction followed standard criteria. Indications for admission due to unstable angina and for revascularization were at the discretion of the physicians in charge of the patients in the different centers. These physicians were unaware of the results of the initial ambulatory ECG monitoring and the treatment assignment. Furthermore, patients were asked about antianginal medication taken since the randomized treatment phase up to 1 year.

On the basis of history and positive exercise ECG, 630 patients were included in the screening phase of TIBBS and underwent 48-hour Holter monitoring. Of these patients, 85 had no, or technically unacceptable, Holter tapes during placebo prephase and were excluded. Follow-up information was not available for 25 patients, giving a follow-up rate of 95.4%. Of the 520 patients evaluated for follow-up information, 203 patients had been screened by Holter ECG, but not randomized; 317 patients had entered the randomized treatment phase of TIBBS. Of the latter group, a subgroup of 283 patients had also shown valid 48-hour Holter tapes during the TIBBS treatment phase, and could thus be evaluated for treatment responses of transient ischemia.

Statistical analysis

All data from the follow-up report forms were continuously entered into a central database. This allowed cross-correlations with information obtained on the same patients during TIBBS.

All data from the case-report forms and the central Holter tape evaluation were continuously entered into a central database. The randomization plan was not disclosed before all the data had been checked for plausibility and any necessary corrections had been carried out. The number and duration of ischemic episodes and the total ischemic burden as they differed from baseline were defined as primary target variables of efficacy. Results are presented as mean value ± sem. Differences from baseline values were checked for significance considering the 95% confidence limits. If the confidence interval did not include zero, the mean baseline difference was regarded as significantly different from zero. The efficacy variables between the two treatment groups were compared using the Wilcoxon rank-sum test. Comparisons within each group between the 4- and 8-week measurements were performed using the Wilcoxon signed-rank test. Responder rates were analyzed using the Fisher's exact probability test. Significance level was alpha 5%, two-tailed.

For comparisons of proportions of patients with events Fischer's exact text or chi-square tests were carried out and for comparisons of event-free survival curves log-rank tests were used. The occurrence of events in the time course was described by life-table curves (Kaplan–Meier). Significance level was alpha 5%, two-tailed.

RESULTS

Study patients

From April 1991 to February 1993, 631 patients fulfilled the inclusion criteria and had a positive result on the exercise ECG. Of these, 330 had two or more transient episodes of ischemia during 48-hour ambulatory ECG monitoring and thus could be randomized to receive bisoprolol (161 patients) or nifedipine (169 patients). The baseline characteristics of the randomized patients are shown in Table 11.1. There were no significant differences in gender, age, smoking history, or other baseline values.

Table 11.1 Baseline characteristics of randomized study patients.

	Bisoprolol (n = 161)	Nifedipine SR (n = 169)	P
Male/female	134/27	146/23	0.45
Smoker and ex-smoker (%)	57.2	62.2	0.31
Age (years)	57.6 (38–77)	57.3 (32–78)	0.75
History of angina (months)	24.8 (1–256)	20.5 (2–195)	0.50
Positive history of myocardial infarction	44	53	0.47
Weight (kg)	77.2 ± 9.3	75.7 ± 9.8	0.16
SBP (mmHg)	139.9 ± 16.2	140.0 ± 18.9	0.92
HR (beats/min)	74.2 ± 10.6	74.0 ± 10.3	0.85
ETT			
Maximal rate-pressure product (mmHg × beats/min)	23 684 ± 5 320	24 147 ± 5 402	0.44
Maximal ST-segment depression (mV)	0.22 ± 0.10	0.22 ± 0.09	0.80

Note: Data presented are mean value ± sd, median value (range) or number of patients. SBP: systolic blood pressure; HR: heart rate; ETT: exercise tolerance test.

Of the patients who started randomized treatment, there were 10 drop-outs in the bisoprolol group and 17 in the nifedipine group, mostly because of adverse drug reactions (described later). Data had to be excluded from analysis because of ineligible tapes or protocol violations for 18 patients in the bisoprolol group and 17 in the nifedipine group. Thus, for phase 1 of the randomized treatments there were 133 patients with eligible tapes in the bisoprolol group and 135 in the nifedipine group. For phase 2 of the randomized treatment, weeks 5 to 8 on the double dose, there were 17 drop-outs and 16 data exclusions in the bisoprolol group and 12 drop-outs and 18 exclusions in the nifedipine group. Patients with eligible tapes for phase 2 included 118 with bisoprolol and 122 with nifedipine (patients with protocol violations or ineligible tapes at the end of phase 1 entered phase 2 of the trial in the normal way). In the bisoprolol group there were 111 patients (nifedipine slow-release, 112 patients) with eligible tapes in both phase 1 and phase 2 of the trial.

Treatment effects on ambulatory ischemia

Number and duration of the ischemic episodes as well as the total ischemic burden showed a marked and statistically significant reduction with both antianginal drugs in the low dosages (confidence intervals do not include zero) (Fig. 11.1). All reductions were significantly greater with bisoprolol than with nifedipine ($P < 0.001$); the effects of bisoprolol were about twice those of nifedipine. Heart rate at onset of ischemic episodes was 99.5 ± 1.17 beats/min in the bisoprolol group and 101.2 ± 1.03 beats/min in the nifedipine group during the placebo prephase. At the end of the low-dose phase, 54 patients in the bisoprolol group and 20 in the nifedipine group had neither silent nor painful ischemic episodes. These patients were not included in the analysis of treatment effects on heart rate at the onset of ischemic episodes. Bisoprolol treatment resulted in a significant reduction in heart rate of 13.7 ± 1.39 beats/min, whereas with nifedipine a small but not significant increase of 1.4 ± 1.08 beats/min was

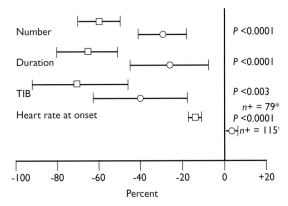

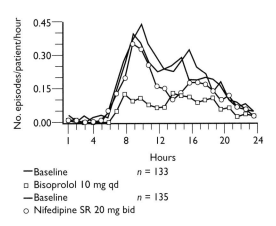

*Patients without ischemic episodes are not included

□ Bisoprolol 10 mg qd *n* = 133
○ Nifedipine SR 20mg bid *n* = 135

Figure 11.1 Effects of bisoprolol and nifedipine slow-release on different measures of transient ischemic episodes (patients evaluable for phases 1 and 2; bisoprolol, *n* = 111; nifedipine, *n* = 112). Number, duration and total ischemic burden (TIB) (mean ± sem) are reduced significantly with both drugs. The difference in reduction between bisoprolol and nifedipine is also significant (at least *P* = 0.01) for all variables compared. The doubling of the dose in phase 2 of the trial showed only a small incremental effect. (Reproduced with permission from reference 19.)

Figure 11.2 Effect of bisoprolol and nifedipine on the circadian distribution of transient ischemic episodes (sum of episodes/hour on two consecutive days as mean value/patient; patients evaluable for phases 1 and 2; bisoprolol, *n* = 111, nifedipine, *n* = 112). From comparable baseline curves, bisoprolol effectively reduces the morning and afternoon peaks of transient ischemic episodes, whereas nifedipine reduces the overall number of episodes but leaves the circadian distribution unchanged. (Reproduced with permission from reference 19.)

observed (*P* = 0.0001, bisoprolol versus nifedipine).

The additional effects of the double dose of bisoprolol and nifedipine were small and significant only for bisoprolol, with a further reduction in the number of ischemic episodes and mean heart rate at the onset of ischemic episodes.

Treatment effects on angina pectoris

Patients were questioned on the frequency of angina during the preceding week both at the start and end of the placebo phase and at the end of the low- and high-dose treatment phases. From 5.4 ± 0.56 and 5.7 ± 0.59 attacks/week, the number of anginal attacks was reduced to 2.8 ± 0.47 and 4.4 ± 0.61 in the bisoprolol and nifedipine groups, respec-

tively. For patients receiving the high dose, the weekly attacks were reduced from a baseline value of 5.8 ± 0.71 to 2.3 ± 0.41 with bisoprolol and from 5.7 ± 0.65 to 3.2 ± 0.48 with nifedipine. Both drugs effectively reduced the frequency of angina pectoris. However, in individual patients the correlation of the number of anginal attacks per week and the number of ischemic episodes per 48 hours was weak (for baseline and difference with treatment, *r* = 0.210–0.251).

Effects on circadian variation of ischemia

Figure 11.2 shows the effects of bisoprolol and nifedipine on the circadian variation of transient ischemic episodes. During phase 1 of the study, the pronounced morning peak of episodes frequency was markedly reduced with

10 mg of bisoprolol. With nifedipine slow-release (2 × 20 mg), the circadian profile was unchanged but showed a clear overall reduction in the number of episodes. The second peak of transient ischemic episodes during the late afternoon hours was more reduced with nifedipine than the morning peak.

Responder rates

During both phases of the trial, the percentage of patients who responded to treatment with a reduction in episodes of transient ischemia was evaluated. For various definitions of response (between 25% and 100% reduction in the number of episodes), there was always a higher responder rate for bisoprolol than for nifedipine. The difference was significant with Fisher's exact test and was similar for duration of episodes and total ischemic burden. During phase 2 of the trial there was some further increase in responder rates. The differences between bisoprolol and nifedipine remained significant: 52.5% of patients achieved 100% reduction of transient ischemic episodes with bisoprolol versus only 15.6% of those with nifedipine.

Adverse drug effects

One patient had an acute myocardial infarction after randomization to nifedipine but before administration of the first medication. During the study, 27 patients taking bisoprolol and 29 taking nifedipine slow-release had to be withdrawn from treatment: adverse events occurred in 20 patients taking bisoprolol and 14 patients taking nifedipine; treatment failure in six patients taking bisoprolol, 10 nifedipine; and other problems in one patient taking bisoprolol, five nifedipine. In most patients the adverse event recorded was of cardiovascular origin. Lack of effect on angina pectoris, occurrence of tachycardia and edema during nifedipine treatment and dyspnea and bradycardia with bisoprolol therapy were the main problems observed.

Event rates

Table 11.2 shows the numbers of patients with events that occurred in the patient population. Of 520 patients at risk, 120 patients had a total of 145 events. If only the severest event per patient is counted, the event rate was 120/520, 23.1% overall, with 49/520 (9.4%) 'hard events' (death, acute MI, admission to hospital due to unstable angina).

Medical treatment at 6 months of follow-up was: platelet aggregation inhibitors 59.4%, beta-blockers 59.4%, long-acting nitrates 57.2%, short-acting nitrates 48.9%, calcium antagonists 47.8%, ACE inhibitors 7.6%, and anticoagulants 7.0%. Beta-blockers were used exclusively (without calcium antagonists) in 37.3%, calcium antagonists exclusively (without beta-blockers) in 27.9% and a combination of both in 19.8% of patients. At 1 year of follow-up there were no significant changes in the frequencies of the different medications used.

Prognostic influence of transient ischemia

Of the 190 patients with less than two ischemic episodes, 13.2% suffered from events compared with 25% of the 164 patients with two to six episodes and 32.5% of the 166 patients with more than six episodes (chi-square, $P < 0.001$). Hard events occurred in 4.7%, 14.0%, and 10.2%, respectively ($P=0.011$). Figure 11.3 shows the event-free survival for patients grouped according to the number of transient ischemic episodes on 48-hour Holter ECG during the placebo prephase of TIBBS. There is a clear separation of the event-free probability between patients with fewer than two episodes and the other two groups with stepwise more severe ischemia.

When only hard events are counted for patients separated into two groups with or without two or more transient ischemic episodes, again there is a significant separation at 1 year, demonstrating the prognostic influence of transient ischemia. When the total ischemic burden or the duration of ischemic episodes are taken as measures of ischemia and two groups separated respectively on either side of the

Table 11.2 Total Ischemic Burden Bisoprolol Study follow-up: number of events (one or more event/patient).

	Cardiac death	Noncardiac death	MI	Hospital admission for unstable angina	CABG	PTCA
All patients ($n = 520$)	4	2	12	35	72	20
Only 1 (severest) event/patient	4	2	11	32	55	16
Ischemic episodes at baseline						
< 2 ($n = 190$)	0	0	2	6	13	5
2–6 ($n = 164$)	2	1	3	19	23	5
> 6 ($n = 166$)	0	0	7	10	36	10
Responders						
100% ($n = 97$)	1	0	1	6	10	3
Non-100% ($n = 186$)	1	1	3	16	42	8
Bisoprolol ($n = 154$)	1	0	2	10	22	5
Nifedipine SR ($n = 163$)	0	2	7	16	36	7

MI: myocardial infarction; CABG: coronary artery bypass graft surgery; PTCA: percutaneous transluminal coronary angioplasty.

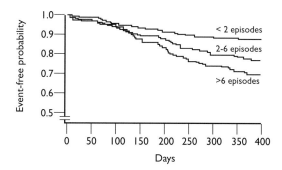

Figure 11.3 Event-free survival to first event in patients screened for TIBBS ($n = 520$). Of these, 190 patients had shown fewer than two transient ischemic episodes in 48-hour ambulatory ECG monitoring, 164 patients had two to six episodes and 166 patients had more than six episodes. A higher number of episodes is clearly followed by an increased event rate. (Reproduced with permission from reference 20.)

median, then the event rates are also significantly higher in the groups with higher total ischemic burden and longer duration of ischemia.

Prognostic influence of response to treatment

Patients who showed 100% reduction of transient ischemic episodes under treatment had an event rate of 17.5%, compared with 32.3% in non-100% responders ($P = 0.008$). Hard events were 7.2% and 11.3%, respectively ($P = 0.276$).

Figure 11.4 shows the event-free survival curves for patients with or without a 100% response to medical treatment, that is, no further transient ischemic episodes on the control Holter tapes (week 4 or 8 of randomized treatment) during TIBBS. Patients who had shown a complete response, and lost all

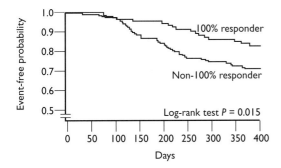

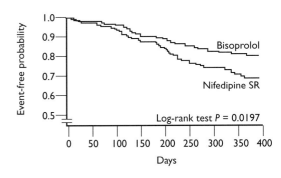

Figure 11.4 Event-free survival in 283 patients treated in the randomized controlled phase of TIBBS (only patients who had technically acceptable tapes throughout the 8-week trial). A 100% reduction of transient ischemic episodes was achieved in 97 patients, who had a reduced risk of subsequent events over non-100% responders ($n = 186$). (Reproduced with permission from reference 20.)

Figure 11.5 Event-free survival for 317 patients treated in the randomized controlled phase of TIBBS. The patients who had received bisoprolol ($n = 154$) during the trial had a significantly lower event rate than patients who had received nifedipine ($n = 163$). (Reproduced with permission from reference 20.)

transient ischemia, had a significantly improved outcome compared with the rest of the randomized patients. When only hard events were counted, the separation was not statistically significant (log rank test, $P = 0.258$). Treatment responses with less than 100% reduction of ischemic episodes did not show an improved prognosis. In fact, the event rates for patients with at least 25% reduction (26.1%), at least 50% reduction (24.7%) and at least 75% reduction (24.3%) were similar and different from patients with 100% reduction (17.5%).

Prognostic influence of initial randomized treatment

Patients randomized to bisoprolol had an event rate of 22.1% versus 33.1% in the patients receiving nifedipine ($P = 0.033$, Fisher's exact test). Figure 11.5 compares the event-free survival curves for patients who had been randomized to either bisoprolol or nifedipine during the initial randomized treatment phase (eight weeks). Patients who had been given bisoprolol during the TIBBS study fared significantly better than those who had been on

nifedipine. Even when only the hard events were counted, a trend (log rank test, $P = 0.104$) remained. Patients who had been randomized to bisoprolol during the initial phase of the study were kept on beta-blockers by their physicians more often than patients who had been randomized to nifedipine (47% versus 32%, $P = 0.008$). Treatment with calcium antagonists during follow-up was comparable for both groups (21% versus 26%, $P = 0.29$).

DISCUSSION

TIBBS was a large study which included selected patients with stable angina pectoris, a positive result on the exercise ECG and evidence of transient ischemia on ambulatory ECG monitoring. Bisoprolol in a single daily dose was an effective antianginal and anti-ischemic treatment. In the reduction of the number and duration of ischemic episodes and total ischemic burden, bisoprolol proved superior to nifedipine, which also showed significant treatment effects. Bisoprolol was also superior to nifedipine with regard to responder rates and effect on angina and on circadian variation or ischemic episodes. Thus, in a large group of patients with stable coronary artery disease, the main determinant of transient myocardial ischemia seems to be increased oxygen demand, which can be reduced by lowering heart rate with a beta-blocker.

Influence of patient selection

The present study followed patients who had undergone a screening phase for a randomized controlled treatment study. It could thus compare patients who had shown episodes of transient ischemia with others who had not. It should be noted that all patients had a history of stable angina pectoris *and* a positive exercise ECG. Thus the results pertain especially to the additive prognostic influence of transient ischemic episodes on ambulatory 48-hour monitoring. The follow-up rate at 1 year was over 95%, and thus the results validate earlier studies showing prognostic significance for transient, predominantly silent ischemia in patients with stable angina pectoris.[15,16,21–23] The study population was also large enough to show a significant prognostic separation for 'hard' events.

These results underscore the prognostic importance of transient ischemia, if demonstrated in addition to a positive exercise ECG. Transient ischemic episodes may represent a sign of underlying 'instability' of the disease in patients who present otherwise with stable angina pectoris. In the study of Mulcahy et al.,[24] a positive exercise test was not a prerequisite for inclusion of patients and this dilution of the patient group may be the reason for the lack of prognostic implications in that study. The present author, however, believes that the prognostic influence of transient ischemia that has been shown here is not only statistically significant, but also clinically relevant.

Prognostic influence of treatment response

The follow-up of patients who had undergone the randomized treatment phase of TIBBS showed a remarkable effect of treatment response on prognosis. Although the treatment was not randomized over 1 year, but only for the 8 weeks of the trial, the results are valid, as the results of the ambulatory monitoring during the trial were not disclosed to the physicians in charge of the patients during the following year. The present study is, of course, observational in this respect, but treatment responses on ambulatory ECG were measured during the controlled randomized phase of the study. Especially for 'hard' events, the effect of initial treatment could only have been 'diluted' during follow-up. The study shows that a complete treatment response confers an improved prognosis for the patients even over 1 year. It is important that the response of ischemia be 100%, as lesser reductions in numbers of episodes were not associated with improved prognosis. The results compare very well with the ASIST trial.[25] In this study patients underwent randomized treatment with atenolol or placebo and the beta-blocker also reduced the amount of ischemia and improved prognosis. As in TIBBS, complete relief of ischemia under medical treatment was important for a positive influence on prognosis. With regard to the marked effect, which the treatment response during the 8-week trial had for the outcome at 1 year, the recent paper of Gill[26] is interesting: in the comparison of 406 patients after an acute myocardial infarction, those with ischemia on ambulatory ECG had a highly increased event rate and the difference occurred almost completely during the first 3 months. Pepine[27] pointed out the possibility of biologically unstable coronary artery disease in a clinically stable patient.

Differences between treatments

In the present study the positive treatment effects, shown by bisoprolol during the randomized phase of the trial, translated into improved outcomes at 1 year. This seems difficult to explain at first, but the initial stabilization of some degree of instability may be a reason. Another important factor may be that the patients who had been randomized to bisoprolol treatment were significantly more likely to be kept on beta-blockers for the following year. Thus the higher rate of complete treatment responses obtained with bisoprolol may have had an extended effect on subsequent prognosis. With the higher dose of 20 mg bisoprolol a 100% response of ischemic episodes was achieved in 52% of patients. Thus, a sizeable proportion of patients remains who are probably not treated to an optimal outcome. Further studies will have to address the question of whether the percentage of complete treatment responses can be improved by combination therapy with a beta-blocker such as bisoprolol and either a calcium antagonist, aggressive lipid-lowering therapy or a strategy including revascularization. The recently published ACIP trial[28] showed revascularization to be somewhat superior to medical treatment in the reduction of subsequent cardiac events.

CONCLUSIONS

The 1-year follow-up of patients with stable angina pectoris, but demonstrable frequent transient ischemia, whether silent or painful, on top of a positive exercise ECG, showed a significantly worse prognosis in patients with less or no transient ischemia. This may represent a degree of hidden instability of coronary artery disease in such patients. Medical treatment can improve the prognosis if it achieves a 100% reduction of ischemic episodes. Patients on bisoprolol during TIBBS fared better than those initially randomized to nifedipine, probably because patients on bisoprolol had a higher rate of 100% responses.

REFERENCES

1. Johnson SM, Mauritson DR, Winniford MD et al. Continuous electrocardiographic monitoring in patients with unstable angina pectoris: identification of high-risk subgroup with severe coronary disease, variant angina, and/or impaired early prognosis. *Am Heart J* 1982; **103**: 4–12.
2. Gottlieb SO, Weisfeldt ML, Ouyang P et al. Silent ischemia as a marker for early unfavorable outcomes in patients with unstable angina. *N Engl J Med* 1986; **314**: 1214–19.
3. Gottlieb SO, Weisfeldt ML, Ouyang P, Mellits ED, Gerstenblith G. Silent ischemia predicts infarction and death during 2-year follow-up of unstable angina. *J Am Coll Cardiol* 1987; **10**: 756–60.
4. Nademanee K, Intarachot V, Josephson MA, Rieders D, Mody FV, Singh BN. Prognostic significance of silent myocardial ischemia in patients with unstable angina. *J Am Coll Cardiol* 1987; **10**: 1–9.
5. von Arnim T, Gerbig HW, Krawietz W, Höfling B. Prognostic implications of transient predominantly silent ischaemia in patients with unstable angina pectoris. *Eur Heart J* 1988; **9**: 435–40.
6. Langer A, Freeman MR, Armstrong PW. ST-segment shift in unstable angina: pathophysiology and association with coronary anatomy and hospital outcome. *J Am Coll Cardiol* 1989; **13**: 1495–502.
7. Bugiardini R, Pozzati A, Borghi A et al. Angiographic morphology in unstable angina and its relation to transient ischemia and hospital outcome. *Am J Cardiol* 1991; **67**: 460–4.
8. Pozzati A, Bugiardini R, Borghi A et al. Transient ischaemia refractory to conventional medical treatment in unstable angina: angiographic correlates and prognostic implications. *Eur Heart J* 1992; **13**: 360–5.
9. Holdright D, Patel D, Cunningham D et al. Comparison of the effect of heparin and aspirin versus aspirin alone on transient myocardial ischemia and in-hospital prognosis in patients with unstable angina. *J Am Coll Cardiol* 1994; **24**: 39–45.
10. Tzivoni D, Gravish A, Zin D et al. Prognostic significance of ischemic episodes in patients with previous myocardial infarction. *Am J Cardiol* 1988; **62**: 661–4.
11. Gottlieb SO, Gottlieb SH, Achuff SC et al. Silent ischemia on Holter monitoring predicts mortality in high risk postinfarction patients. *JAMA* 1988; **259**: 1030–5.

12. Langer A, Minkowitz J, Dorian P et al. (TPAT Study Group). Pathophysiology and prognostic significance of Holter-detected ST-segment depression after myocardial infarction. *J Am Coll Cardiol* 1992; **20**: 1313–17.

13. Currie P, Ashby D, Saltissi S. Prognostic significance of transient myocardial ischemia on ambulatory monitoring after acute myocardial infarction. *Am J Cardiol* 1993; **71**: 773–7.

14. Bonaduce D, Petretta M, Lanzillo T et al. Prevalence and prognostic significance of silent myocardial ischaemia detected by exercise test and continuous ECG monitoring after acute myocardial infarction. *Eur Heart J* 1991; **12**: 186–93.

15. Deedwania P, Carbajal EV. Silent ischemia during daily life is an independent predictor of mortality in stable angina. *Circulation* 1990; **81**: 748–56.

16. Yeung AC, Barry J, Orav J, Bonassin E, Rabyu KE, Selwyn AP. Effects of asymptomatic ischemia on long-term prognosis in chronic stable coronary disease. *Circulation* 1991; **83**: 1598–604.

17. Rehnquist N, Hjemdahl P, Billing E et al. Effects of metoprolol vs verapamil in patients with stable angina pectoris. The Angina Prognosis Study in Stockholm (APSIS). *Eur Heart J* 1996; **17**: 76–91.

18. Dargie HJ, Ford I, Fox KM, on behalf of the TIBET study group. Total Ischaemic Burden European Trial (TIBET): effects of ischaemia and treatment with atenolol, nifedipine SR and their combination on outcome in patients with chronic stable angina. *Eur Heart J* 1996; **17**: 104–12.

19. von Arnim T. Medical treatment to reduce total ischemic burden: Total Ischemic Burden Bisoprolol Study (TIBBS), a multicenter trial comparing bisoprolol and nifedipine. *J Am Coll Cardiol* 1995; **25**: 231–8.

20. von Amim T. Prognostic significance of transient ischemic episodes: response to treatment shows improved prognosis. Results of the Total Ischemic Burden Bisoprolol Study (TIBBS) follow-up. *J Am Coll Cardiol* 1996; **28**: 20–24.

21. von Arnim T, Szeimies-Seebach U, Erath A, Schreiber MA, Höfling B. Ischemia detected on ambulatory monitoring: has it prognostic implications? *Adv Cardiol* 1990; **37**: 236–43.

22. Rocco MB, Nabel EG, Campbell S et al. Prognostic importance of myocardial ischemia detected by ambulatory monitoring in patients with stable coronary artery disease. *Circulation* 1988; **78**: 877–84.

23. Tzivoni D, Weisz G, Gavish A, Zin D, Keren A, Stern S. Comparison of mortality and myocardial infarction rates in stable angina pectoris with and without ischemic episodes during daily activities. *Am J Cardiol* 1989; **63**: 273–6.

24. Mulcahy D, Knight C, Patel D et al. Detection of ambulatory ischaemia is not of practical clinical value in the routine management of patients with stable angina. A long-term follow-up study. *Eur Heart J* 1995; **16**: 317–24.

25. Pepine CJ, Cohn PF, Deedwania PC et al. Effects of treatment on outcome in mildly symptomatic patients with ischemia during daily life. The Atenolol Silent Ischemia Study (ASIST). *Circulation* 1994; **90**: 762–8.

26. Gill JB, Cairns JA, Roberts RS et al. Prognostic importance of myocardial ischemia detected by ambulatory monitoring early after acute myocardial infarction. *N Engl J Med* 1996; **334**: 65–70.

27. Pepine CJ. Prognostic implications of silent myocardial ischemia. *N Engl J Med* 1996; **334**: 113–14.

28. Rogers WJ, Bourassa MG, Andrews TC et al. Asymptomatic Cardiac Ischemia Pilot (ACIP) study: outcome at 1 year for patients with asymptomatic cardiac ischemia randomized to medical therapy or revascularization. *J Am Coll Cardiol* 1995; **26**: 594–605.

12

Asymptomatic selected populations with silent ischemia

Serge GLG Degré

Silent myocardial ischemia may occur in completely asymptomatic selected populations as in other groups of patients with coronary artery disease which are generally symptomatic in stable or unstable conditions. It is nevertheless a difficult task to assess the frequency of occurrence of silent myocardial ischemia in a completely asymptomatic, apparently healthy population considering the absence of a real 'gold standard' for detection in such populations.

PREVALENCE OF SILENT MYOCARDIAL ISCHEMIA IN PATIENTS WITHOUT DOCUMENTED ISCHEMIC HEART DISEASE

The prevalence of painless myocardial ischemia in totally asymptomatic individuals is unknown and varies with the level of risk factors for ischemic heart disease. Even in presumably healthy men the prevalence of asymptomatic ischemia is controversial. Baseline medical screening in the 2363 participants recruited from various places of work in the Belgian Physical Fitness Study identified 1701 presumably healthy men, aged 40–55 years, who underwent a submaximal bicycle exercise test (increasing loads of 30 watts by 3 minutes). In this population, smoking habits, body mass index, and total and high density lipoprotein (HDL) cholesterol were measured; according to the European Society of Cardiology guidelines for prevention

of coronary artery disease the average risk was mild at between 5 and 10%. Of the total, 662 subjects were excluded from exercise testing for suspected coronary artery disease based on medical history, resting electrocardiogram abnormalities, or blood pressure higher than 170/105 mmHg. An asymptomatic positive exercise electrocardiogram characterized by an ST-segment depression higher than 0.1 mV at 0.06 or 0.08 seconds after the peak of the R-wave was observed in 199 subjects (11%). Compared with the subjects without ST-segment depression no differences were observed in systolic blood pressure, smoking habits, serum cholesterol, HDL cholesterol, body mass index, and leisure time physical activity.[1,2] Deanfield et al. reported that less than 2% of the apparently normal population has ischemic-type ST-segment depression on ambulatory electrocardiographic monitoring.[3] The lower frequency in ST-segment depression observed by Deanfield et al. compared with the author's data could be partly explained by the lower level of energy expenditure reached during daily activities registered on Holter monitoring than during submaximal exercise tests used in the latter study. Anatomical studies in subjects who died from noncardiac causes, angiographic data collected in patients free of chest pain, a history of coronary artery disease, and positive exercise testing with subsequent coronary angiography have led Cohn to propose a prevalence of less than 5% for hemodynamically significant asymptomatic anatomic disease in men.[4] In the Multiple Risk Factor Intervention Study (MRFIT) the prevalence of individuals with a positive electrocardiogram exercise stress test and no angina was 2.5%, but in the top decile of coronary risk the figure was 12.5%.[5] It could thus be concluded that in an apparently healthy middle-aged population completely asymptomatic myocardial ischemia could be estimated at between 2.5 and 12.5% according to the coronary risk, with an average estimation of 5%.

In patients with peripheral vascular diseases and without angina or history of myocardial infarction the prevalence of silent myocardial ischemia detected by Holter monitoring was 9.4% according to Kirwin et al.[6] In a population of 208 older patients including 68 men and 140 women (81 ± 8 years) with 40–100% extracranial carotid arterial disease, with or without prior atherothrombotic brain infarction, Aronow et al. reported that 33% of the patients had silent myocardial ischemia at 24-hour ambulatory electrocardiogram monitoring.[7]

HYPERTENSION AND SILENT ISCHEMIA

In patients with mild to moderate hypertension and left ventricular hypertrophy detected by an excessive ventricular index, silent myocardial ischemia at maximal exercise test was observed by Otterstad in 2.5% of patients.[8] It is now clearly shown that definite left ventricular hypertrophy on electrocardiogram identifies a cohort of patients with more prevalent silent ischemia.[9,10] In this regard, thallium scintigraphy appears to be superior to exercise testing and the ambulatory electrocardiogram for identifying latent coronary artery disease in high-risk hypertensive patients.[9,10] The mechanisms underlying the development of myocardial ischemia in hypertensive patients remain controversial, particularly in patients with normal epicardial coronary arteries. Sympathetic neural dysfunction has been implicated as a causal factor,[11] as well as a more recently discovered elevated level of plasma norepinephrine.[12] Excessive noradrenergic tone might contribute to myocardial

ischemia by enhancing coronary vasoconstriction and myocardial oxygen demand.[12] Impaired coronary flow reserve has been proposed as a mechanism of myocardial ischemia when the epicardial coronary arteries are normal.[13] Inadequate enlargement in coronary artery cross-sectional area, giving rise to functional stenosis, may be responsible for the development of ischemia in the setting of left ventricular hypertrophy, as might be suspected from the observation of abnormally high coronary flow velocity in the coronary vessels of hypertensive patients with left ventricular hypertrophy and silent myocardial ischemia.[14] Abnormal coronary vasomotor response is an additional possible mechanism responsible for myocardial ischemia in hypertensive patients: coronary vasoconstriction occurred in response to cold pressure test in hypertensive patients with myocardial ischemia who were free from coronary artery disease while vasodilatation was observed in those patients without myocardial ischemia.[15] Abnormal endothelium-dependent coronary vasomotion may, in part, provide the explanation for these observations.[16,17] It was recently demonstrated that endothelial-dependent, flow-mediated coronary vasodilatation was lost in hypertensive patients, whereas endothelial-independent vasomotor mechanisms, such as the nitrates response, are preserved.[18] As far as silent myocardial infarctions are concerned, a few distinguishing characteristics appear to be important. According to the Framingham study,[19] in more than 25% of those who sustained a myocardial infarction over 30 years of follow-up, the infarct was discovered only because of new abnormalities on the resting electrocardiogram. Of these unrecognized events, almost half in men and women were completely silent and without even atypical symptoms. In this study only one coronary risk factor seems specifically related to unrecognized myocardial infarction, and that is hypertension. As many as 50% of myocardial infarctions in hypertensive women and 35% in hypertensive men went unrecognized, a clear excess.[19] This is unexpected, as hypertensive individuals are likely to be under closer surveillance and to have more severe disease. This finding seems to be genuine, as the excessive occurrence persists when excluding diabetics, those receiving beta-blockers, and those with electrocardiographic left ventricular hypertrophy, which is occasionally confused with anteroseptal infarction.[20]

SILENT ISCHEMIA IN PATIENTS WITH DIABETES

In recent years many authors have demonstrated that asymptomatic myocardial infarction or asymptomatic myocardial ischemia occur more frequently in diabetic patients.[21–24] Others have shown a similar prevalence of asymptomatic ischemia in diabetic and nondiabetic patients during exercise tests.[25,26] Silent myocardial ischemia was detected in 5.5% of diabetic patients in a study undertaken in 13 African countries.[27] In diabetic and uremic patients waiting for kidney and pancreas transplants, silent ischemia was observed by exercise thallium scintigraphy in 44% of patients.[28] The New York Veterans Administration Medical Center and Clinics reported that 61% of asymptomatic diabetic patients demonstrated exertional silent myocardial ischemia.[29] Nesto et al.[24] demonstrated that only 28% of diabetic patients with positive thallium scintigraphy experienced angina pectoris during the treadmill test compared with 68% of nondiabetic patients.

In contrast with these data, in a low-risk group of patients with known ischemic heart disease exercise testing was positive in 38% of cases and more than 50% of those episodes of ischemia were silent.[30] The increased number of episodes of silent myocardial ischemia in diabetic patients with coronary heart disease compared with that observed in other coronary patients may be explained by various factors including different thresholds of pain sensitivity, psychological denial, or the presence of autonomic neuropathy leading to sensory denervation. Autonomic neuropathy is a common feature of diabetes, and abnormalities of the autonomic nerve fibers were demonstrated histologically in diabetic patients who died after painless myocardial infarction.[31] Moreover, diabetic patients with or without signs of autonomic neuropathy have a decreased vagal activity during the night hours and in the afternoon during which time a higher frequency of cardiovascular incidents has been reported.[32] For example, Zarich et al. reported an absence of peak incidence of myocardial ischemia in the morning hours contrary to the observations collected in nondiabetic coronary patients.[33] All these observations are nevertheless in contradiction with the recent paper of Caracciolo et al., which stated: 'Diabetics with coronary disease have a prevalence of asymptomatic ischemia during exercise treadmill testing and ambulatory ischemia monitoring similar to that of nondiabetic patients (an ACIP database study)'.[34] It is nevertheless important to observe that, in this latter study, the relative sample size of diabetic and nondiabetic patients was unbalanced: more nondiabetic patients were treated by beta-blocking agents and basal heart rate was higher in nondiabetic patients.[35] That these peculiarities acted in favor or not of the number of asymptomatic episodes in diabetic or nondiabetic patients, or on the statistical power of the study, could partly explain the conclusions of that paper.[35] As stated by Chiariello and Indolfi, further studies should be performed to evaluate prospectively the frequency and duration of silent ischemic events in a larger number of well characterized diabetic patients compared with well matched nondiabetic patients. It will also be of great interest for clinicians to determine whether the presence of residual silent ischemia documented during daily life constitutes an independent predictor of cardiac death in diabetic patients.[35] The unexpected appearance of myocardial infarction on a routine electrocardiogram provides, in the majority of cases, evidence of silent coronary disease. The incidence of myocardial infarction becomes important beyond the age of 45 years in men and 55 in women. According to the

Framingham study,[19] in more than 25% of those who sustained a myocardial infarction over 30 years of follow-up, the infarct was discovered only because of new abnormalities on the resting electrocardiogram. Of these unrecognized events, almost half in men and women were completely silent and without even atypical symptoms.

PROGNOSTIC SIGNIFICANCE OF SILENT MYOCARDIAL ISCHEMIA IN ASYMPTOMATIC SELECTED POPULATIONS

The significance of silent ischemia is as varied as that of symptomatic ischemia.[36]

In the Belgian Physical Fitness Study, at 5-year follow-up, 9.4% (6/64) developed angina compared with 3.2% (44/1379) observed in subjects without abnormal evolution of ST-segment at exercise ($P < 0.008$). No difference in the incidence of sudden death and myocardial infarction was detected. This observation further supports the hypothesis that the pathophysiological mechanisms leading to sudden death and myocardial infarction in asymptomatic subjects may be different from those leading to angina.[2] This nevertheless corresponds to a smaller total number of angina patients (6) in the 64 individuals with positive exercise stress test than in the 1379 with negative tests (44) over the same 5-year follow-up period.

In the MRFIT study[5] in individuals between 37 and 57 years of age who were in the top decile of coronary risk, a positive exercise test conferred about a threefold greater risk (5.0%) of cardiac death than a negative test (1.6%) over a 7-year follow-up period. As in the Belgian Physical Fitness Study, this corresponds also with a smaller total number of deaths in the 1601 individuals with positive exercise test than in the 10 417 individuals with negative tests. In a meta-analysis including 14 studies and 26 000 normal individuals, Yusuf calculated an average 4.2-fold excess risk of cardiac death occurring among those with positive results, but twice as many events occurred in those with negative results.[37] Calculated sensitivity of test was 37% and its specificity was 69% with a positive predictive value of only 7.5%. Exercise electrocardiogram screening in completely healthy, asymptomatic individuals, even with high levels of risk factors for coronary heart disease, thus appears to be extremely limited. In daily clinical practice, a highly positive exercise electrocardiogram with a more than 2 mm ST-segment depression, observed at a low level of exercise and in a large number of leads has nevertheless to be considered with a high probability of coronary heart disease and managed accordingly.

WOMEN AND SILENT ISCHEMIA

This subject has recently been reviewed by Stern and Gottlieb.[38] These authors identified 11 investigations[39–48] from which the frequency of silent ischemia in women with suspected or proven coronary artery disease, postmyocardial infarction, angina pectoris etc. could be calculated. Seven of the 11 studies have shown similar frequency of silent ischemia in men and women, three showed less in women, and only one showed that women had more silent ischemia. Pooling the data, taking into consideration the size of the different cohorts, a small, but significant difference (29% versus 33%, p=0.01) was documented, women having less silent ischemia (odds ratio 0.85; 95% confidence interval 0.75, 0.96).

In a recent study Mulcahy and coworkers[49] found that women with coronary artery disease have a pattern and behavior of transient myocardial ischemia similar to those in men. There was a similar and significant circadian variation in ischemia activity in both women and men, with a trough at night, a surge in the morning and a peak between 1 and 2 pm. The ischemia threshold had similar variability in women and men and no gender difference was found in the pattern of preonset to onset heart rate changes over time.

MANAGEMENT OF SILENT MYOCARDIAL ISCHEMIA IN COMPLETELY ASYMPTOMATIC HEALTHY POPULATIONS

As shown above, exercise electrocardiogram screening in completely healthy populations has a very poor predictive value and cannot be taken into consideration in the detection of individuals at risk for coronary heart disease nor used to indicate specific management. In clinical practice, in men aged over 45 years and women aged over 55 without known coronary heart disease, the occurrence of ST-segment depression during routine exercise stress testing should lead to the following question: are the electrocardiographic changes caused by ischemia? Known risk factors, ST-segment depression more than 2 mm at a low exercise level (heart rate lower than 120 bpm), improvement in a test performed after sublingual nitrates, other markers of myocardial ischemia demonstrated at stress echo (dobutamine) or at stress myocardial scintigraphy (exercise, dipyridamol), will largely increase the positive predictive value of the test. In this highly selected group, coronary angiography should be performed and treatment managed in accordance with the severity of the illness, bearing in mind that the prognostic value of myocardial ischemia, symptomatic or asymptomatic, is similar.

REFERENCES

1. Degré S, Fang ZY, Sobolski J, Abramowicz M, Unger Ph, Berkenboom G. Detection of silent myocardial ischemia in asymptomatic selected populations and in unstable angina. In: Kellermann JA, Braunwald E, eds. *Silent Myocardial Ischemia: A Critical Appraisal* (Basel: Karger, 1990): 215–22.
2. Sobolski J, Kornitzer M, De Backer G, Dramaix M, Degré S, Denolin H. Silent ST segment depression predicts angina but not sudden death and myocardial infarction in asymptomatic middle-aged men. *Acta Cardiol* 1991; **2**: 52 (abst).
3. Deanfield JE, Ribiero P, Oakley K et al. Analysis of ST-segment changes in normal subjects: implications for ambulatory monitoring in angina pectoris. *Am J Cardiol* 1984; **54**: 1321–5.
4. Cohn PF. Silent myocardial ischemia. *Ann Intern Med* 1988; **109**: 312–17.
5. Rautaharji PM, Prineas RJ, Eifler WJ et al. Prognostic value of exercise electrocardiogram in men at high risk of future coronary heart disease: Multiple Risk Factor Intervention Trial experience. *J Am Coll Cardiol* 1986; **8**: 1.
6. Kirwin JD, Ascer E, Gennaro M et al. Silent myocardial ischemia is not predictive of myocardial infarction in peripheral vascular surgery patients. *Ann Vasc Surg* 1993; **7**: 27–32.
7. Aronow WS, Ahn C, Mercando AD, Epstein S, Gutstein H, Schoenfeld MR. Association of silent myocardial ischemia with new atherothrombotic common carotid arterial disease with and without previous atherothrombotic brain infarction. *J Am Geriatr Soc* 1995; **43**: 1272–4.
8. Otterstad JE. Is left ventricular hypertrophy in hypertension a marker for coronary risk factor? *Tidsskr Nor Laegeforen* 1993; **113**: 609–13.
9. Pringle SD, Dunn FG, Tweddel AC et al. Symptomatic and silent myocardial ischemia in hypertensive patients with left ventricular hypertrophy. *Br Heart J* 1992; **67**: 377–82.
10. Massie MB, Szlachcic Y, Tubau JF, O'Kelly BF, Ammon S, Chin W. Scintigraphic and electrocardiographic evidence of silent coronary artery disease in asymptomatic hypertension: a case–control study. *J Am Coll Cardiol* 1993; **22**: 1598–606.
11. Lee DP, Rigonan K, Quattro V. Increased blood pressure and neural tone in the silent ischemia of hypertension: disparate effects of immediate release of nifedipine. *J Am Coll Cardiol* 1993; **22**: 1438–45.
12. Pell ACH, Dunn FG. The interface of hypertension and ischemic heart disease. *Curr Opin Cardiol* 1995; **10**: 473–9.
13. Opherk D, Mall G, Zebe H et al. Reduction of coronary reserve: a mechanism for angina pectoris in patients with arterial hypertension and normal coronary arteries. *Circulation* 1984; **69**: 1–7.
14. Issaz K, Bruntz JF, Paris D, Ethevenot G, Aliot E. Abnormal coronary flow velocity profile in patients with left ventricular hypertrophy,

angina pectoris and normal coronary arteries: a transoesophageal Doppler echocardiographic study. *Am Heart J* 1994; **128**: 500–50.

15. Antony I, Aptecar E, Lerebours G, Nitenberg G. Coronary artery constriction caused by the cold pressor test in human hypertension. *Hypertension* 1994; **24**: 212–19.

16. Brush JE, Faxon DP, Salmon S, Jacobs AK, Ryian TJ. Abnormal endothelium-dependent coronary vasomotion in hypertensive patients. *J Am Coll Cardiol* 1992; **19**: 809–15.

17. Treasure CB, Klein JR, Vita JA et al. Hypertension and left ventricular hypertrophy are associated with impaired endothelium-mediated relaxation in human coronary resistance vessels. *Circulation* 1993; **87**: 86–93.

18. Antony I, Lerebours G, Nitenberg A. Loss of flow-dependent coronary artery dilatation in patients with hypertension. *Circulation* 1995; **91**: 1624–8.

19. Kannel WB. Silent myocardial ischemia and infarction: insights from the Framingham study. *Cardiol Clin* 1986; **4**: 583–91.

20. Margolis JR, Kannel WS, Feinleib M, Dawber TR, McNamara PM. Clinical features of unrecognized myocardial infarction: silent and asymptomatic: eighteen-year follow-up study: the Framingham study. *Am J Cardiol* 1973; **32**: 1–7.

21. Kannel WB, Abbott RD. Incidence and prognosis of unrecognized myocardial infarction: an update of the Framingham study. *N Engl J Med* 1984; **311**: 1144–7.

22. Cabin HS, Roberts WC. Quantitative comparison of extent of coronary narrowing and size of healed myocardial infarct in 33 necropsy patients with clinically recognized and in 28 clinically unrecognized (silent) previous acute myocardial infarction. *Am J Cardiol* 1982; **50**: 677–81.

23. Chiariello M, Indolfi C, Cotecchia MR, Sifola C, Romano M, Condorelli M. Asymptomatic transient changes during ambulatory ECG monitoring in diabetic patients. *Am Heart J* 1985; **110**: 529–34.

24. Nesto RW, Phillips RT, Kett KG et al. Angina and exertional myocardial ischemia in diabetic and nondiabetic patients: assessment by exercise thallium scintigraphy. *Ann Intern Med* 1988; **108**: 170–5.

25. Callaham PR, Froelicher VF, Klein J, Risch M, Dubach P, Frijs R. Exercise-induced silent ischemia: age, diabetes mellitus, previous myocardial infarction and prognosis. *J Am Coll Cardiol* 1989; **14**: 1175–80.

26. Chipkin SR, Frid D, Alpert JS, Baker SP, Dalen JE, Aronin N. Frequency of painless myocardial ischemia during exercise tolerance testing in patients with and without diabetes mellitus. *Am J Cardiol* 1987; **59**: 61–5.

27. Bertrand E. Coronary disease in black Africans: epidemiology risk factors, clinical symptomatology and coronarography, evolution. *Bull Acad Natl Med* 1992; **176**: 311–23.

28. Trochu JN, Cantarovich D, Renaudeau J, Patra O, Du Roscoat P, Helias J. Assessment of coronary artery disease by thallium scintigraphy in type 1 diabetic uremic patients awaiting combined pancreas and renal transplantation. *Angiology* 1991; **42**: 302–7.

29. Rubler S, Fischer VJ. The significance of repeated exercise testing with thallium 201 scanning in asymptomatic diabetic males. *Clin Cardiol* 1985; **8**: 621–8.

30. Ignone G, Vona M, Scardi S, on behalf of the participants. Multicenter Study on Silent Ischemia during Exercise Testing (SMISS). Clinical and ergometric parameters in 4389 patients with proven ischemic heart disease. *G Ital Cardiol* 1984; **24**: 349–57.

31. Faerman I, Faccio E, Milei J et al. Autonomic neuropathy and painless myocardial infarction in diabetic patients. *Diabetes* 1977; **26**: 1147–58.

32. Bernardi L, Ricordi I, Lazzari P et al. Impaired circadian modulation of sympathovagal activity in diabetes: a possible explanation for temporal onset of cardiovascular disease. *Circulation* 1992; **86**: 1443–52.

33. Zarich S, Waxman S, Freeman RT, Mittleman M, Hegarty P, Nesto RW. Effect of autonomic system dysfunction on the circadian pattern of myocardial ischemia in diabetes mellitus. *J Am Coll Cardiol* 1994; **24**: 956–62.

34. Caracciolo EA, Chaitman BR, Forman SA et al. for the ACIP Investigators. Diabetics with coronary disease have a prevalence of asymptomatic ischemia during exercise treadmill testing and ambulatory ischemia monitoring similar to that of nondiabetic patients: an ACIP database study. *Circulation* 1996; **93**: 2097–105.

35. Chiariello M, Indolfi C. Silent myocardial ischemia in patients with diabetes mellitus. *Circulation* 1996; **93**: 2089–91.

36. Maseri A. *Ischemic Heart Disease*. Edinburgh: Churchill Livingstone, 1995.

37. Yusuf S. Design of studies to critically evaluate if detection of asymptomatic ST-segment deviation

(silent ischemia) is of medical or public health importance. In: Singh BN, ed. *Silent Myocardial Ischemia and Angina. Prevalence, Prognostic and Therapeutic Significance.* New York: Pergamon Press, 1988 pp 206–19.

38. Stern S, Gottlieb S. Silent myocardial ischemia in women, In: *Women and Heart Disease*, eds Julian DG, Wenger NK, London, Martin Dunitz Ltd, 1997: 125–33.

39. Kemp GL, Ellestad MH. The incidence of 'silent' coronary heart disease. *California Medicine* 1968; **109**: 363–7.

40. Stern S, Weisz G, Gavish A, Keren A, Tzivoni D. Comparison between silent and symptomatic ischemia during exercise testing in patients with coronary artery disease. *J Cardiopulmonary Rehabil* 1988; **12**: 507–12.

41. Mark DB, Hlatky MA, Califf RM et al. Painless exercise ST deviation on the treadmill: Long-term prognosis. *J Am Coll Cardiol* 1989; **14**: 885–92.

42. Gasperetti CM, Burwell LR, Beller GA. Prevalence of and variables associated with silent ischemia on exercise thallium-201 stress testing. *J Am Coll Cardiol* 1990; **16**: 115–23.

43. Heller LI, Tresgallo M, Sciacca RR, Blood DK, Seldin DW, Johnson LL. Prognostic significance of silent myocardial ischemia on a thallium stress test. *Am J Cardiol* 1990; **65**: 718–21.

44. Bolognese L, Rossi L, Sarasso G, et al. Silent versus symptomatic dipyridamole-induced

ischemia after myocardial infarction: clinical and prognostic significance. *J Am Coll Cardiol* 1992; **19**: 953–9.

45. Hecht HS, DeBord L, Sotomayor N, Shaw R, Ryan C. Truly silent ischemia and the relationship of chest pain and ST segment changes to the amount of ischemic myocardium: Evaluation by supine bicycle stress echocardiography. *J Am Coll Cardiol* 1994; **23**: 369–76.

46. Klein J, Chao SY, Berman DS, Rozanski A. Is 'silent' myocardial ischemia really as severe as symptomatic ischemia? The analytical effect of patient selection disease. *Circulation* 1994; **89**: 1958–66.

47. Weiner DA, Ryan TJ, Parsons L, et al. Significance of silent myocardial ischemia during exercise testing in women: Report from the Coronary Artery Surgery Study. *Am Heart J* 1995; **123**: 465–70.

48. Elhendy A, Geleijnse ML, Roelandt RTC, Cornel JH, van Domburg RT, Fioretti PM. Stress-induced left ventricular dysfunction in silent and symptomatic myocardial ischemia during dobutamine stress test. *Am J Cardiol* 1995; **75**: 1112–15.

49. Mulcahy D, Dakak N, Zalos G, Andrews NP, et al. Patterns and behavior of transient myocardial ischemia in stable coronary disease are the same in both men and women: A comparative study. *J Am Coll Cardiol* 1996; **27**: 1629–36.

13

Drug suppression of silent myocardial ischemia

Bramah N Singh

BACKGROUND

In the 1970s it became possible to monitor the electrocardiogram (ECG) over long periods of time in ambulatory patients as well as in those who were hospitalized.[1-5] The Holter technique reproducibly and reliably detected and quantified the number and frequency of episodes of silent ST-segment deviations consistent with myocardial ischemia. The technique as used by numerous investigators has now confirmed that such episodes of silent ischemia do not differ significantly from those that are associated with symptoms. Objective anatomic, functional and hemodynamic as well as metabolic correlates of silent myocardial ischemia have been shown to be similar, if not identical, to those of the symptomatic episodes, barring minor differences.[6-13]

There is now growing evidence that various pharmacologic agents, percutaneous transluminal coronary angioplasty (PTCA), or coronary artery bypass graft (CABG) surgery are variably effective in suppressing episodes of myocardial ischemia documented on Holter recordings in patients with coronary artery disease (CAD). However, few comparative studies defining the effects of different classes of anti-ischemic agents and of invasive interventions have been reported. It should be emphasized that while this discussion pertains largely to silent ischemia, it is impossible to provide a critical perspective on the subject without allusion to symptomatic ischemia. In this context, two fundamental observations

should be remembered: (1) the largest number of episodes of silent ischemia occur in patients with symptomatic coronary artery disease, and (2) symptomatic ischemia needs suppression for relief of symptoms but suppression of silent ischemia should be undertaken only for the purposes of prolonging survival and/or the prevention of fatal and/or nonfatal infarction. Theoretically, these objectives can be attained either by pharmacologic means or by myocardial revascularization. It has become increasingly clear that both issues need to be addressed by stringently controlled clinical trials.

In terms of pharmacologic properties, agents which improve myocardial blood flow and those which reduce myocardial workload have the capability to reduce silent as well as symptomatic ischemia. Three broad categories of these agents have been identified: nitrates, calcium-channel blockers and beta-blockers. Few or no data exist on agents that reduce ischemia by producing the isolated reduction of heart rate (specific sinus node inhibitors such as zatebradine) or specific metabolic inhibitors (for example trimetazidine or ranolazine). The bulk of the available data deal with the effects of beta-blockers and calcium-channel blockers and the role of nitrates will be mentioned in brief. Even in the earliest studies, in which silent myocardial ischemic episodes were identified with Holter recordings in patients with CAD, nitrates were found to reduce significantly the number of episodes and their duration. Few systematic studies have been carried out to determine the precise efficacy of these agents in eliminating silent myocardial ischemia and there are few data that pertain to mortality.

In the case of beta-adrenergic-blocking drugs, the bulk of the pharmacologic effects can ultimately be attributed to the ability of these compounds to antagonize beta-adrenoreceptors competitively. Structurally, these compounds are reasonably homogeneous: minor structural differences have produced compounds of variable beta-blocking potencies, varied pharmacokinetics, and associated features such as intrinsic sympathomimetic activity, cardioselectivity, and membrane-depressant propensities. However, while such features may influence the overall profile of side-effects of an individual agent, they have little or no effect on their therapeutic efficacy, which results essentially from blockade of beta-adrenoreceptors. The sole exception is the presence of intrinsic sympathomimetic activity which appears to attenuate efficacy. In contrast, calcium antagonists constitute a structurally heterogeneous group of compounds that share two significant properties: (1) the ability to block the slow calcium channel in cardiac muscle and (2) the capacity to inhibit transmembrane fluxes of calcium in smooth muscle, especially in the coronary and peripheral circulations.[13]

Because of their often striking structural differences, individual calcium-channel blockers may exhibit other pharmacologic actions (for example verapamil and diltiazem have noncompetitive sympatholytic actions) that may lead to a complex interplay between their intrinsic properties (demonstrable in isolated tissues) and the reflex changes they may produce as a result of sympathetic activation due to peripheral vasodilatation.[13] Because of resulting reflex effects and the varying potencies of different calcium antagonists to induce peripheral vasodilatation, the actions of calcium antagonists in vitro and in vivo may differ markedly. This is particularly striking in the case of atrioventricular (AV) nodal conduction and refractoriness. For example, as in the case of beta-blockers, calcium antagonists such as verapamil, diltiazem, tiapamil, and gallopamil predictably lengthen AV conduction and refractoriness both in vivo and in vitro. In contrast, the dihydropyridines (for example nifedipine and nicardipine) are potent depressants of AV nodal conduction in isolated hearts, but this effect is nullified or even reversed by their reflex effects.[13] However, it must be emphasized that while calcium antagonists alter AV nodal conduction by blocking the slow channel potentials in this structure, beta-blockers produce their negative dromotropic effects by altering the sympathetic impulse traffic in the AV node. Thus, the AV nodal effects of the two classes of compounds are likely to summate if they have similar effects individually (for example propranolol versus verapamil or diltiazem); in the case of the dihydropyridines, concomitant beta-blockade is likely to convert a potentially facilitatory action on the AV node to a depressant one. These electrophysiologic features of the various compounds are of therapeutic significance in the choice of an agent or combination of agents for the control of ischemic syndromes in patients who may have pre-existing conduction system disease. However, from the standpoint of control of ischemia, the comparative cardiocirculatory effects of calcium antagonists and beta-antagonists are the most relevant pharmacologic effects.

It is now well established that most beta-antagonists, when administered intravenously or orally, depress heart rate, cardiac output, and indices of ventricular contractility and increase the filling pressures of the ventricle. Thus, the major mechanism of their anti-ischemic action is via a reduction in oxygen demand. These drugs may also reduce coronary blood flow commensurate with the reduction in myocardial oxygen demand. From studies utilizing quantitative angiography, it is also known that beta-blockers may produce coronary vasoconstriction, an effect that may aggravate the tendency to coronary vasospasm, especially in the setting of Prinzmetal's angina in patients with normal coronary vessels. For this reason, beta-blockers are unlikely to eliminate episodes of ischemia that are triggered by coronary vasospasm. On the other hand, in patients whose episodes of ischemia are triggered by vasospasm in the setting of advanced CAD, the increases in heart rate and blood pressure in response to ischemia are likely to augment the overall duration of ischemia. Beta-blockers are likely to curtail the duration of such ischemic episodes[14] and perhaps prevent them from reaching the threshold of pain perception. In contrast to the action of beta-blockers, the most striking hemodynamic effect of calcium antagonists consists of a predictable and consistent reduction in systemic vascular resistance accompanied by either no change or an increase in cardiac output.[14] Furthermore, unlike beta-blockers, calcium antagonists reduce coronary vascular resistance, with a tendency for coronary sinus flow to increase. Furthermore, these agents have the propensity to dilate resistance as well as capacitance vessels in the coronary circulation;[15,16] while such an effect is modest in extent, lesion dilatation even of such a degree is hemodynamically significant.[17] It may be an important component of the anti-ischemic actions of calcium-channel blockers.

The differing pharmacologic effects of beta-blockers and calcium-channel blockers therefore provide a rational basis for a combined regimen in the amelioration of transient myocardial ischemia to test the hypothesis that reduction or suppression of silent ischemia improves prognosis (see later).

Beta-blockers and suppression of silent ischemia

At present, there appear to be only limited data on this subject but experience is increasing. However, a recent study[18] has documented that beta-blockade exerts a salutary effect on silent myocardial ischemia in patients with chronic stable angina. Imperi and colleagues[18] studied the effects of titrated doses of metoprolol (50–200 mg bid) in patients with positive electrocardiographic evidence of asymptomatic ischemia but angiographically confirmed CAD. The frequency and duration of episodes of silent myocardial ischemia were quantified over 72 hours of Holter monitoring in each patient at baseline and after steady-state therapy at each dose of the beta-blocker. A significant reduction was accomplished at each dose with a clear-cut dose–response effect.

The well-known circadian pattern of ischemia distribution[13,19] over 24 hours was markedly attenuated by metoprolol. The blunting of the circadian pattern of silent ischemia in patients with CAD may be one mechanism that reduces the rate of sudden death and reinfarction in survivors of acute myocardial infarction (MI) given prophylactic beta-blockade. Imperi et al.[18] reported that metoprolol also reduced the total ischemia time per 24 hours; it attenuated the heart rate at the onset of ischemia while reducing the increases in heart rate associated with individual episodes, the durations of which were also shortened. A detailed discussion of the role of beta-blockers in suppressing silent myocardial ischemia is presented elsewhere in this volume.[20]

Suppression of silent myocardial ischemia by calcium-channel blockers

In the setting of vasospastic angina, the effects of all calcium-channel blockers, in silent as well as symptomatic ischemia, appear comparable, reflecting their somewhat similar coronary vasodilator propensities. The effects in chronic stable angina undoubtedly stem from a much more complex action of different classes of these agents in relation to the possibly equally complex mechanisms underlying different episodes of transient ischemia in this setting.

As previously emphasized, there are few systematic data regarding the effects of calcium-channel blockers on silent myocardial ischemic episodes in chronic stable angina. The earliest observations dealt with the effects of bepridil, a calcium antagonist with a complex pharmacologic profile.[21] When 300 mg/day of the compound was given to patients with chronic stable angina and an exercise stress test positive for ischemia, the drug increased the time to angina and to the development of 1 mm ST-segment depression. Twenty-four-hour Holter recordings obtained before and during drug therapy and analyzed by the compact analog technique indicated that bepridil significantly reduced the cumulative duration of silent myocardial ischemia per 24 hours. Schnellbacher et al.[22] studied the effects of diltiazem (60 mg three times daily) on silent and symptomatic episodes of myocardial ischemia in 19 patients. Holter monitoring revealed no episodes of ischemia in seven patients. In the remainder, after the first day of therapy with the calcium-channel blockers, the frequency and duration of ischemic episodes (over 90% silent) were reduced by 65 and 77%, respectively, and by 69 and 65%, respectively, on the seventh day. Verapamil is likely to exert a similar action on silent myocardial ischemic episodes in chronic stable angina, but systematic data must be obtained in controlled clinical trials.

Combined beta-blockers and calcium-channel blocker therapy in silent ischemia

Lynch et al.[23] objectively evaluated the antianginal and anti-ischemic effects of propranolol, nifedipine, and their combination in 16 patients with severe exertional angina. The study was conducted in a double-blind fashion with multiple end-points including parameters of exercise stress tests, subjective features (chest pain, nitroglycerin consumption), and electrocardiographic data obtained from 48-hour Holter recordings (the total area and amount of ST-segment depression on the precordial exercise map and the total number of episodes of ST-segment depression). Two doses of each drug were used in the study: nifedipine 30 and 60 mg/day, and propranolol 240 and 480 mg/day, each drug given in three divided doses. Both drugs exerted a beneficial effect on the conventional subjective and objective indices of angina and ischemia. The effects of the combination therapy in general were more striking than the effects of either drug given alone at both doses. With respect to the effects and doses of the two drugs and their combination, at both doses, nifedipine and propranolol given alone significantly reduced the number of

episodes of ST-segment depression per 48 hours (most episodes being silent); propranolol was somewhat more potent in this regard. The combination therapies at both dosages were significantly more potent than either drug given alone, with evidence for a synergistic effect. The data (not shown) were also similar for the effects on exercise-induced ST-segment depression during treadmill stress testing.

The authors conducted a double-blind study[24] of the anti-ischemic effects of propranolol and a new dihydropyridine type of calcium antagonist, nicardipine, singly and in combination versus placebo using a protocol with an extended Latin square design. The goal was to evaluate the relative efficacy of these agents in terms of standard clinical parameters and treadmill variables. The major focus was on the effects of the two classes of drugs and their combination on episodes of silent myocardial ischemia as determined by ST-segment deviations occurring during ambulatory Holter monitoring in patients with chronic stable angina.

The mean data demonstrated the effects of propranolol, nicardipine, and the combination therapy on the number of episodes of ischemia (over 80% being silent) per 24 hours documented on ambulatory electrocardiographic recordings. Although both propranolol (−29%) and nicardipine (−18%) given alone reduced the number of episodes of ischemia, the change was not statistically significant. In contrast, combination therapy was effective in significantly ($P < 0.05$) reducing the number of ischemic episodes (−86%) compared with the placebo, the blockers or the calcium antagonist given alone. The combination regimen reduced the frequency of ischemic episodes by over 90% ($P < 0.05$), the maximum duration by 90% ($P < 0.05$), and the total duration per 24 hours by 92% ($P < 0.05$). Combination therapy had a significantly greater effect than either propranolol or nicardipine given alone.

Deedwania and Carbajal[25] found that patients receiving beta-blockers alone or in combination with other drugs had fewer episodes of silent ischemia in the morning hours and the duration of ischemia per 24 hours was significantly shorter compared with patients not receiving beta-blockers. These results are similar to those reported previously in a group of 348 patients with stable angina who were receiving nitrates or a beta-blocking agent.[26] Forty-three percent of patients in that study had one or more episodes of transient ischemic ST depression (>80% silent) during the 48-hour ambulatory ECG monitoring (AEM). The high prevalence of residual ischemia reported in these studies suggests that whereas some drugs may be more effective than others, in general, conventional antianginal drug therapy directed for control of angina pectoris does not abolish the silent ischemic events recorded on AEM during routine daily activities.

Recently, in a placebo-controlled, double-blind, randomized, crossover study Deedwania et al.[27] compared the effects of atenolol and nifedipine in 25 patients with stable CAD, exercise-induced ischemia and 5 minutes' or longer duration of silent ischemia during the 48-hour AEM. The results showed that, although both atenolol and nifedipine treatments reduced the frequency and duration of transient ischemic episodes, atenolol was significantly more effective than nifedipine in reducing the magnitude of ischemic activity as well as total abolition of ischemic episodes (50% versus 25% suppression rate, respectively). During the placebo phase there was a morning surge in ischemic activity which was adequately controlled during therapy with atenolol.

Parmley et al.[28] recently investigated the effects of long-acting nifedipine (nifedipine gastrointestinal therapeutic system (GITS)) alone and in combination with a beta-blockade on episodes of myocardial ischemia detected by 48-hour ambulatory ECG recordings. A total of 207 patients completed all phases of the study. Overall, nifedipine GITS significantly reduced weekly angina attacks (from 5.7 to 1.8; $P < 0.0001$) and the number of ischemic events from 7.28 to 4.0 (mostly silent; $P < 0.0001$) reported during 48-hour monitoring periods. Nifedipine GITS significantly reduced ischemia during the 48-hour period when administered as monotherapy or in combination with a beta-blocker. The morning surge of ischemia was attenuated most effectively by the combination regimen.

Reduction of transient myocardial ischemia by pravastatin

A number of studies recently have reported that cholesterol-lowering therapy reduces morbidity and mortality in subjects at high risk as well as in patients with established coronary artery disease.[29,30] It has been suggested that such benefit stems either from regression of atheromatous plaques[31] and/or a reduction in endothelial function as a result of the direct action of the drugs.[32] Van Boven et al.[33] recently tested the hypothesis that lipid-lowering therapy, when used in association with usual anti-ischemic therapy, might lead to a reduction in the number of episodes of transient myocardial ischemia documented on Holter recordings in patients with chronic stable angina. In this 2-year prospective, randomized, placebo-controlled study, the effect of pravastatin given in a dose of 40 mg/day was evaluated.

The study was conducted in 768 male patients with chronic stable angina pectoris and documented coronary artery disease, and a range of serum cholesterol levels between 155 and 310 mg/dl. The patients received their usual antianginal therapy during the trial. In the randomized patients on pravastatin, ischemic episodes were present in 28% at baseline compared with 19% after treatment; the corresponding figures for the placebo group were 20% and 23%. The difference in the change between the two groups was statistically significant ($P < 0.021$). Pravastatin reduced the ischemic episodes by 1.23 ± 0.25 (sem); the corresponding reduction on placebo was 0.53 ± 0.25 ($P = 0.047$). The total ischemic burden under the influence of pravastatin decreased (Fig. 13.1) from 41 ± 5 to 22 ± 5 mm.min ($P = 0.0058$) and from 34 ± 6 to 26 ± 6 mm.min on placebo ($P = 0.24$). The effect of pravastatin on risk for ischemia remained statistically significant even when adjusted for independent risk factors. In this report the investigators did not indicate the number of ischemic episodes which

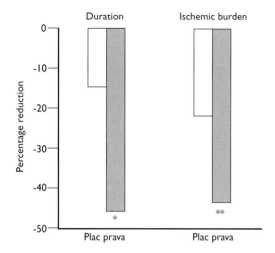

Figure 13.1 Diagram of the percentage reduction in components of transient myocardial ischemia during the study in placebo patients (plac, open bars) and in pravastatin patients (prava, shaded bars). *P = 0.017 and **P = 0.0058. Note the very significant percentage reduction in transient myocardial ischemia induced by pravastatin therapy. (Reproduced with permission from van Boven et al.[33])

were clinically silent. However, from the consistent pattern of previously published data, it is reasonable to assume that over 80% of the episodes in the 48-hour Holter recordings were clinically silent. Their data are the first of their kind which indicate that pravastatin reduces transient myocardial ischemia which may occur independently of changes in the level of serum cholesterol. Whether this might also occur with other statins or other forms of lipid-lowering drugs remains to be defined.

MODIFYING SUBSTRATE VERSUS SUPPRESSING MANIFESTATIONS OF THE SUBSTRATE

As indicated above, the relevant question about silent myocardial ischemia is whether one can fundamentally alter the incidence of myocardial infarction, and especially death related to it, simply by suppressing silent or symptomatic myocardial ischemia in a patient with coronary artery disease. In this context, data from large, uncontrolled and controlled clinical studies are of particular relevance. These will be considered in brief as a preamble to the discussion of the issue of whether the focus should be on silent ischemia as an approach to defining the extent and severity of coronary artery disease or to quantifying it as a prelude to its suppression aimed at reducing morbid coronary events. A study of particular importance in this regard is the Atenolol Silent Ischemia Study (ASIST). This is the first study in which the hypothesis that suppression of silent myocardial ischemia leads to a reduction in mortality, lower infarction rate, less heart failure and fewer serious ventricular arrhythmias has been tested.[34] In ASIST, patients with coronary artery disease and minimal symptoms, but with significant episodes of silent ischemia on Holter recordings, were randomized to atenolol and placebo in a double-blind, multicenter study in which the primary end-point was event-free survival at 1 year. The events quantified were death, resuscitated ventricular tachycardia/fibrillation, MI, and hospitalization for unstable angina or revascularization. The secondary outcome was ischemia documented on Holter recordings at 4 weeks from the initiation of therapy. Three hundred and six outpatients with mild or no angina, abnormal exercise tests, and ischemia on ambulatory monitoring were randomized to 100 mg/day atenolol and placebo.

Compared with placebo, atenolol exerted a marked suppressant effect on silent ischemia, and at the 12-month follow-up period there were fewer coronary events (11% versus 25%; $P < 0.001$) on atenolol, a longer event-free survival (120 versus 79 days, with a 56% reduction in relative risk; $P = 0.001$). On atenolol, there was a nonsignificant trend for reduction in death, nonfatal MI, ventricular tachycardia or ventricular fibrillation (resuscitated) and hospitalization for unstable angina (as a composite end-point). Of note, the most powerful univariate and multivariate correlate of coronary event-free survival was absence of silent ischemia on Holter recordings after 4 weeks of therapy, a finding that appears consistent with the observations that both in unstable angina and in chronic stable angina, silent ischemia is the single most powerful predictor of morbid coronary events during follow-up, as was noted by Deedwania.[20] However, in the case of the ASIST trial results, does it logically follow that the observed benefit in some outcomes and trends in benefit in others stem from suppression of ischemia and that suppression and benefit are causally related? Atenolol is a potent beta-blocker and it is known that this class of drugs reduces mortality and reinfarction rate in survivors of infarcts and total mortality in certain other subsets of patients, such as those with congestive heart failure. The observed benefit in these settings cannot be attributed solely to the suppression of ischemia or arrhythmias. Suppression of ischemia and an impact on coronary events responsible for total mortality in this setting might be dissociated in the case of certain anti-ischemia agents. For example, it is known that certain dihydropyridine-type calcium-channel blockers, especially those with a short half-life (for example nifedipine) can be powerful anti-ischemic agents while having the proclivity to *increase* mortality and infarction rate, presumably by other mechanisms.[35] Such a dichotomy in mortality and suppression of one of the manifestations of diseased substrate is not unique for ischemia and was demonstrated in a striking fashion in the case of ventricular arrhythmias in the Cardiac Arrhythmia Suppression Trial (CAST).[36] Viewed in this way, it is possible that the marked suppressant effect of atenolol on silent ischemia in ASIST may simply represent a drug effect that is not responsible for the beneficial effect on coronary events which the drug might produce by other, possibly indirect, mechanisms.

Therapeutic implications

The data discussed in this chapter suggest that both beta-blockers and calcium-channel blockers have the potential to reduce silent myocardial ischemic episodes in patients with chronic stable angina and in many other ischemic myocardial syndromes. Nitrates are also effective but seemingly at a lower order of potency. The fact that the suppressant effects of calcium-channel blockers and beta-blockers on silent myocardial ischemia in the setting of chronic stable angina are most pronounced when these agents are combined might be of therapeutic significance. Such an effect appears to be synergistic rather than simply additive. It may reflect the complementary effects of two classes of anti-ischemic agents on myocardial oxygen supply and demand relative to their differing hemodynamic effects.

In contrast, much prognostic data has been obtained with the exercise treadmill in patients with CAD and chronic stable angina. A positive test for myocardial ischemia in these patients is clearly associated with an augmented risk for a morbid coronary event (infarction or sudden death), whether such patients are symptomatic or asymptomatic.[37] It is also well established[37] that in patients whose exercise treadmill test is electrocardiographically positive, the prognosis is identical, whether or not such patients develop chest pain during the treadmill test. These data indicate that ischemia (as closely correlated with the extent of coronary artery disease, as reflected in the severity of stenoses and/or the number of the vessels stenosed) rather than its symptomatic manifestations is prognostically important. Therefore, it is reasonable to assume that a patient with a strongly positive treadmill test should undergo evaluation and treatment of myocardial ischemia whether it is symptomatic or silent.[38–40]

As previously indicated, in unstable angina the persistence of silent myocardial ischemia documented on Holter after symptomatic episodes have been eliminated by medical therapy appears to be highly predictive of an adverse short-term prognosis.[41,42] Newer

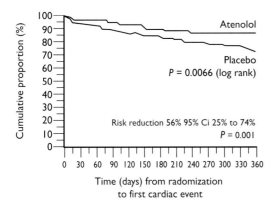

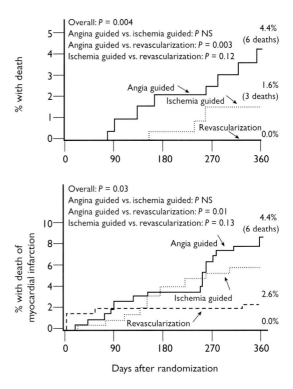

Figure 13.2 Event-free survival in patients with chronic stable angina with evidence of silent myocardial ischemia randomized to placebo and atenolol in a double-blind protocol. The Kaplan–Meier curves compare the cumulative probabilities of not experiencing an adverse event during follow-up for patients with ambulatory electrocardiogram-monitored silent myocardial ischemia. (Reproduced with permission from Pepine et al.[34])

data[40,43,44,45] provide evidence that the same holds for chronic stable angina. These observations have raised a number of practical questions. For example, does it imply that a concerted effort should be made to reduce silent myocardial ischemia further by intensifying medical therapy? Or are we, with rigorous triple-drug regimens, already at the upper end of the dose–response curve of medical therapy? The phenomenon of residual ischemia in this setting may simply be an expression of the fact that drug therapy merely distinguishes 'responders' from 'nonresponders', the latter having an inherently worse prognosis that is unlikely to be influenced significantly by further attempts with more aggressive medical therapy. The implication here might be that the failure of drug therapy to effect a substantive change simply reflects the presence of a substrate not amenable to the influence of pharmacologic regimens. The decisive resolution of this issue is possible only by stringently controlled,

Figure 13.3 Effects of three forms of therapy on death and myocardial infarction in patients with chronic stable angina. Although the number of fatal events was small, the percentage of patients who died during the 1-year follow-up was significantly lower for patients assigned to the revascularization strategy than those assigned to the angina-guided therapy, but not for patients assigned to the ischemia-guided strategy (top). The mortality rate was similar between the angina-guided and ischemia-guided strategies. The combination of death or myocardial infarction was significantly less common among patients assigned to the revascularization strategy than among patients assigned to the angina-guided or ischemia-guided strategy (bottom). (Reproduced with permission from Rogers et al.[46])

adequately designed clinical trials of a larger sample size. However, such trials are unlikely to be carried out, in the case of unstable angina, because most patients with unstable angina routinely undergo coronary angiography.

A strong correlation between the angiographic findings and the frequency and duration of silent myocardial ischemia on Holter recordings has now been demonstrated.[40] Most unstable patients now undergo PTCA or surgical myocardial revascularization and the results from the ACIP study[46], preliminary as it is, indicates, in another subset of patients, that revascularization might be superior to either angina-guided or ischemia-guided medical therapy (Fig 14.3). Thus, the use of silent myocardial ischemia as an end-point to gauge adequacy of therapy in this setting currently appears to have limited practical appeal or applicability. The data suggest that the focus needs to be more directly on the substrate, which in the case of most, if not all, ischemic myocardial syndromes is clearly the coronary vessels—the number, severity, and location of their stenoses and occlusions. In this context, it is pertinent to consider that aspirin, thrombolytics, pravastatin and presumably other statins and lipid-lowering drugs reduce ischemia by an indirect effect on the myocardium via a primary change in the coronary lumen.

The issue of a controlled clinical trial may nevertheless be of fundamental importance in chronic stable angina; however, the difficulties of carrying out meaningful clinical trials of a controlled-design in this setting are formidable for a number of reasons. First, as already mentioned, patients with chronic stable angina in whom silent ischemia is readily abolished by drug therapy ('responders') may have an inherently good prognosis. Ideally, they need to be randomized in a blinded fashion to placebo versus active therapy. This may not be possible on ethical grounds. In any event, the agents which have the most consistent suppressant effect on silent myocardial ischemia—beta-blockers—may exert an effect on mortality independently of their action on ischemia, as suggested by the data in the beta-blocker trials in the survivors of acute myocardial infarction. The group with residual ischemia despite aggressive medical therapy ('nonresponders') are those in which the effects of interventions with an end-point of mortality or recurrent infarction theoretically are the most logical group to study. In this group the issue of a change in prognosis consequent upon reduction of silent ischemia could be the focus of a trial. On the other hand, these are the very patients in whom drug therapy has essentially failed to produce a satisfactory response, and they may need to be considered as candidates for revascularization.

CONCLUSIONS

For the present, it appears reasonable to conclude that the sole reason for the treatment of silent myocardial ischemia is to improve prognosis. There is now substantial evidence suggesting that silent myocardial ischemia is a distinct clinical entity and that its presence may be related to adverse clinical outcome, at least in certain subsets of patients. Numerous reports indicate that medical therapy with nitrates, beta-blockers, and calcium-channel blockers, as single agents or in combination, is effective in reducing silent myocardial ischemia and its duration. In the case of both unstable as well as chronic stable angina, therapy with single or combination regimens indicates that over 30% of patients continue to experience silent episodes of ischemia after symptomatic ones have been abolished. Silent ischemia on Holter or exercise treadmill testing can be significantly and more consistently reduced by revascularization. However, it remains unclear whether these treatments will influence prognosis when they are effective in suppressing silent ischemia. Nor is it known what degrees of reduction in silent myocardial ischemic episodes or in cumulative durations over a finite period may be necessary in order to effect a favorable change in prognosis. A resolution of these uncertainties by controlled clinical trials will be necessary before the presumed implications of silent myocardial ischemia can be translated confidently into routine clinical practice. On the other hand, is this a compelling clinical question for which decisive answers need to be generated with a high priority?

Recent data suggest that it might not be illogical to view ischemia (silent or symptomatic) as simply, and no more than, a manifestation of a diseased substrate, the severity of which needs to be determined accurately for clinical decision-making as to the most appropriate therapy.[42] Therapy may then be keyed, not to the suppression of graded degrees of ischemia (unless for symptom relief) but to a meaningful reduction in end-points such as death, infarction, life-threatening ventricular arrhythmias, heart failure, or other morbid coronary events. Within this framework, silent ischemia suppression appears to be no more a surrogate end-point than the suppression of spontaneously occurring but silent ventricular arrhythmias in cardiac disease. The parallelism is inescapable. Silent ischemia and asymptomatic ventricular arrhythmias are both powerful predictors of serious prognosis and assist the physician in identifying patients at risk for life-threatening morbid events, the occurrence of which are critically dependent on the myocardial and vascular substrates. Their suppression might be specific to the drugs and interventions, but the use of suppression as a surrogate for improvement in mortality has not been validated. A direct and independent link between suppression and a defined clinically meaningful outcome has not been substantiated. Until such a validation is forthcoming it would appear sound clinical practice to suppress ischemia to alleviate symptoms and to recommend the use of drug regimens (which must now include certain hypolipidemic agents) and nonpharmacologic interventions (especially CABG) which, in controlled clinical trials, have been shown to prolong survival and to reduce nonfatal and fatal complications of coronary artery disease whether or not associated with silent myocardial ischemia.

ACKNOWLEDGMENTS

A number of colleagues have allowed me access to their knowledge and wisdom which have shaped my appreciation and thinking about the complex subject of silent myocardial ischemia. A number of them have been collaborators. I would particularly like to thank Drs Koonlawee Nademanee, Freny Vaghaiwalla Mody, John Deanfield, William W Parmley, Prakash Deedwania, James Muller, Alberto Malliani, Vincent de Quattro, and Jaime Figueras. Their contributions to the ideas expressed in this chapter are gratefully acknowledged, but those aspects that might appear frankly egregious are solely my responsibility. In part, the information presented here is taken from my paper entitled 'Silent myocardial ischemia: to treat or not to treat?'[38]

REFERENCES

1. Stern S, Tzivoni D. Early detection of silent ischemic heart disease by 24-hour electrocardiographic monitoring of active subjects. *Br Heart J* 1974; **36**: 481–8.

2. Stern S, Tzivoni D. Early detection of silent ischemic heart disease by 24-hour electrocardiographic monitoring, as validated by coronary arteriography. *Circulation* 1975; **52**: 1045–52.

3. Allen RD, Gettes LS, Phalan C et al. Painless ST-segment depression in patients with angina pectoris. *Chest* 1976; **60**: 467–73.

4. Schang SJ, Pepine CJ. Transient asymptomatic ST-segment depression during daily activity. *Am J Cardiol* 1977; **39**: 297–303.

5. Tzivoni D, Gavish A, Benhorin J et al. Myocardial ischemia during daily activities and stress. *Am J Cardiol* 1982; **58**: 47B–52B.

6. Nademanee K, Intarachot V, Singh BN et al. Characteristics and clinical significance of silent myocardial ischemia in unstable angina. *Am J Cardiol* 1986; **58**: 26B–34B.

7. Singh BN, Nademanee K, Figueras J et al. Hemodynamic and electrocardiographic correlates of symptomatic and silent myocardial ischemia: pathophysiologic and therapeutic implications. *Am J Cardiol* 1986; **38**: 3B–12B.

8. Nademanee K, Singh BN, Guerrero J et al. Accurate rapid compact analog method for the quantification of frequency and duration of myocardial ischemia by semi-automated analy-

sis of 24-hour Holter ECG recordings. *Am Heart J* 1982; **103**: 802–12.

9. Wolf E, Tzivoni D, Stern S. Comparison of exercise stress tests and 24-hour ambulatory electrocardiographic monitoring of ST-T changes. *Br Heart J* 1980; **86**: 501–12.

10. Deanfield JE, Maseri A, Selwyn AP et al. Myocardial ischemia during daily life in patients with stable angina. Its relation to symptoms and heart rate changes. *Lancet* 1983; **2**: 753–9.

11. Cecchi A, Dovellini EV, Morchi F et al. Silent myocardial ischemia during ambulatory electro-cardiographic monitoring in patients with effort angina. *J Am Coll Cardiol* 1983; **1**: 934–40.

12. Chierchia S, Brunelli C, Simonetti I et al. Sequence of events in angina at rest: primary reduction in coronary flow. *Circulation* 1980; **61**: 759–65.

13. Nademanee K, Intarachot V, Josephson MA et al. Circadian variation in occurrence of transient overt and silent myocardial ischemia in chronic stable angina and comparison with Prinzmetal angina in men. *Am J Cardiol* 1987; **60**: 494–502.

14. Singh BN, Nademanee K. Beta-adrenergic blockade and unstable angina. *Am J Cardiol* 1986; **57**: 992–5.

15. Hossack KF, Brown BG, Stewart DK et al. Diltiazem-induced effects on sympathetically mediated constriction of normal and diseased coronary arteries: lack of epicardial coronary dilatory effect in humans. *Circulation* 1984; **70**: 465–71.

16. Brown BG, Bolson EL, Dodge HT. Dynamic mechanisms in human coronary stenosis. *Circulation* 1984; **70**: 917–22.

17. Singh BN, Chew CYC, Josephson MA. Pharmacologic and hemodynamic mechanisms underlying the antianginal actions of verapamil. *Am J Cardiol* 1982; **50**: 886–92.

18. Imperi GA, Lambert CR, Coy K et al. Effects of titrated beta-blockade (metoprolol) on silent myocardial ischemia in ambulatory patients with coronary artery disease. *Am J Cardiol* 1987; **60**: 519–24.

19. Rocco MB, Barry J, Campbell S et al. Circadian variation of transient myocardial ischemia in patients with coronary artery disease. *Circulation* 1987; **75**: 395–402.

20. Deedwania PC. Effects of beta-adrenergic blocking drugs in silent myocardial ischemia. In: Stern S, ed. 1997 (in press).

21. Nademanee K, Singh BN, Piontek M et al. Antianginal efficacy of bepridil, a novel calcium antagonist: double-blind evaluation by quantitating myocardial ischemia by compact Holter analog technique in chronic stable angina. *J Am Coll Cardiol* 1984; **3**: 551–60.

22. Schnellbacher K, Droste C, Roskamm H. Medical and surgical therapy of patients with asymptomatic ischemia. In: Arnim TV, Maseri A, eds. *Silent Ischemia*. (New York: Springer-Verlag, 1987): 154–61.

23. Lynch P, Dargie H, Krikler S et al. Objective assessment of anti-anginal treatment: a double-blind comparison of propranolol, nifedipine and their combination. *BMJ* 1980; **281**: 184–9.

24. Khan S, Nademanee K, Intarachot V, Singh BN. Effects of nicardipine and propranolol, alone and in combination, on silent myocardial ischemia in patients with chronic stable angina. *Am Heart J* 1997 (submitted).

25. Deedwania P, Carbajal E. Prevalence and patterns of silent myocardial ischemia during daily life in stable angina patients receiving conventional antianginal drug therapy. *Am J Cardiol* 1990; **65**: 1090–6.

26. Cohn P, Vetrovec G, Nesto R, Gerber F. The nifedipine-total ischemia awareness program: a national survey of painful and painless myocardial ischemia including results of antiischemic therapy. *Am J Cardiol* 1989; **63**: 534–9.

27. Deedwania PC, Carbajal EV, Nelson JR, Hait H. Anti-ischemic effects of atenolol versus nifedipine in patients with coronary artery disease and ambulatory silent ischemia. *J Am Coll Cardiol* 1990; **17**: 963–9.

28. Parmley W, Deanfield J, Gottlieb S, Nesto R, Singh B. Attenuation of the circadian patterns of myocardial ischemia with nifedipine GITS in chronic stable angina patients. *J Am Coll Cardiol* 1992; **19**: 1380–9.

29. Multiple Risk Factor Interventions Trial Research Group. Exercise electrocardiogram and coronary heart disease mortality in the Multiple Risk Factor Intervention Trial. *Am J Cardiol* 1985; **55**: 16–24.

30. Gordon D, Ekelund L, Karon J et al. Predictive value of the exercise tolerance test for mortality in North American men: the lipid research clinics mortality follow-up study. *Circulation* 1986; **74**: 252–61.

31. Jukema JW, Bruschke AVG, van Bove AJ et al. on behalf of the REGRESS Study Group. Effects of lipid-lowering by pravastatin on progression

and regression of coronary artery disease in symptomatic men with normal to moderately elevated serum cholesterol levels: the Regression Growth Evaluation Statin Study (REGRESS). *Circulation* 1995; **91**: 2528–40.

32. Treasure CB, Klein JL, Weintraub WS, Talley JD et al. Beneficial effects of cholesterol-lowering therapy on the coronary endothelium in patients with coronary artery disease. *N Engl J Med* 1995; **332**: 481–7.

33. van Boven AJ, Jukema W, Zwinderman AH et al. Reduction of transient myocardial ischemia with pravastatin in addition to the conventional treatment in patients with angina pectoris. *Circulation* 1996; **94**: 1053–58.

34. Pepine C, Cohn P, Deedwania P et al. Effects of treatment on outcome in mildly symptomatic patients with ischemia during daily life. The Atenolol Silent Myocardial Ischemia Study (ASIST). *Circulation* 1994; **90**: 762–8.

35. Conti CR. Re-examining the clinical safety and roles of calcium antagonists in cardiovascular medicine. *Am J Cardiol* 1996; **78**: 13–18.

36. The Cardiac Arrhythmia Suppression Trial (CAST) Investigators. Effect of encainide and fleicainide on mortality in a randomized trial of arrhythmia suppression after myocardial infarction. *N Engl J Med* 1992; **327**: 227–33.

37. Weiner DA, Ryan TJ, McCabe CH et al. Significance of silent myocardial ischemia during exercise testing in coronary artery disease. *Am J Cardiol* 1987; **59**: 725–31.

38. Singh BN. Silent myocardial ischemia: to treat or not to treat? In: Messerli FH, ed. *Cardiovascular Drug Therapy*. (Philadelphia, PA: WB Saunders, 1990): 254–64.

39. Mody F, Singh BN. Silent ischemia in the elderly: overview. *Cardiol Elderly* 1995; **3**: 321–5.

40. Mody FV, Nademanee K, Intarachot V et al. Severity of silent myocardial ischemia on ambulatory ECG monitoring in patients with stable angina pectoris: relation between prognostic determinants during exercise stress testing and coronary angiography. *J Am Coll Cardiol* 1988; **12**: 1169–77.

41. Nademanee K, Intarachot V, Josephson MA et al. Prognostic significance of silent myocardial ischemia in patients with unstable angina. *J Am Coll Cardiol* 1987; **10**: 1–8.

42. Gottlieb SO, Weisfeldt ML, Ouyang P et al. Silent ischemia as a marker for early unfavorable outcomes in patients with unstable angina. *N Engl J Med* 1986; **314**: 1214–24.

43. Deedwania P, Carbajal E. Silent ischemia during daily life is an independent predictor of mortality in stable angina. *Circulation* 1990; **81**: 748–56.

44. Reeves T. Relation and independence of angina pectoris and sudden death in persons with coronary atherosclerotic heart disease. *J Am Coll Cardiol* 1985; **5**: 167B–174B.

45. Warnes CA, Roberts WC. Sudden coronary death: relation of amount and distribution of coronary narrowing at necropsy to previous symptoms of myocardial ischemia, left ventricular scarring and heart weight. *Am J Cardiol* 1984; **65**: 6–13.

46. Rogers W, Bourassa M, Andrews T, Bertolet B, Blumenthal R, Chaitman B et al. Asymptomatic cardiac ischemia pilot study: outcome at one year for patients with ischemia randomized to medical therapy or revascularization. *J Am Coll Cardiol* 1995; **26**: 594–605.

14

Circadian variation in myocardial ischemia: pathophysiologic mechanisms

Arshed A Quyyumi

INTRODUCTION

It is now well recognized that the distribution according to time of day of many cardiovascular phenomena is uneven. These circadian variations have been described in recent years for certain cardiac parameters such as heart rate,[1,2] blood pressure,[3] and premature ventricular contractions[4,5] and, more importantly, for cardiovascular events including sudden cardiac death,[6] myocardial infarction,[7] transient myocardial ischemia,[1,2,5,8] and stroke. In order to facilitate understanding of the pathophysiology of cardiac events, attempts have been made to relate the morning preponderance of these vascular events to underlying parameters that can easily be measured with the ultimate aim of discovering strategies for prevention. This review will examine the pathophysiology of transient myocardial ischemia, its susceptibility to circadian variation, the reasons for this distribution, and the potential therapeutic implications.

PATHOPHYSIOLOGY OF TRANSIENT MYOCARDIAL ISCHEMIA

Several investigators have demonstrated that there is a marked circadian variation in transient myocardial ischemia, with a peak number of episodes occurring in the morning hours, sometimes with a reduction at midday with a second evening peak, and with a trough during the night (Fig. 14.1).[1,2,5,8] Recent analysis has determined that this pattern of ischemia occurs in both men and women.[9] A similar circadian rhythm has been observed with myocardial infarction and sudden cardiac death.[6,7] Although subgroups of patients with myocardial infarction, for example people with diabetes, the elderly, and smokers, have been shown to have a different or absent circadian variation in infarction frequency,[10] such differences have not been described in patients with transient myocardial ischemia. An opposite circadian variation, resulting in peak ischemic activity during the night is classically observed in patients with variant angina.

With the advent of ambulatory monitoring of heart rate, blood pressure, electro-cardiographic ST-segments and left ventricular function, it is now possible to study ischemic activity and its surrogates over the long term. Ambulatory ST-segment monitoring in patients with stable coronary artery disease has demonstrated that approximately one-third of the patients have transient ischemic episodes during daily living, and that more than 80% of these episodes are unrecognized or silent and have been shown by perfusion techniques to represent myocardial ischemia.[2] These episodes tend to occur relatively frequently in patients with more severe underlying coronary artery disease and in those with normal left ventricular function in whom the R-wave in the electrocardiogram is well preserved.

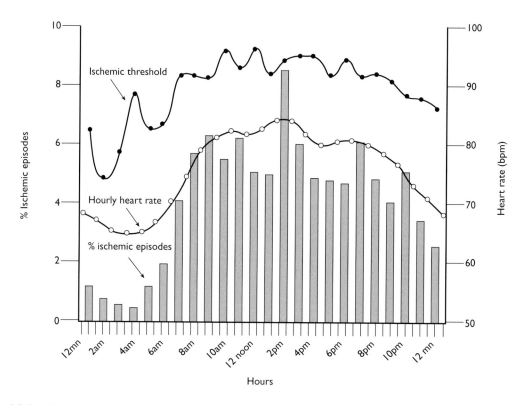

Figure 14.1 Circadian variation in transient ischemic episodes, mean hourly heart rate and the ischemic threshold (heart rate at 1 mm ST depression). (Adapted from Mulcahy et al.[9])

Factors determining myocardial oxygen demand

Ambulatory blood pressure and heart rate monitoring has shown that there is a distinct circadian variation in these parameters, paralleling the diurnal change in ischemia frequency.[1-3,8] Indirect determinants of contractility (also a determinant of myocardial oxygen demand) such as plasma catecholamines also have a similar circadian variation with a morning rise (Fig. 14.2).[11]

Several trials have linked the changes in heart rate and blood pressure to myocardial ischemia, proving that in most episodes, the increases in myocardial oxygen demand precede the development of ischemia during normal daily activities.[12-16] Increases in heart rate may occur over

a protracted period—up to 30 minutes[14] before ischemia occurs—although the major increase appears to occur in the immediate 5-minute period before ischemia.[12,14] Indeed, it appears that the likelihood of ischemia is related to the magnitude and duration of increase in heart rate, ranging from a 4% likelihood with a heart rate increase of 5–9 beats per minute (bpm), and lasts less than 10 minutes, to 60% likelihood when heart rate increases by more than 20 bpm and lasts for more than 40 minutes.[16] Thus, in patients with stable disease who have episodes of transient myocardial ischemia, whether silent or accompanied by chest pain, between 80% and 90% of all ischemic episodes occur with preceding increases in heart rate. Even when heart rate changes related to episodes occurring during the night were analyzed, a time when

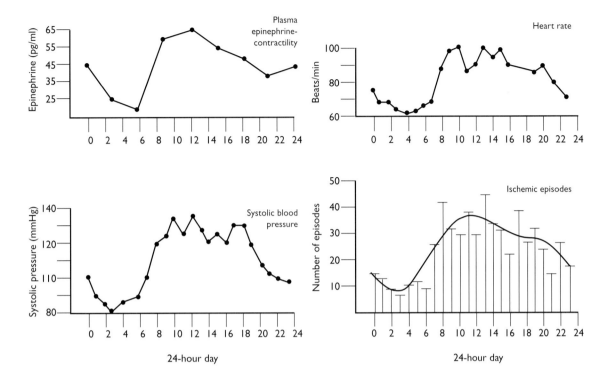

Figure 14.2 Circadian variation in indices of myocardial oxygen demand. (Adapted from Quyyumi.[26])

physical activity is minimal, it was found that the majority were preceded by increases in heart rate, often occurring as a result of awakening from deep stages of sleep, body movements, and occasionally during rapid eye movement (REM) sleep and sleep apnea.[15,17] Studies examining changes in systemic blood pressure in relation to the onset of ischemia have yielded similar results: increases in systolic but not diastolic blood pressure occur before the onset of ST-segment depression in the majority of cases; the maximum increase in blood pressure occurs before the maximum ST depression; and the ST depression returns to baseline after the systolic pressure has normalized.[13,18]

The striking and sudden increase in ischemic activity between 7 and 8 a.m. in the mornings led to investigations that addressed the question of activity as a trigger for ischemia. Parker et al. have demonstrated that awakening, arousal, and activities constituted the most important trigger,[19] because allowing patients to arise later in the day delayed the peak in ischemic activity to a later time. Adjusting the ischemic frequency to wake-up time demonstrated a more discrete peak (during which 24% of all ischemic episodes occurred) in the first 2–3 hours after awakening in contrast to a more diffuse increase observed in population studies where the time of awakening varies between individuals.[8]

Thus, it seems reasonable to conclude that an important and perhaps predominant trigger for myocardial ischemia, and for its distribution during the day, is a change in myocardial oxygen demand.

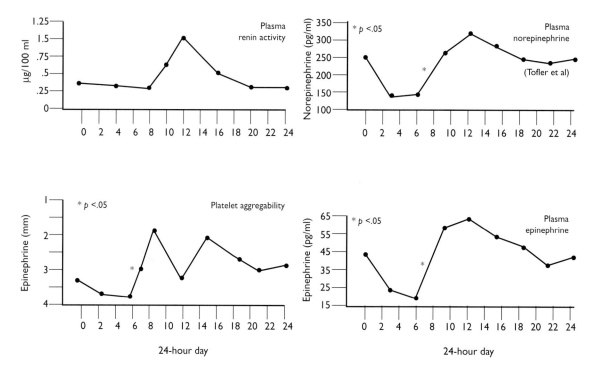

Figure 14.3 Circadian variation in plasma renin activity, plasma norepinephrine and epinephrine levels, and platelet aggregability. (Adapted from Quyyumi.[26])

Factors determining coronary blood flow

Clearly the major limitation to myocardial oxygen supply that results in ischemia in patients with coronary artery disease is determined by the degree of coronary stenosis and the state of the collateral circulation which together determine the magnitude or ease with which ischemia will develop. There is much clinical and experimental evidence which favors the role of vasomotion causing changes in the caliber of the coronary arteries thus resulting in variability in the ischemic threshold.

Clinical observations have provided important evidence in favor of changes in vasomotor tone. For example, psychologic stress and exposure to cold are frequent environmental triggers for precipitation of myocardial ischemia. Hypoperfusion during mental stress, demonstrated by positron emission tomography, is identical to the defects produced by exercise.[20] Wall motion abnormalities occur during a mentally challenging speech test at a considerably lower rate–pressure product than that achieved during physical exercise; these episodes of ischemia are more frequently silent than painful.[21] Finally, exercise in the cold significantly reduces ischemic threshold.

Variations in the heart rate ischemic threshold were confirmed during ambulatory ST-segment monitoring. For example, in some patients, ischemia occurs not only during physical activities, but also during less challenging circumstances such as eating, sleeping, or during mental stress. Analysis of heart rate changes before the onset of ischemic episodes shows that approximately 15% of episodes are not preceded by any appreciable increase in heart rate.[12,14,16,22] A possible explanation for these findings is that alterations in the caliber of coronary arteries, particularly at the site of coronary narrowing, may transiently lower coronary blood flow to such an extent that myocardial ischemia occurs with little or no change in myocardial oxygen demand.

SYSTEMIC FACTORS IN PRECIPITATING ISCHEMIA

There are several systemic and local mediators of coronary and peripheral vasomotion, some of which have a circadian variation similar to that of ischemic events (Fig. 14.3). For example, catecholamine levels surge in the morning hours resulting in dramatic increases in norepinephrine and epinephrine.[11] Alpha-adrenergic receptor stimulation with consequent increases in coronary vascular tone may therefore contribute to the morning increase phenomenon. Another powerful endogenous vasoconstrictor, the renin-angiotensin system, is activated in the morning hours.[23] Whether this merely constitutes an increase in plasma renin activity or a simultaneous activation of the tissue renin-angiotensin system is not known. Both these vasoconstrictor mechanisms appear to be triggered by assumption of upright posture and exercise.[24] Moreover, a morning increase in plasma cortisol acts synergistically with catecholamines in altering vasomotor tone.[25] Thus, vascular tone may be increased in the morning hours, especially after arousal and assumption of upright posture as a result of increases in systemic noradrenergic and renin activities.[26]

It is also well known that platelet activation occurs in the morning hours, an event that appears to be particularly related to assumption of upright posture and exercise.[24] This activation may be a much more important trigger for thrombotic coronary events than it is for myocardial ischemia. It has, however, been speculated that platelet activation and aggregation on atherosclerotic plaques can increase local levels of constrictors such as thromboxane and contribute to vasoconstriction of the plaque. Against this is evidence indicating that no systemic activation of platelet surface receptors (indicative of in vivo aggregation) occurs on standing and with mild exercise. Furthermore, there was no systemic increase in platelet activity during ambulatory episodes of myocardial ischemia.[27]

CIRCADIAN VARIATION IN VASOCONSTRICTOR TONE

To investigate the possibility that the morning increase in myocardial ischemia is due not only to an increase in demand at that time, but also to an increase in coronary vasoconstrictor tone, patients were exercised four times during the day and the heart rate at onset of ST-segment depression (ischemic threshold) was measured.[28] The ischemic threshold, or the ease with which myocardial ischemia developed, was lower in the morning and at night compared with other times of the day, a change that paralleled the simultaneous circadian variation in postischemic forearm vascular resistance. These findings suggest that there is a circadian variation in coronary vascular resistance such that it is lower in the early morning and at night compared with other times of the day, and that this change in resistance is likely to be generalized and is likely to affect other vascular beds.

Other studies also support the concept of an elevated coronary vascular resistance in the night and early morning compared with other times of the day. Thus, heart rate at onset of spontaneously occurring episodes of ischemia during ambulatory monitoring is significantly lower at night than the heart rate at onset of ischemia during the day (Fig. 14.1).[9,29] Cardiac pacing during ischemia in patients with rest angina produced similar results.[30] Angiography demonstrated narrower coronary arteries in the morning (7 a.m.) in patients with normal coronary arteries than later in the day.[31] In dogs, coronary blood flow was significantly greater in the afternoon than in the morning.[32] Together, these studies support the concept that the coronary vasculature is responsive to vasomotor influences, and that the constrictor tone predominates at night and in the early morning hours compared with the rest of the day.

There is accumulating evidence to suggest that microvascular coronary tone is also abnormal during stress in patients with atherosclerosis. For example, patients with coronary atherosclerosis without a critical narrowing of the epicardial coronary artery, or those exposed to risk factors for atherosclerosis,[33,34] appear to have depressed coronary vasodilatation in response to mental stress, cold-pressor test, or cardiac pacing, suggesting impairment of microvascular vasodilatation during stress.[33–35]

The contribution of systemic vasoconstrictors, especially the activation of the sympathetic nervous system has been studied.[36,37] Norepinephrine-induced constriction through activation of α-1 and α-2 adrenoceptors in the human coronary circulation has been demonstrated during exercise, cold-pressor, and mental stresses. Exercise-induced ST-segment depression was ameliorated by intracoronary phentolamine,[38] and in atherosclerotic patients, mental-stress-induced increases in coronary vascular resistance, suggesting microvascular constriction, were also reversed by intracoronary phentolamine.[39]

To investigate whether the circadian pattern of change in coronary and systemic vascular resistance is also determined by changes in alpha-adrenergic sympathetic tone, the effect of phentolamine on the circadian variation of forearm vascular resistance, previously shown to be higher in the early morning hours compared with later times of the day, was investigated.[40] Phentolamine produced a greater reduction in forearm vascular resistance during the morning hours compared with other times of the day, leading to abolition of the circadian variation in vascular resistance. In contrast, sodium nitroprusside, that also reduced forearm vascular resistance, did so equally at all times of the day. These observations may have immense therapeutic implications. Although there appears to be no convincing evidence that alpha-adrenergic blockade is of therapeutic benefit in patients

with variant angina in whom alterations in coronary vasomotor tone are severe,[41–44] increase in exercise capacity has been reported in patients with stable coronary artery disease with an α-1 adrenergic antagonist, indoramin.[45] Whether α-1 blockade will be helpful in attenuating the morning increase in vascular resistance, and thus the surge in ischemic activity, needs to be investigated.

Proposed mechanisms for circadian variation in transient ischemia

Based on these findings, Fig. 14.4 illustrates potential mechanisms at play in the genesis of transient myocardial ischemia in patients with stable coronary artery disease.[9] The ischemic threshold reaches a lower level at night when compared with the day, as a result of the circadian variation in coronary vasomotor tone which is increased at night. The mean basal hourly heart rate also has a very similar circadian variation, with a trough at night, and thus the *relative* increase in heart rate required to produce ischemia is similar at night compared

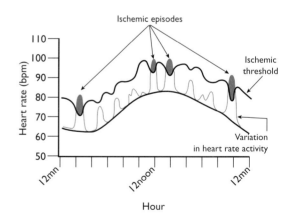

Figure 14.4 Proposed pattern and mechanisms of ischemia, showing circadian variation in basal heart rate, heart rate at onset of ischemia (ischemic threshold) and transient ischemic activity during both nocturnal and daytime hours. (Adapted from Mulcahy et al.[9])

with all other times of the day, despite the fact that the heart rate at which ischemia occurs is lower at night. This underscores the importance of heart rate increases in the genesis of ischemia throughout the 24-hour period, even allowing for variations in coronary tone. Furthermore, every time there is increase in myocardial work, there is paradoxical vasoconstriction of the stenosis leading to a transient decrease in ischemic threshold. It appears, therefore, that both vasoconstriction of stenotic coronary arteries, leading to dramatic increases in coronary vascular resistance, and increases in myocardial oxygen demand, occur simultaneously during physical exercise, or during emotional and environmental stresses. It is also clear from the ambulatory monitoring data, which shows considerable variation in heart rate threshold during different ischemic episodes, that the variation in vasomotor tone does indeed influence the ease with which myocardial ischemic episodes, silent or with angina, occur at different times in the same individual.

Local factors and coronary vasomotion

The concept that atherosclerotic coronary arteries which exhibit severe encroachment of the lumen by fibrotic, often calcified, atherosclerotic material[46,47] are incapable of vasomotion was overturned by data demonstrating significant capacity of these segments for alterations in size in response to a variety of physiologic and pharmacologic stimuli. Brown and colleagues[47,48] studied epicardial coronary artery diameter changes of atherosclerotic segments at rest and after hand-grip exercise. Despite a 20% increase in heart rate, a 24% increase in blood pressure, and a 66% increase in coronary blood flow during hand-grip exercise, there was 15–22% narrowing of angiographically 'normal'-appearing segments and 5–33% narrowing of stenosed segments. Additionally, paradoxic vasoconstriction in atherosclerotic coronary arteries has been demonstrated during physical exercise, mental stress, and cold-pressor test,[35,49–52] whereas patients with normal coronary arteries, in

contrast, vasodilate epicardial coronary arteries during these stimuli.

VASCULAR BIOLOGY OF CORONARY ARTERY VASOMOTION

Recent years have seen development in our understanding of why exercise-induced vasoconstriction or 'collapse' of atherosclerotic coronary arteries occurs. Hydrodynamic principles described by Bernouille state that the pressure across a significantly narrowed lesion falls due to turbulence, and when this occurs in the setting of a compliant lesion it may lead to its partial collapse. Nevertheless, it is now clear that other, locally active factors may contribute substantially to this vasoconstriction, and the contributory role of the vascular endothelium to these phenomena is described below.

Endothelium and coronary vasomotion

In the cardiovascular system, the endothelium is involved in the regulation of lipids, transport and permeability of solutes and fluids, participation in immune and inflammatory responses, and control of cell growth and proliferation.[53–55] Here, the endothelial control of vascular smooth muscle tone and in platelet function will be discussed.

The endothelium regulates tone and platelet aggregation by releasing a variety of constricting and dilating substances (Fig. 14.5). Constricting factors include arachidonic acid metabolites such as thromboxane A2, endoperoxidase, and a potent 21-amino acid peptide called endothelin (Fig. 14.6).[56] The endothelium also converts angiotensin-I to angiotensin-II by the membrane-bound angiotensin converting enzyme, that also metabolizes the endogenous endothelium-dependent vasodilator, bradykinin.[57] Dilators from the endothelium include endothelium-derived relaxing factors (EDRE) (nitric oxide and endothelium-derived hyperpolarizing factor) and prostacyclin (PGI_2).[58]

The role of constricting factors in the control of coronary vasomotor tone, their circadian variation, and their influence during physiologic stresses is poorly understood. Nitric oxide

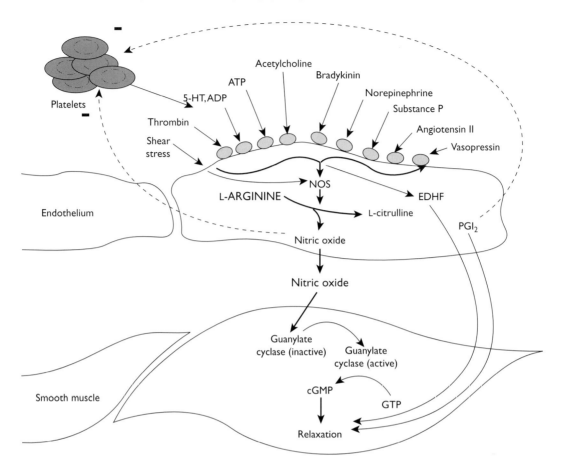

Figure 14.5 Factors causing endothelium-dependent vasodilatation. A variety of exogenous pharmacologic probes, platelet-derived factors, and shear stress can promote release of nitric oxide by stimulating nitric oxide synthase (NOS). Some of these factors also release endothelium-derived hyperpolarizing factor (EDHF). Nitric oxide leads to relaxation by cyclic GMP (guanylate monophosphate)-dependent mechanism. Prostacyclin (PGI_2) causes relaxation of vascular smooth muscle cell by a cyclic AMP-dependent mechanism and both nitric oxide and PGI_2 inhibit platelet aggregation. (5-HT: serotonin; ADP; adenosine diphosphate; AMP (adenosine monophosphate) ATP: adenosine triphosphate; GTP: guanosine triphosphate.)

(NO), the most important and ubiquitous endothelium-derived relaxing factor, is tonically produced in picomole quantities by the endothelium from L-arginine by the action of a constitutive calcium and calmodulin-dependent enzyme, nitric oxide synthase.[53-55] NO is rapidly oxidized and inactivated by oxygen-free radicals, an event that appears to be important in genesis of endothelial dysfunc-tion. Several pharmacologic and physiologic factors promote release of NO. These include acetylcholine, substance P, bradykinin, adeno-sine diphosphate (ADP), adenosine triphos-phate (ATP), thrombin, serotonin, and histamine. Tonically produced NO can be enhanced by physiologic events that stimulate NO production including increasing shear stress and aggregating platelets.[58-60] Other than

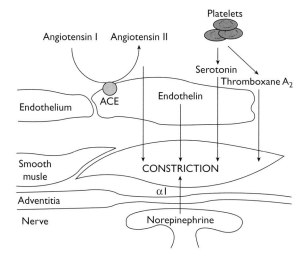

Figure 14.6 Endothelium-dependent and platelet-derived factors causing smooth muscle constriction. (ACE: angiotensin converting enzyme.)

its smooth-muscle dilating action, NO also inhibits platelet aggregation (antithrombotic) and inhibits cell proliferation (antiatherosclerotic).

In normal blood vessels, there exists a balance between shear-stress-induced, endothelium-dependent relaxation and pressure or stretch-induced contraction (myogenic contraction), such that shear stress leads to myogenic contraction that is offset by endothelium-dependent relaxation due to release of NO and other EDRFs. In patients with endothelial dysfunction (see below) the myogenic vasoconstriction would remain unopposed because of the deficient shear-stress-induced release of EDRF, leading to constriction. Thus, in the morning hours, when vascular shear stress is increased because of surges in blood pressure and heart rate, atherosclerotic vessels constrict, causing reduction in myocardial blood flow, and consequent exacerbation of ischemia.

The term endothelial dysfunction refers to an imbalance between relaxing and contracting factors, between pro- and anticoagulant mediators, or between growth-inhibiting and growth-promoting factors. It may not be pathologically visible but represents a biochemical and functional abnormality or injury. Endothelial function appears to be impaired in patients with a variety of cardiovascular risk factors.[61–65] Cholesterol-fed animal models have depressed endothelial NO production, observations that have been confirmed in human hypercholesterolemia.[66–68] Acetylcholine causes endothelium-dependent epicardial vessel dilatation in normal smooth coronary arteries but produces constriction in patients with hypercholesterolemia or atherosclerosis. Vasodilatation with acetylcholine is also depressed in hypertension, especially in patients with left ventricular hypertrophy.[65,69] Diabetes and heart failure are also accompanied by depressed endothelium-dependent vasodilatation.[70] Exposure to multiple risk factors for coronary artery disease such as hypercholesterolemia, hypertension, diabetes, age, and smoking can compound the injury to the endothelium.[61,64,71,72]

The author's studies have also clarified the link between endothelial dysfunction of the coronary vessels and reduced vasodilatation in response to physiologic stress. Patients with reduced coronary vasodilatation in response to acetylcholine also had depressed dilatation in response to atrial pacing.[73] In a subsequent study, it was also demonstrated that NO contributes to pacing-induced coronary vasodilatation, a contribution that is reduced in patients with risk factors for atherosclerosis,[74] indicating that there is impaired pharmacologic and physiologic activity of NO in these patients. Patients with risk factors and endothelial dysfunction failed to dilate their epicardial coronary arteries in response to pacing whereas those without risk factors dilated epicardial coronary arteries in response to pacing as well as with acetylcholine. Similar responses have been reported with several other physiologic stimuli such as exercise, mental stress, cold, and increased flow.[35,51,52,75] These stimuli cause epicardial vessel vasodilatation in patients with angiographically smooth, normal coronary arteries. However, in patients with atherosclerosis and in segments with angiographic irregularities, these same stimuli lead to vasoconstriction. These studies further demonstrate that segments which constrict in response to physiologic stimuli also constrict in response to acetylcholine, whereas normal smooth segments of coronary arteries that dilate during physiologic stimulation also dilate in response to acetylcholine. Thus, there is a strong correlation between endothelium-dependent and physiologic vasomotion in human coronary vessels.

Over the long term, reduced activity of NO in the vascular wall may promote the atherogenic process.[76–78] Animals on atherogenic diets and L-NMMA Nmonomethyl-L-argiunine) (which inhibits endothelial production of NO) had more rapid development of intimal thickening than those fed high-cholesterol diet alone, suggesting that endothelium-derived NO prevents the development and progression of atherosclerosis.

THERAPEUTIC IMPLICATIONS

Studies in patients with myocardial infarction have demonstrated that patients who were on beta-adrenergic antagonists had an absence of the peak in myocardial infarction episodes in the morning hours.[79] A similar blunting of the morning peak in myocardial infarction was observed in patients treated with aspirin. However, patients on calcium antagonists did not have abolition of the morning increase in myocardial infarction frequency.[79] The protective value of beta-blockers in reducing mortality and reinfarction after myocardial infarction has been well established.[80,81] Whether the observed abolition of the morning increase in first myocardial infarction with beta-receptor antagonists is representative of a true decrease in frequency of myocardial infarction remains to be proven. Similarly, whether the observed similarity between transient myocardial ischemia on the one hand and of myocardial infarction and sudden cardiac death on the other implies a direct causal relationship between transient ischemia and acute coronary events, that is, that ischemia acts as a trigger for thrombotic coronary events, is far from proven.

LINK BETWEEN ISCHEMIA AND ACUTE THROMBOTIC EVENTS

It must be appreciated that thrombotic coronary events such as unstable angina, myocardial infarction, and sudden cardiac death usually result from plaque disruption or rupture with superimposed thrombosis.[82,83] This usually occurs at the site of an insignificant coronary lesion and, rarely, at the site of a severe coronary lesion, whereas the latter severe lesion is often responsible for myocardial ischemia.[84] Thus, the location of the lesion producing ischemia is often different from that of the lesion that causes a subsequent acute coronary event, and therefore it is unlikely that transient myocardial ischemia predisposes to acute coronary events. Although patients known to have transient myocardial ischemia and underlying severe coronary artery disease may have a higher incidence of acute coronary events, transient ischemia appears not to be the cause of these events but is merely a marker of underlying severe coronary artery disease.

Conventional drug therapy

Several antianginal agents have been investigated for their effects on the circadian variation in transient ischemia. Beta-adrenergic receptor antagonists are able to abolish efficiently the morning increase in transient myocardial ischemia, a finding that has been uniformly observed with most agents without intrinsic sympathomimetic activity.[1] Short-acting dihydropyridine calcium antagonists (nifedipine) failed to abolish the morning increase in transient ischemia; however, there was blunting of the morning increase with diltiazem, long-acting nifedipine, and with verapamil.[85–87]

Recognition of the circadian nature of transient myocardial ischemia emphasizes the importance of 24-hour protection in patients with long-acting antianginal agents. It appears that agents which exercise chronotropic control are likely to be the most effective in attenuating myocardial ischemia. Trials using antianginal medications should therefore emphasize the timing of drug administration. This is particularly important when considering that most patients with coronary artery disease observe a nitrate-free interval at night. Patients on monotherapy with nitrates may be unprotected in the morning hours after arousal and assumption of upright posture, a time when ischemic activity increases dramatically, if they have not been protected with a short-acting nitrate beforehand.

Drugs to improve vascular function

There are potential therapeutic avenues for treating endothelial dysfunction that may stabilize the vessel wall in atherosclerotic patients and thus reduce the incidence of future thrombotic coronary events in this population. These approaches include use of tissue plasminogen activator (tPA), stable analogs of prostacyclin, and nitric oxide donors[88,89] such as nitroglycerin or nitroprusside that yield NO directly in smooth muscles or in the platelets. There is increasing evidence that L-arginine, the substrate for endothelial NO synthesis can reverse the abnormal endothelium-dependent responses in hypercholesterolemia,[90,91] heart failure, and atherosclerosis.[92,93] Angiotensin converting enzyme inhibitors that antagonize vascular constriction by angiotensin-II and increase bradykinin-dependent, endothelium-mediated relaxation have recently been demonstrated to reduce thrombotic events in patients with coronary artery disease and left ventricular dysfunction. They have also been shown to improve acetylcholine responses in the atherosclerotic coronary arteries.[94]

Increased oxidant stress in the vessel wall may be responsible for the reduced activity of NO in certain pathologic conditions.[95] Antioxidants such as superoxide dismutase,

oxypurinol, and vitamin E are being investigated as potential ways of reversing the endothelial dysfunction.

Finally, cholesterol-lowering agents, known to reduce mortality in patients with hypercholesterolemia and atherosclerosis dramatically, also improve endothelial dysfunction.[96] Plaque stabilization may be an important explanation for their beneficial effects, because the degree of regression in atherosclerotic lesions is negligible.

Thus, understanding the physiology and pathophysiologic role of the vascular endothelium as a modulator of smooth-muscle vasomotion, intravascular thrombosis, and intimal growth, will greatly enhance future possibilities for treatment of the atherosclerotic process, and its effects on vascular function.

CONCLUSION

With dramatic advances in our understanding of the pathophysiology of coronary artery disease ranging from the cellular to the clinical level, we can now advance the concept of myocardial ischemia from the simple 'demand versus supply' equation to a more complex interplay of local and systemic factors. These interactions result in a combination of coronary vasoconstriction and increase in myocardial oxygen demand when the patient is subjected to physical or psychological stress, and the degree to which each of these compromises blood delivery to the myocardium varies and is responsible for the observed variability. Further, the understanding of vascular biology of the vessel wall allows us to treat patients with myocardial ischemia, whether silent or accompanied by pain, both with conventional ischemia-reducing drugs and other agents that improve endothelial function, stabilize plaque, and reduce the incidence of sudden cardiac events.

REFERENCES

1. Mulcahy D, Keegan J, Cunningham D et al. Circadian variation of total ischaemic burden and its alteration with antianginal agents. *Lancet* 1988; **ii**: 755–9.
2. Quyyumi AA, Mockus L, Wright C, Fox KM. Morphology of ambulatory ST-segment changes in patients with varying severity of coronary artery disease: investigation of the frequency of nocturnal ischaemia and coronary spasm. *Br Heart J* 1985; **53**: 186–93.
3. Millar-Craig MW, Bishop CN, Raftery EB. Circadian variation of blood pressure. *Lancet* 1978; **i**: 795–7.
4. Raeder EA, Hohnloser SH, Graboys TB, Podrid P, Lampert S, Lown B. Spontaneous variability and circadian distribution of ectopic activity in patients with malignant ventricular arrhythmia. *J Am Coll Cardiol* 1988; **12**: 656–61.
5. Lampert R, Rosenfeld L, Batsford W, Lee F, McPherson C. Circadian variation of sustained ventricular tachycardia in patients with coronary artery disease and implantable cardioverter defibrillators. *Circulation* 1994; **90**: 241–7.
6. Muller JE, Ludmer PL, Willich SN et al. Circadian variation in the frequency of sudden cardiac death. *Circulation* 1987; **75**: 131–8.
7. Muller JE, Stone PH, Turi ZG et al. Circadian variation in the frequency of onset of acute myocardial infarction. *N Engl J Med* 1985; **313**: 1315–22.
8. Rocco MB, Barry J, Campbell S et al. Circadian variation of transient myocardial ischemia in patients with coronary artery disease. *Circulation* 1987; **75**: 395–400.
9. Mulcahy D, Dakak N, Zalos G et al. Patterns and underlying mechanisms of transient myocardial ischemia in stable coronary artery disease are the same in both sexes: a comparative study. *J Am Coll Cardiol* 1996; **27**: 1629–36.
10. Hjalmarson A, Gilpin EA, Nicod P et al. Differing circadian patterns of symptom onset in subgroups of patients with acute myocardial infarction. *Circulation* 1989; **80**: 267–75.
11. Turton MB, Deegan T. Circadian variations of plasma catecholamine, cortisol, and immunoreactive insulin concentrations in supine subjects. *Clin Chim Acta* 1974; **55**: 389–97.
12. Panza JA, Diodati JG, Callahan TS, Epstein SE, Quyyumi AA. Role of increases in heart rate in determining the occurrence and frequency of myocardial ischemia during daily life in patients with stable coronary artery disease. *J Am Coll Cardiol* 1992; **20**: 1092–8.
13. Deedwania PC, Nelson JR. Pathophysiology of silent myocardial ischemia during daily life: hemodynamic evaluation by simultaneous electrocardiographic and blood pressure monitoring. *Circulation* 1990; **82**: 1296–304.
14. McLenachan JM, Weidinger FF, Barry J et al. Relations between heart rate, ischemia, and drug therapy during daily life in patients with coronary artery disease. *Circulation* 1991; **83**: 1263–70.
15. Quyyumi AA, Wright C, Mockus LJ, Fox KM. Mechanisms of nocturnal angina pectoris: importance of increased myocardial oxygen demand in patients with severe coronary artery disease. *Lancet* 1984; **ii**: 1207–9.
16. Andrews TC, Fenton T, Toyosaki N et al. Subsets of ambulatory myocardial ischemia based on heart rate activity: circadian distribution and response to anti-ischemic medications. *Circulation* 1993; **88**: 92–100.
17. Quyyumi AA, Efthimiou J, Quyyumi A, Mockus LM, Spiro SG, Fox KM. Nocturnal angina: precipitating factors in patients with coronary artery disease and those with variant angina. *Br Heart J* 1986; **56**: 346–52.
18. Rehman A, Zalos G, Andreus NP, Mulcahy D, Quyyumi AA. Blood pressure changes during transient myocardial ischemia: insights into mechanisms. *J Am Coll Cardiol* (in press).
19. Parker JD, Testa MA, Jimenez AH et al. Morning increase in ambulatory ischemia in patients with stable coronary artery disease. Importance of physical activity and increased cardiac demand. *Circulation* 1994; **89**: 604–14.
20. Deanfield JE, Selwyn AP, Chierchia S et al. Myocardial ischaemia during daily life in patients with stable angina: its relation to symptoms and heart rate changes. *Lancet* 1983; **i**: 753–8.
21. Rozanski A, Bairey N, Krantz DS et al. Mental stress and induction of silent myocardial ischemia in patients with coronary artery disease. *N Engl J Med* 1988; **318**: 1005–12.
22. Mulcahy D, Keegan J, Fox KM. Characteristics of silent and painful ischaemia during ambulatory monitoring in patients with coronary arterial disease. *Int J Cardiol* 1990; **28**: 377–9.
23. Gordon RD, Wolfe LK, Island DP, Liddle GW. A diurnal rhythm in plasma renin activity in man. *J Clin Invest* 1966; **45**: 1587–92.

24. Brezinski DA, Tofler GH, Muller JE et al. Morning increase in platelet aggregability: association with assumption of the upright posture. *Circulation* 1988; **78**: 35–40.

25. Weitzman ED, Fukushima D, Nogeire C, Roffwarg H, Gallagher TF, Hellman L. Twenty-four hour pattern of the episodic secretion of cortisol in normal subjects. *J Clin Endocrinol Metab* 1971; **33**: 14–22.

26. Quyyumi AA. Circadian rhythms in cardiovascular disease. *Am Heart J* 1990; **120**: 726–33.

27. Andrews NP, Gralnick H, Quyyumi AA. Mechanisms underlying the morning increase in platelet aggregation: a flow cytometry study. *J Am Coll Cardiol* 1996; **28**: 1789–95.

28. Quyyumi AA, Panza JA, Diodati JG, Lakatos E, Epstein SE. Circadian variation in ischemic threshold. A mechanism underlying the circadian variation in ischemic events. *Circulation* 1992; **86**: 22–8.

29. Benhorin J, Banai S, Moriel M, Gavish A, Keren A, Stern S, Tzivoni D. Circadian variation in ischemic threshold and their relation to the occurrence of ischemic episodes. *Circulation* 1993; **87**: 808–14.

30. Figueras J, Cinca J, Balda F, Moya A, Rius J. Resting angina with fixed coronary artery stenosis: nocturnal decline in ischemic threshold. *Circulation* 1986; **74**: 1248–54.

31. Yasue H, Omote S, Takizawaw A, Nagao M, Miwa K, Tanaka S. Circadian variation of exercise capacity in patients with Prinzmetal's variant angina: role of exercise-induced coronary arterial spasm. *Circulation* 1979; **59**: 938–48.

32. Fugita M, Franklin D. Diurnal changes in coronary blood flow in conscious dogs. *Circulation* 1987; **76**: 488–91.

33. Seiler C, Hess OM, Buechi M, Suter TM, Krayenbuehl HP. Influence of serum cholesterol and other coronary risk factors on vasomotion of angiographically normal coronary arteries. *Circulation* 1993; **88**: 2139–48.

34. Zeiher AM, Schächinger V, Hohnloser SH, Saurbier B, Just H. Coronary atherosclerotic wall thickening and vascular reactivity in humans. *Circulation* 1994; **89**: 2525–32.

35. Gordon JB, Ganz P, Nabel EG et al. Atherosclerosis influences the vasomotor response of epicardial coronary arteries to exercise. *J Clin Invest* 1989; **83**: 1946–52.

36. Heusch G. α-Adrenergic mechanisms in myocardial ischemia. *Circulation* 1990; **81**: 1–13.

37. Mudge GH, Grossman W, Mills RM Jr, Lesch M, Braunwald E. Reflex increase in coronary vascular resistance in patients with ischemic heart disease. *N Engl J Med* 1976; **295**: 1333–7.

38. Berkenboom GM, Abramowicz M, Vandermoten P, Degre SG. Role of alpha-adrenergic coronary tone in exercise-induced angina pectoris. *Am J Cardiol* 1986; **57**: 195–8.

39. Dakak N, Quyyumi AA, Eisenhoffer G, Goldstein DS, Cannon RO III. Sympathetically-mediated effects of mental stress on cardiac microcirculation of patients with coronary artery disease. *Am J Cardiol* 1995; **76**: 125–30.

40. Panza JA, Epstein SE, Quyyumi AA. Circadian variation in vascular tone and its relation to alpha sympathetic vasoconstrictor activity. *N Engl J Med* 1991; **325**: 986–90.

41. Yasue H, Touyama M, Kato H, Tanaka S, Akiyama F. Prinzmetal's variant form of angina as a manifestation of alpha-adrenergic receptor-mediated coronary artery spasm: documentation of coronary arteriography. *Am Heart J* 1976; **91**: 148–55.

42. Tzivoni D, Keren A, Benhorin J, Gottlieb S, Atlas D, Stern S. Prazosin therapy for refractory variant angina. *Am Heart J* 1983; **105**: 252–66.

43. Robertson RM, Bernard YD, Carr RK, Robertson D. Alpha-adrenergic blockade in vasotonic angina: lack of efficacy of specific alpha1-receptor blockade with prazosin. *J Am Coll Cardiol* 1983; **2**: 1146–50.

44. Chierchia S, Davies G, Berkenboom G, Crea F, Crean P, Mersi A. α-Adrenergic receptors and coronary spasm: an elusive link. *Circulation* 1984; **69**: 8–14.

45. Collins P, Sheridan D. Improvement in angina pectoris with alpha adrenoceptor blockade. *Br Heart J* 1985; **53**: 488–92.

46. Quyyumi AA, Al-Rufaie H, Olsen EGJ, Fox KM. Coronary anatomy in patients with varying manifestations of three vessel coronary artery disease. *Br Heart J* 1985; **54**: 362–6.

47. Brown BG. Coronary vasospasm: observations linking the clinical spectrum of ischemic heart disease to the dynamic pathology of coronary athero-sclerosis. *Arch Intern Med* 1981; **141**: 716–22.

48. Brown BG, Lee AB, Bolson EL, Dodge HT. Reflex constriction of significant coronary stenosis as a mechanism contributing to ischemic left ventricular dysfunction during isometric exercise. *Circulation* 1984; **70**: 18–24.

49. Nabel EG, Selwyn AP, Ganz P. Paradoxical narrowing of atherosclerotic coronary arteries induced by increases in heart rate. *Circulation* 1990; **81**: 850–9.

50. Nabel EG, Ganz P, Gordon JB, Alexander RW, Selwyn AP. Dilation of normal and constriction of atherosclerotic coronary arteries caused by the cold pressor test. *Circulation* 1988; **77**: 43–52.

51. Yeung AC, Vekshtein VI, Krantz DS et al. The effect of atherosclerosis on the vasomotor response of coronary arteries to mental stress. *N Engl J Med* 1991; **325**: 1551–6.

52. Gage JE, Hess OM, Murakami T, Ritter M, Gramm J, Krayenbuehl HP. Vasoconstriction of stenotic coronary arteries during dynamic exercise in patients with classic angina pectoris: reversibility by nitroglycerin. *Circulation* 1986; **73**: 865–76.

53. Furchgott RF, Zawadski JV. The obligatory role of endothelial cells in the relaxation of arterial smooth muscle by acetylcholine. *Nature* 1980; **288**: 373–6.

54. Snyder SH, Bredt DS. Biological roles of nitric oxide. *Sci Am* 1992; **266**: 68–71, 74–7.

55. Moncada S, Higgs A. The L-arginine-nitric oxide pathway. *N Engl J Med* 1993; **329**: 2002–12.

56. Yanagisawa M, Kurhara H, Kimura S et al. A novel potent vasoconstrictor peptide produced by vascular endothelial cells. *Nature* 1988; **332**: 411–15.

57. Dzau VJ. Vascular wall renin angiotensin pathway in control of the circulation. *Am J Med* 1984; **77**: 31–6.

58. Vanhoutte PM, Shimokawa H. Endothelium-derived relaxing factor and coronary vasospasm. *Circulation* 1989; **80**: 1–9.

59. Holtz J, Forstermann U, Pohl U, Giesler M, Bassenge E. Flow-dependent, endothelium-mediated dilatation of epicardial coronary arteries in conscious dogs: effects of cyclooxygenase inhibition. *J Cardiovasc Pharmacol* 1984; **6**: 1161–9.

60. Rubanyi GM, Romero JC, Vanhoutte PM. Flow-induced release of endothelium-derived relaxing factor. *Am J Physiol* 1986; **250**: H1145–9.

61. Vita JA, Treasure CB, Nabel EG et al. Coronary vasomotor response to acetylcholine relates to risk factors for coronary artery disease. *Circulation* 1990; **81**: 494–7.

62. Casino PR, Kilcoyne CM, Quyyumi AA, Hoeg JM, Epstein SE, Panza JA. Role of nitric oxide in the endothelium-dependent vasodilation of hypercholesterolemic patients. *Circulation* 1992; **86**: I-618.

63. Creager MA, Cooke JP, Mendelsohn ME et al. Impaired vasodilation of forearm resistance vessels in hypercholesterolemic humans. *J Clin Invest* 1990; **86**: 228–34.

64. Quyyumi AA, Dakak N, Andrews NP et al. Nitric oxide activity in the human coronary circulation: impact of risk factors for coronary atherosclerosis. *J Clin Invest* 1995; **95**: 1747–55.

65. Quyyumi AA, Mulcahy D, Andrews NP, Husain S, Panza JA, Cannon RO III. Coronary vascular nitric oxide activity in hypertension and hypercholesterolemia: comparison of acetylcholine and substance P. *Circulation* 1997 **95**: 104–10.

66. Takahasi M, Yui Y, Yasumoto H et al. Lipoproteins are inhibitors of endothelium-dependent relaxation of rabbit aorta. *Am J Physiol* 1990; **258** (*Heart Circ Physiol* 27): H1–H8.

67. Bossaller C, Yamamoto H, Lichtlen PR, Henry PD. Impaired cholinergic vasodilation in the cholesterol-fed rabbit in vivo. *Basic Res Cardiol* 1987; **82**: 396–404.

68. Osborne JA, Siegman MJ, Sedar AW, Mooers SU, Lefer AM. Lack of endothelium-dependent relaxation in coronary resistance arteries of cholesterol-fed rabbits. *Am J Physiol* 1989; **256**: C591–C597.

69. Treasure CB, Klein JL, Vita JA et al. Hypertension and left ventricular hypertrophy are associated with impaired endothelium-mediated relaxation in human coronary resistance vessels. *Circulation* 1993; **87**: 86–93.

70. Katz SD, Schwarz M, Yuen J, LeJemtel TH. Impaired acetylcholine-mediated vasodilation in patients with congestive heart failure. *Circulation* 1993; **88**: 55–61.

71. Williams SB, Cusco JA, Roddy M, Johnstone MT, Creager MA. Impaired nitric oxide-mediated vasodilation in patients with non-insulin-dependent diabetes mellitus. *J Am Coll Cardiol* 1996; **27**: 567–74.

72. Egashira K, Inou T, Hirooka Y et al. Effects of age on endothelium-dependent vasodilation of resistance coronary artery by acetylcholine in humans. *Circulation* 1993; **88**: 77–81.

73. Quyyumi AA, Cannon RO, Panza JA, Diodati JG, Epstein SE. Endothelial dysfunction in patients with chest pain and normal coronary arteries. *Circulation* 1992; **86**: 1864–71.

74. Quyyumi AA, Dakak N, Andrews NP, Gilligan DM, Panza JA, Cannon RO III. Contribution of nitric oxide to metabolic vasodilation in the human heart. *Circulation* 1995; **92**: 320–6.

75. Cox DA, Vita JA, Treasure CB et al. Atherosclerosis impairs flow-mediated dilatation of coronary arteries in humans. *Circulation* 1989; **80**: 458–65.

76. Garg UC, Hassid A. Nitric oxide-generating vasodilators and 8-bromo-cyclic guanosine monophosphate inhibit mitogenesis and proliferation of cultured rat vascular smooth muscle cells. *J Clin Invest* 1989; **83**: 1774–7.

77. Cayatte AJ, Palacino JJ, Horten K, Cohen RA. Chronic inhibition of nitric oxide production accelerates neointima formation and impairs endothelial function in hypercholesterolemic rabbits. *Arterioscler Thromb* 1994; **14**: 753–9.

78. Naruse K, Shimizu M, Muramatsu M et al. Long-term inhibition of NO synthesis promotes atherosclerosis in the hypercholesterolemic rabbit thoracic aorta. *Arterioscler Thromb* 1994; **14**: 746–52.

79. Willich SN, Linderer T, Wegscheider K, Leizorowicz A, Alamercery I, Schroder R. Increased morning incidence of myocardial infarction in the ISAM study: absence with prior beta-adrenergic blockade. *Circulation* 1989; **80**: 853–8.

80. The Norwegian Multicenter Study Group. Trimolol-induced reduction in mortality and re-infarction in patients surviving acute myocardial infarction. *N Engl J Med* 1981; **304**: 801–7.

81. Yusuf S, Peto R, Lewis J et al. Beta blockade during and after myocardial infarction: an overview of the randomized trials. *Prog Cardiovasc Dis* 1985; **27**: 335–71.

82. DeWood MA, Spores J, Notske R et al. Prevalence of total coronary occlusion during the early hours of transmural myocardial infarction. *N Engl J Med* 1980; **303**: 897–902.

83. Davies MJ, Thomas AC. Thrombosis and acute coronary-artery lesions in sudden cardiac ischemic death. *N Engl J Med* 1984; **310**: 1137–40.

84. Little WC, Constatinescu MS, Applegate RJ et al. Can coronary angiography predict the site of subsequent myocardial infarction in patients with mild-to-moderate coronary artery disease? *Circulation* 1988; **78**: 1157–66.

85. Quyyumi AA, Crake T, Wright CM, Mockus LJ, Fox KM. Medical treatment of patients with severe exertional and rest angina: double-blind comparison of B blocker, calcium antagonist, and nitrate. *Br Heart J* 1987; **57**: 505–11.

86. Parmley WW, Nesto RW, Singh BN, Deanfield J, Gottlieb SO (N-CAP Study Group). Attenuation of the circadian patterns of myocardial ischemia with nifedipine GITS in patients with chronic stable angina. *J Am Coll Cardiol* 1992; **19**: 1380–9.

87. Stone PH, Gibson RS, Glasser SP et al. (ASIS Study Group). Comparison of propranolol, diltiazem, and nifedipine in the treatment of ambulation ischemia in patients with stable angina: differential effects on ambulatory ischemia, exercise performance, and anginal symptoms. *Circulation* 1990; **82**: 1962–72.

88. Diodati JG, Quyyumi AA, Hussain N, Keefer LK. Complexes of nitric oxide with nucleophiles as agents for the controlled biologic release of nitric oxide: anti-platelet effect. *Thromb Hem* 1993; **70**: 654–8.

89. Diodati JG, Quyyumi AA, Hussain N, Keefer LK. Complexes of nitric oxide with nucleophiles as agents for the controlled biologic release of nitric oxide: hemodynamic effect. *J Cardiovasc Pharmacol* 1993; **22**: 287–92.

90. Creager MA, Gallagher SJ, Girerd XJ, Coleman SM, Dzau VJ, Cooke JP. L-arginine improves endothelium-dependent vasodilation in hypercholesterolemic humans. *J Clin Invest* 1992; **90**: 1248–53.

91. Drexler H, Zeiher AM, Meinertz T, Just H. Correction of endothelial dysfunction in coronary microcirculation of hypercholesterolemic patients by L-arginine. *Lancet* 1991; **338**: 1546–50.

92. Panza JA, Casino PR, Badar DM, Quyyumi AA. Effect of increased availability of endothelium-derived nitric oxide precursor on endothelium-dependent vascular relaxation in normals and in patients with essential hypertension. *Circulation* 1993; **87**: 1475–81.

93. Casino PR, Kilcoyne CM, Quyyumi AA, Hoeg JM, Panza JA. Investigation of decreased availability of nitric oxide precursor as the mechanism responsible for impaired endothelium-dependent vasodilation in hypercholesterolemic patients. *J Am Coll Cardiol* 1994; **23**: 844–50.

94. Mancini GBJ, Henry GC, Macaya C et al. Angiotensin-converting enzyme inhibition with quinapril improves endothelial vasomotor dysfunction in patients with coronary artery disease: the TREND (Trial on Reversing Endothelial Dysfunction) study. *Circulation* 1996; **94**: 258–65.

95. Minor RL Jr, Myers PR, Guerra R Jr, Bates JN, Harrison DG. Diet-induced atherosclerosis increases the release of nitrogen oxides from rabbit aorta. *J Clin Invest* 1990; **86**: 2109–16.

96. Scandinavian Simvistatin Survival Study Group. Randomized trial of cholesterol lowering in 4444 patients with coronary heart disease: the Scandinavian Simvistatin Survival Study (4S). *Lancet* 1994; **344**: 1383–9.

15

Mental stress and silent myocardial ischemia: evidence, mechanisms, and clinical implications

John S Gottdiener, Willem J Kop and David S Krantz

INTRODUCTION

Mental and emotional stress have long been considered to be etiologically linked to adverse cardiac outcomes including angina, myocardial infarction, hypertension, and sudden death. A dramatic example of the potential effect of acute mental stress as a trigger of ischemic cardiac death is afforded by the celebrated English surgeon Sir John Hunter, who in describing the effects of mental stress on his angina said, 'My life is in the hands of any rascal who chooses to tease and annoy me.' In 1793, after attending a contentious hospital board meeting, he clutched his chest and fell dead.[1]

While the lay public has long held the notion that there is an important linkage between mental stress and cardiac disease,[2,3] such a connection has been regarded with some doubt by the cardiology community.[3] Until relatively recently, evidence for this connection existed primarily in the form of anecdotal and case reports,[4] sparse epidemiologic research,[5] and mechanistic studies in humans and in animals demonstrating physiologic and pathophysiologic effects of mental stress on the heart.[6,7] Some of the difficulties in studying the relationship between mental stress and myocardial ischemia have been difficulties in the definitions and measurement of both. In particular, 'mental stress', a term to describe mental and/or emotional activation perceived in a negative manner, has been difficult to measure in naturalistic studies, as well as to utilize as a reproducible intervention in laboratory studies. However, investigators of psychosocial stress now emphasize the crucial role of interpretation or appraisal of events or stimuli for the perception of stress and the elicitation of physiologic response.[8,9] Accordingly, mental stress can be broadly defined as a negative internal state of the individual that is dependent on interpretation or appraisal of threat, harm, or demand. Unfortunately, many confounding factors affect associations between mental stress and cardiac events. Although epidemiology studies may be successful in defining such associations, they cannot uncover the mechanisms by which psychosocial mechanisms are associated with disease or expressions of disease. However, recent developments have revived the interest of clinicians in the role of mental stress as a 'trigger' of myocardial ischemia and events including myocardial infarction and sudden death.

CARDIOVASCULAR TRIGGERS

The concept of cardiovascular 'triggers', that is, events or activities capable of converting a stable pathophysiological state into an acute, and sometimes catastrophic, clinical occurrence has become a popular and potentially useful one.[10] In addition to the importance of physical stress as a trigger of ischemia, sedentary triggers[10,11] such as smoking, exposure to cold, and mental stress[12] are also of importance. Using diary self-reports during Holter monitoring, it was shown[13] that most ischemic episodes, in addition to being asymptomatic, occur at rest or with only light physical activity, for example sitting or slow walking. Other diary studies have extended these findings in noting that the greatest proportion of total ischemic time during Holter monitoring occurs while sedentary.[13,14] Moreover, during the activities of daily life, mental activities appear to be as potent as exercise as ischemic triggers, and are more frequent precipitants of transient ischemia than physical exertion.[13] Intense anger,[14] in particular, is a potent ischemic trigger. The circadian distribution of physical and mental triggers of painless ischemia also appears to differ.[15] The effect of physical activities as triggers of ischemia is greatest in the morning and somewhat less so in the afternoon, while mental activity is a significant trigger in the morning and evening, but not in the afternoon.

PAINFUL VERSUS PAINLESS ISCHEMIA WITH MENTAL STRESS

Initial studies of ischemia during Holter monitoring have found that most episodes are painless and occur during lower heart rates and, presumably, myocardial oxygen consumption than ischemia during exercise testing.[16–19] Since these findings suggested that myocardial metabolic demand was lower than with painful ischemia, it was reasonable to infer that painless ischemia may have been the consequence of diminished myocardial oxygen supply, possibly due to coronary vasoconstriction. Additionally, studies have shown decreased myocardial perfusion[20] and coronary vasoconstriction[21] during silent ischemia induced by mental stress. However, since oxygen demand is related to the double product of heart rate and blood pressure, blood pressure measurement at the time of ischemia is important to characterize more fully oxygen demand. When ambulatory blood

pressure monitoring was performed concomitant with Holter ECG, it was found that increases in heart rate and blood pressure preceded the majority of silent ischemic events.[22] Nonetheless, a substantial minority of patients (39%) had no increase in heart rate greater than 5 bpm preceding ischemia. Using a more gradual exercise protocol than generally utilized clinically, it was demonstrated that the heart rate at the onset of ischemia ('ischemic threshold') with exercise was in fact similar to that during ambulatory monitoring during the activities of daily life.[23] However, ECG changes may fail to detect the earliest onset of ischemia during exercise or during daily life activities. Hence, it remains uncertain whether vasospasm is a more common mechanism of silent than of painful ischemia. Likely, both myocardial supply and metabolic demand-related factors play a role.[24]

Contrary to what might be suggested by the experience of Sir John Hunter, most episodes of ischemia triggered by mental stress are also painless. For example, 45 men with active ischemia were evaluated using echocardiography to detect new (and presumably ischemic) wall motion during mental stress testing in the laboratory. The findings were cross-tabulated with those of Holter recordings obtained with diary entries of mental and physical activities.[25] Of 40 patients who had ischemia with exercise, 17 (43%) had chest pain at the time of ischemia. In contrast, of 24 patients with ischemia during mental stress testing, only one (4%) had chest pain. Similarly, in another study,[26] using radionuclide cineangiography to detect ischemia during mental stress, 83% of episodes were symptomatically 'silent'. To assess possible mechanisms for this effect, Sheps et al.[27] measured beta-endorphin levels and thermal pain thresholds in 20 patients with coronary artery disease (CAD) immediately after psychological stress produced by a public-speaking task requiring discussion of personal difficulties. Their finding of a correlation between beta-endorphin levels with increased thermal pain thresholds following mental stress may be relevant to the finding that ischemia during psychological stress is usually painless.

PHYSIOLOGIC RESPONSES TO MENTAL STRESS: NEUROHUMORAL AND CARDIOVASCULAR REACTIVITY

The physiologic consequences of behavioral stress were recognized by the prominent physiologist Walter Cannon, who noted that fear and anger elicited a massive sympathetic 'fight-or-flight' response marked by increases in circulating catecholamines.[28] Subsequently, a generalized physiological stress response to several noxious stimuli marked by activation of the pituitary-adrenal cortical axis was described by Selye.[29] The magnitude of physiologic responses to a mental stressor can be considered measures of cardiovascular reactivity to stress.

Neurohormonal response to mental stress

The stress response most often includes release of catecholamines and corticosteroids.[30,31] Epinephrine has been considered to be a more sensitive indicator of behavioral arousal than norepinephrine.[32,33] In normal men it was found[34] that the cold pressor test and mental arithmetic performed during harassment produced equivalent increases in venous plasma norepinephrine, while increases in epinephrine were greater with mental arithmetic than with cold pressor.

Cardiodynamic responses to mental stress

Previous studies have shown that mental stress is associated with increases in heart rate, and with systolic and diastolic blood pressure[27,30,34–36] which is dependent upon the presence of intact cardiac innervation.[37] Additionally, mental-stress-induced increases in cardiac output and stroke volume have been documented by impedance cardiography[38] and echocardiography.[34,39,40] Increased ejection fraction with stress has been demonstrated by radionuclide angiography.[41,42] Studies of normal men and women in the laboratory using 2D-Doppler echocardiography to measure beat-by-beat alterations in cardiac function during

mental arithmetic, in comparison with cold pressor and with exercise stress, have shown increased ejection fraction with mental arithmetic consequent to decreased end-systolic volume with no change in end-diastolic volume.[34] With cold pressor there was a trend towards decrease in ejection fraction (Fig. 15.1). The systolic time velocity integral in the left ventricular (LV) outflow tract, a Doppler measure of stroke volume, increased with mental stress (Fig. 15.2, upper panel) but not with cold pressor. Peak early (E) diastolic filling velocity and peak velocity with atrial (A) contraction increased with mental arithmetic (Fig. 15.2, lower panel), while cold pressor was associated with decrease in E velocity but increased A velocity, hence decreased E/A ratio. Of note, even silent mental attention to instructions for the mental arithmetic task is associated with hemodynamic alterations. Notably, self-perceived magnitude of stress during the task was not associated with the magnitude of the reactivity response.[43]

As part of the Psychophysiological Investigations of Myocardial Ischemia (PIMI) study, Becker et al.[44] reported on cardiac, peripheral vascular and neurohormonal responses to simulated public speaking and the Stroop color–word test administered to 29 middle-aged and older (age 45–73 years) subjects who had low prior probability of clinically significant coronary disease. There was a marked sympathetic response with both stressors, as evidenced by increases in blood pressure, heart rate, and cardiac index as well as increases in plasma levels of epinephrine and norepinephrine. No changes in beta-endorphin or plasma cortisol were noted. Responses of LV ejection fraction to mental stress varied among individuals. However there were decreases in ejection fraction of greater than 5% in 12 (of whom five decreased by more than 8%) of these presumably normal individuals. Regional wall motion abnormalities were observed in three individuals. Ejection fraction changes were associated inversely with baseline ejection fraction and with increases in afterload.

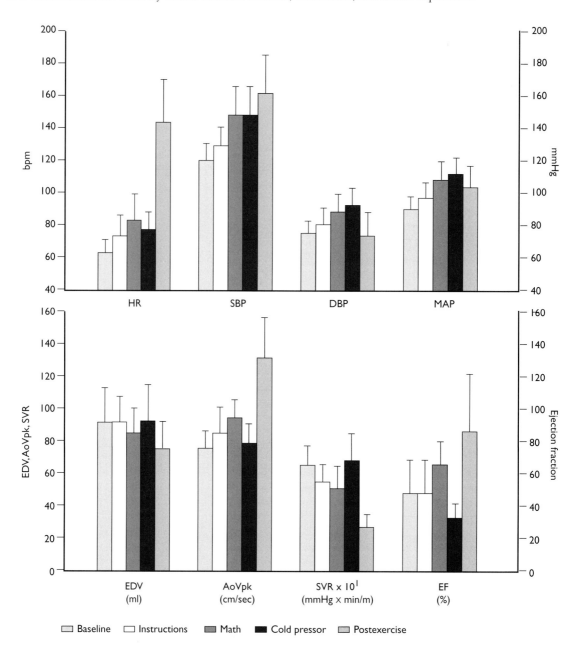

Figure 15.1 Upper panel: effects of silent attention (to task instructions), mental arithmetic (math) task, cold pressor stress and exercise (immediately post-treadmill) stress on heart rate (HR), systolic blood pressure (SBP), diastolic blood pressure (DBP), and mean arterial blood pressure (MAP). Lower panel: echocardiographic end-diastolic volume (EDV), peak aortic Doppler flow velocity (AoVpk), systemic vascular resistance (SVR), and ejection fraction (EF). Note hemodynamic responses produced by silent attention to verbal instructions, as well as increased EF and aortic ejection velocity with mental stress.

Aortic Outflow Velocity

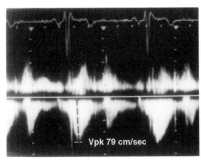
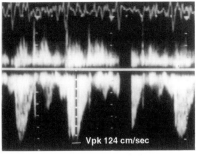

LV Inflow Velocity

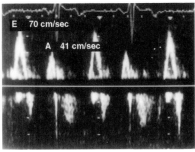
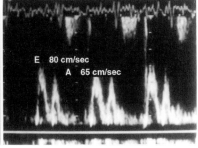

Baseline   Mental Arithmetic Task

Figure 15.2 Upper panel: effects of mental arithmetic on Doppler aortic flow velocity profile. Note increased peak velocity and systolic velocity integral indicative of increased stroke volume. Lower panel: effects of mental arithmetic on Doppler LV diastolic filling profile. Note marked increase in atrial (A) filling velocity with mental stress (lower right) compared with baseline (lower left).

Effects of mental stress on blood rheology, hemostasis, and thrombosis

Recent research suggests that acute stress can also affect processes that are relevant to hemostasis and thrombosis. For example, acute mental stress results in increased platelet activation,[31,45–47] increased thromboxane B2 (a metabolite of thromboxane A2—a coronary vasoconstrictor),[48] increased blood viscosity[49,50] and acute decreases in circulating plasma volume.[51–53]

These are of relevance in that platelet activation may potentiate ischemia both by leading to coronary thrombosis as well as by platelet-mediated vasoconstriction.[54] Moreover, decreases in plasma volume and increases in blood viscosity potentiate ischemia and myocardial infarction (MI).[55,56] Studies performed in the laboratory in normal subjects demonstrated substantial increases in platelet

factor 4 and beta-thromboglobulin (Fig. 15.3) which persisted even after correction for mental-stress-induced contraction of intravascular volume.[52,57] In addition, a recent study[58] noted hemostatic alterations attributable to the stress induced by an earthquake in Japan.

Mental stress and the autonomic nervous system

Utilizing analysis of heart rate variability and microneurography it was shown that stress[59–62] is associated with increased sympathetic contribution to autonomic tone even during reflex sympathetic inhibition by baroreceptor stimulation.[61] It has been shown[63] that mental stress testing produces increases in muscle sympathetic nerve activity, measured by peroneal nerve microneurography, in normotensive offspring of hypertensive parents but not in offspring of normotensive

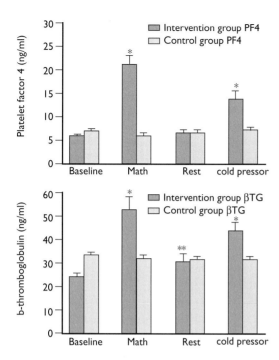

Figure 15.3 Comparison of effects of mental arithmetic (math) with cold pressor stress on platelet factor 4 (PF4) (upper panel) and beta-thromboglobulin (βTG) (lower panel) in normal subjects. To determine effects of prolonged supine position and repeat phlebotomy on PF4 and βTG, control group comprises individuals studied with same number and volume of blood withdrawals, lying flat for same time duration as intervention group. (Reproduced with permission from Patterson et al.[52])

parents. Moreover, increases in sympathetic nerve activity in the offspring of hypertensive parents were accompanied by increases in plasma norepinephrine and in endothelin. Endothelin is a substance released by vascular endothelium which at low concentrations enhances vasoconstrictor effects of norepinephrine, and at higher concentrations has direct vasoconstrictor properties.[64] Since normotensive offspring of normotensive and of hypotensive parents both had equal increases in plasma norepinephrine and muscle sympathetic activity to hypoxic stress, the effects of mental stress appear to be specific. Further,

studies in experimental animals[65] have shown that endothelin itself may increase sympathetic outflow. Hence, effects of mental stress on sympathetic tone may potentiate ischemia both by sympathetically mediated increases in oxygen demand, primarily from systolic pressor responses to systemic vasoconstriction, as well as by decreases in myocardial flow consequent to coronary vasoconstriction. Moreover, genetic susceptibility may play an important part.

Another study found that positive emotions, in contrast, are associated with enhanced vagal/sympathetic ratio.[59] Cardiac autonomic tone may therefore be a marker of stress response and vulnerability to stress.

In the authors' laboratory,[66] studies performed in a closed chest dog model have demonstrated the importance of tonic vagal tone for the maintenance of coronary dilatation. Withdrawal of vagal tone either surgically or pharmacologically was associated with marked decreases in the diameter of the normal circumflex coronary artery, measured by intracoronary ultrasound.

Additionally, CAD patients with lower vagal tone have been shown to have greater pressor reactivity[59,67] and systemic vasoconstriction to mental stress than patients with higher vagal tone.[59] This is of clinical relevance in that enhanced cardiovascular reactivity is associated with the magnitude of ischemia induced by mental stress,[35] as well as with a greater likelihood of ischemia during daily life and mental stress.[68] Moreover, enhanced reactivity is of prognostic value in postinfarction patients.[69] Conversely, enhanced cardiovascular reactivity is also associated with decreased vagal tone on Holter monitoring[70] and decreases in vagal tone precede ischemia during the activities of daily life.[71,72]

PATHOPHYSIOLOGICAL EFFECTS OF STRESS ON THE CARDIOVASCULAR SYSTEM

Relationships between brain and heart: autonomic activation

Current models suggest a role of behaviorally induced autonomic nervous system activation

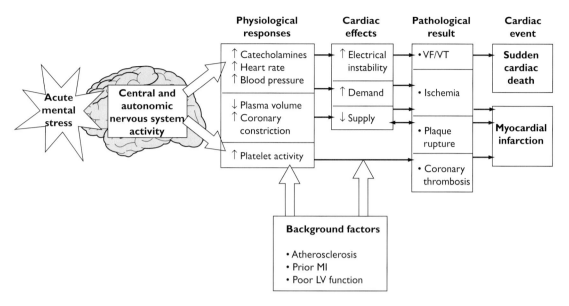

Figure 15.4 Pathophysiological model of the effects of acute stress as a trigger of cardiac clinical events including myocardial ischemia in patients with coronary artery disease. Acting via the central and autonomic nervous system, stress can produce a cascade of physiological responses that may lead to myocardial ischemia, potentially fatal arrhythmia, plaque rupture, and/or coronary thrombosis. (Reproduced with permission from Krantz et al.[131])

as the mediator of at least some of the effects of mental and physical stress on cardiac pathophysiology.[6,73] Autonomic nervous system activation might predispose to clinical cardiovascular events at several levels, including promotion of atherosclerosis and/or coronary endothelial dysfunction, by influencing intermediate pathological and pathophysiological processes which increase vulnerability to clinical events such as myocardial ischemia, coronary thrombosis, plaque rupture, and by directly triggering lethal arrythmias through alterations of neural transmission to the heart.[6,51] A model for these pathophysiological pathways linking acute mental stress to myocardial ischemia and other acute cardiac events is presented in Fig. 15.4. These pathways are presumed to operate among individuals who are predisposed to clinical events by virtue of pre-existing atherosclerosis.

Using positron emission tomography (PET) to measure regional cerebral blood flow

changes in patients with coronary artery disease, Rosen et al.[74] found that ischemia produced by pharmacologic stress was accompanied by increased bilateral thalamic blood flow in patients with painless as well as in patients with painful ischemia. Patients with angina, however, had greater blood flow increases than patients with painless ischemia in the left temporal pole and some other cortical regions. While myocardial ischemia, even in the absence of pain, is associated with activation of the brain, it is uncertain what effects brain stimulation has on myocardial blood flow or physiologic functions of the heart. However, evidence from a variety of sources suggests the influence of selected brain regions on LV dysfunction. It has long been observed that subarachnoid hemorrhage is associated with marked ECG abnormalities.[75] Moreover, Kono et al.[76] observed LV regional wall motion abnormalities on left ventriculography and echocardiography with subarachnoid hemorrhage in the absence of fixed coronary obstructive lesions or coronary vasospasm on angiography. Wall motion abnormalities tended to improve with time, suggesting that neurogenic stunning of the myocardium occurred rather than infarction. Also supporting the importance of brain function to cardiac physiology has been the experimental finding of decreased systolic and diastolic LV function following brain death in canines.[77]

Pathologic stress responses

There are several specific components of the physiological responses to stress that may be pathologic given the appropriate clinical substrate. In patients with atherosclerotic coronary disease, stress responses may promote coronary vasoconstriction, platelet aggregation, or plaque rupture. For example, mental stress can produce arterial pressure surges, often comparable to those elicited by acute exercise.[26] In patients with vulnerable plaque this surge may cause a plaque rupture and lead to occlusive or nonocclusive coronary thrombosis.[10] In the presence of flow-limiting coronary obstructive lesions, stress-induced increases in blood pressure, heart rate, and contractility may produce increases in myocardial oxygen demand sufficient to result in acute myocardial ischemia. With mental-stress-induced hypercoagulability, even a small thrombus may trigger the clotting cascade, resulting in acute coronary occlusion and subsequent MI, ischemia, or vulnerability to arrythmias or sudden death. Moreover, mental-stress-induced hypercoagulability[31,54,56,78] may potentiate vasoconstriction, which can probably also occur via neuroparacrine mechanisms.[78]

Effects of mental stress on coronary vasoconstriction

Yeung et al.[21] (Fig. 15.5) found that diseased coronary segments constricted during mental arithmetic while nondiseased, smooth segments

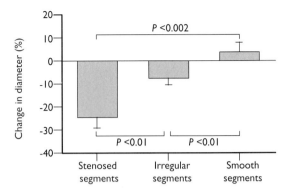

Figure 15.5 Effects of mental arithmetic on epicardial coronary artery diameters in stenosed, irregular, and smooth segments. Stenosed segments constricted a mean of –24 ± 4%; irregular segments constricted –9 ± 3%, while smooth segments were unchanged (+3 ± 3%). (Reproduced with permission from Yeung et al.[21])

either vasodilated or showed no change in diameter. Coronary vasoconstriction and/or dilatation in response to mental stress was significantly correlated with the response to intracoronary infusions of acetylcholine, suggesting that coronary endothelial dysfunction is a mechanism for paradoxical vasoconstriction. Using an anger recall as a laboratory stressor in patients with symptomatic myocardial ischemia, Boltwood et al.[79] noted coronary vasoconstriction only with high levels of reported anger. Preliminary studies in the authors' laboratory have shown a range of responses of coronary artery diameter to mental stress measured by quantitative coronary angiography, ranging from physiologic vasodilatation to paradoxical vasoconstriction. However, in angiographically smooth segments, elevated low-density lipoproteins (LDL) appears to be associated with a propensity to coronary vasoconstriction with mental stress.[80] In one dramatic case,[81] mental stress testing provoked total, but fortunately transient, occlusion at the site of a 70% occlusive lesion of the left anterior branch of the coronary artery (Fig. 15.6).

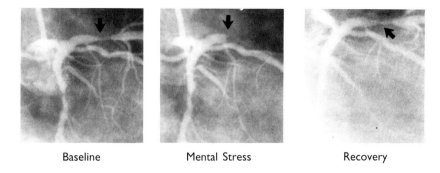

Baseline   Mental Stress   Recovery

Figure 15.6 Transient total occlusion (middle panel, arrow) of left anterior descending branch of the left coronary artery after mental stress (mental arithmetic task). After nitrates and nifedipine, artery reopened (right-hand panel) to same diameter as baseline (left-hand panel). (Reproduced with permission from Papademetriou et al.[81])

Pathophysiology of mental stress ischemia

Although mental stressors produce reliable increases in heart rate and blood pressure, the magnitude of heart rate responses is less during mental tasks than during exercise in the same patient. Blood pressure changes, however, are comparable between exercise and mental tasks.[25,26] Most studies have shown that the double product (systolic blood pressure × heart rate) at the onset of ischemia is less with mental stress than with exercise. This suggests the possibility that ischemia with mental stress results from reduced oxygen delivery (vasoconstriction) while exercise produces ischemia via increased oxygen demand. The findings of Yeung et al.,[21] who noted epicardial coronary arterial constriction in response to mental stress, are in support of this notion. However, since there was no significant decrease in epicardial coronary blood flow, mental stress ischemia could not be attributed to epicardial coronary constriction alone. However, microcirculatory effects of mental stress on the coronary circulation were found by Dakak et al.[82] They found evidence of impaired dilatation of coronary resistance vessels in patients with minimal angiographic evidence of CAD, but microvasculature dilatation with mental stress in patients without angiographic abnormality of the coronary arteries.

Despite evidence for flow-mediated ischemia with mental stress, the substantial blood pressure responses with mental stress suggest that increased myocardial oxygen demand also contributes to mental-stress-induced ischemia. The greater pressor reactivity found in several studies[68,35,83] in patients who evidence ischemia with mental stress is consistent with this supposition.

BEHAVIORAL CHARACTERISTICS AND ISCHEMIA

Burg et al.[84] demonstrated that CAD patients with mental-stress-induced depression of LV function had higher scores of 'aggressive responding', trait anger, hostile effect, behavioral reactivity, and a lower score on anger control. In studies performed in our laboratory,[85] it was found that the combination of high scores for defensiveness and for hostility was associated with greater frequency and duration of ischemia episodes on Holter monitoring, as well as more marked ischemic LV dysfunction on echocardiogram during

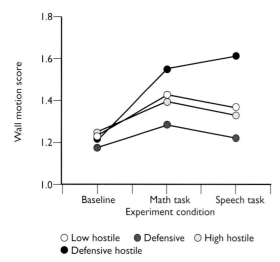

Figure 15.7 Relationship of defensiveness, hostility, and their combination to magnitude of ischemic regional wall motion abnormality on echocardiogram induced by mental stress testing. Higher wall motion score represents worse regional wall motion abnormality. (Reproduced with permission from Helmers et al.[85])

mental stress testing (Fig. 15.7). Moreover, these behavioral characteristics were also associated with the functional severity of ischemia with exercise as determined by the extent of perfusion abnormality on thallium scintigraphy during upright treadmill exercise. The relationships between behavioral characteristics and ischemia with mental and exercise stress are of interest in that the prevalence of clinically significant coronary occlusive lesions on angiography is also related to behavioral characteristics, most notably hostility.[86]

EPIDEMIOLOGICAL EVIDENCE FOR MENTAL STRESS AS A TRIGGER OF ACUTE CARDIOVASCULAR EVENTS

There is extensive epidemiological literature on mental stress and the morbidity and mortality of heart disease.[6,87,88] Although 'mental stress' is usually thought of as a relatively acute event,

chronic 'psychosocial' stressors are also of relevance to coronary outcomes. These include social isolation and lack of social support,[89–91] the effects of stressful occupations on CAD risk,[92] the effects of emotional distress and depression on prognosis in post-MI patients,[89,93,94] psychosocial prodromata preceding lethal arrythmias and sudden cardiac death,[6,95–97] and the triggering effects of acutely stressful events on myocardial infarction or sudden cardiac death.[4,98–102] For the purposes of this review, however, we will confine ourselves to mental stress as an acute trigger of MI in individuals presumed to have pre-existing CAD.

SITUATIONAL CRISES, PSYCHOLOGICAL TRAUMA, AND ACUTE CARDIOVASCULAR EVENTS

Population crises

An increase in cardiovascular deaths and increased rates of MI have been reported after several general disasters and personal traumas. The effect of Iraqi missile attacks on Israel during the initial days of the 1991 Gulf War on fatal and nonfatal cardiac events among the population living close to Tel Aviv was described by Meisel et al.[99] who noted increased incidence of acute MI treated in the intensive care unit of a Tel Aviv medical center in the week following the missile attacks (17–25 January, 1991), compared with the week prior to the attacks as well as with an index period of the same week one year earlier. Mean age and sex distribution were similar in all study periods. Further, there was an increase in the sudden death rate during January, 1991 (41 deaths) compared with the same period a year earlier (22 deaths). These findings were extended by a second study which examined mortality statistics among the entire Israeli population during the time of the Iraqi missile attacks. Mortality in excess of control periods was greater among women than among men (77% versus 41%, $P < 0.01$).[102] Moreover, most excess mortality, which was attributable to cardiovascular causes, occurred in the Tel Aviv area where the missile attacks took place. Two possible causes of increased cardiovascular mortality include the stressful conditions posed by fear of the missile attacks and/or respiratory difficulties resulting from confinement to sealed, unventilated rooms. Supporting the former explanation is the fact that women, who reported proportionately more distress resulting from confinement in the sealed room than men, also experienced a higher excess of event rates. On the other hand, confinement was significantly longer during the first, compared with subsequent missile attacks, during which time the Israeli population appears to have adapted to the situation.

Excess cardiac mortality attributed to acute psychological stress has also been reported following earthquakes and other natural disasters. Following the 1981 Athens earthquake, the incidence of cardiac deaths nearly doubled within 5 days of the event[103] and there was a 22% increase in ischemic heart disease deaths following blizzards in Massachusetts.[104] Additionally, there was an increased incidence of acute MI following the 1994 Los Angeles earthquake. Coronary care unit admissions for acute MI (odds ratio 2.4), but not for unstable angina, increased in the week following the earthquake compared with the week before the disaster, particularly for hospitals within 15 miles of the earthquake epicenter.[105] A recent paper by Kario et al.[58] evaluated physically uninjured elderly patients with controlled hypertension following the 17 January, 1995 earthquake in Hyogo Prefecture, Japan, following which excess cardiovascular deaths were also noted. All patients who were selected for study experienced maximum psychological stress on a standardized scoring system, although 19 of the 42 patients studied were considered to be in a particularly high-stress group because of homelessness or serious injury or death of at least one family member. Compared with measurements before the earthquake, there were substantial elevations of blood pressure, hematocrit (along with fibrinogen a determinant of blood viscosity), and d-dimer (a marker of fibrin

turnover) in both stress groups. Moreover, patients in the high-stress group also had increases in fibrinogen, von Willebrand factor (an endothelial cell-derived marker), as well as tissue-type plasminogen activator antigen and plasmin-alpha2-plasmin inhibitor complex (fibrinolytic factors). Lipid profiles were unchanged after the earthquake. With the exception of von Willebrand factor, all these hemodynamic and hemostatic risk factors decreased to pre-quake levels by 4–6 months after the earthquake. Notably, in elderly normotensive subjects in whom pre-quake measurements were not available, systolic blood pressure, heart rate, hematocrit, d-dimer, and von Willebrand factor also decreased from post-quake values within 3–9 months. Hence, this study provides potential mechanistic associations between the psychological stress of a natural disaster, and biological factors which are potential triggers of cardiovascular events.

However, it is difficult in studies of population disasters to determine the etiologic roles of mental stress versus increases in physical exertion as triggers of MI. This criticism seems particularly relevant in the case of snowstorms, where physical exertion from shoveling snow or walking through deep snow seems likely. However, increased physical exertion is also possible during earthquakes, as stricken inhabitants carry belongings, move debris, or flee from risk.

Personal crises

A relationship of stressful life-events to sudden cardiac death was found in an uncontrolled study[5] in which stressful life-events were reported to have occurred among 40 of 100 sudden-death victims in the 24 hours preceding death. Cottington et al.[106] found that temporally related personal loss occurred to sudden-death victims more frequently than to controls. These and similar studies, however, rely on biased recall of stressful events by relatives or friends of sudden-death victims. Overcoming this criticism are prospective studies of the link between emotional trauma and MI sudden death which have evaluated individuals after severe life crises. A 40% increase in mortality, mostly cardiovascular, was found in a large cohort of middle-aged widowers in the first 6 months following bereavement.[97] However, it is not possible to exclude the role of changes in lifestyle during the grieving process, or unfavorable environments shared by the widower and the deceased in increased mortality, as opposed to the stress of bereavement per se.

The relationship of psychological and behavioral antecedents to acute MI may also be studied by determining the occurrence of potential triggers prior to the events. Psychologically stressful events have been implicated as possible external triggers of infarction in several studies of patients hospitalized for acute MI. Among 849 patients with acute MI, 48% reported one or more possible triggers, the most common of which was emotional upset.[107] In another study,[98] possible external triggers of acute MI were identified in 10% of patients. These included heavy physical exertion, a bitter quarrel at work or home, and unusually marked mental stress within 24 hours preceding the onset of pain. The lower percentage of possible triggers reported in the latter study may be due to methodologic differences between the two studies.[98]

An ingenious approach, employed by Mittleman et al.[100,108] utilized a case-crossover design, a relatively new epidemiologic methodology that compares each patient's pre-MI activities with his or her usual levels of activities. Hence, the proximate physical and mental triggers of onset of MI may be assessed in a controlled fashion. In a multicenter study, 39 of 1623 (2.4%) patients interviewed a median of 4 days post-MI, reported anger within the 2 hours prior to the onset of MI (RR 2.3). The relative risk of acute infarction following anger was significantly lower among regular users of aspirin, and there was a trend for the relative risk to be lower in women than men, and in regular users of beta-adrenergic medications versus non-users. Unfortunately, this methodology cannot

overcome retrospective bias, since awareness of MI may have affected reporting of emotional responses.

MENTAL STRESS AS A TRIGGER OF MYOCARDIAL ISCHEMIA

While MI and sudden cardiac death are of primary importance for the prevention of cardiac morbidity and mortality, laboratory and field studies using myocardial ischemia as an intermediate measure have provided a pathophysiologic model for understanding mechanisms by which mental stress may trigger clinical events. Moreover, since most episodes of ischemia in both field and laboratory studies are symptomatically 'silent', an important advantage of studying ischemia is that it permits studies of environmental triggers of cardiac events without confounding by reporting biases.

In contrast to ischemia elicited with exercise testing, out-of-hospital ischemia occurs during a wide variety of physical and mental activities, and not just during strenuous exertion. Ischemia during the activities of daily life is predominantly asymptomatic and occurs at relatively low heart rate elevations compared with ischemia triggered by exercise testing.[11] Moreover, there is a typical circadian rhythm for myocardial ischemia,[109,110] and in contrast to exercise testing which is relatively reproducible, there is an unexplained variability in the frequency of ischemic episodes when patients are repeatedly monitored over time.[111]

Graded exercise testing seems to be an effective means of testing the functional severity of stable coronary obstructive lesions. However, it is likely that the observed features of myocardial ischemia out of hospital are produced by the interaction of patient behaviors, including mental stress and possibly health damaging behavior, as well as other environmental factors with the dynamic pathobiology of coronary artery disease. Unlike the controlled circumstances of graded exercise testing, patients out of hospital encounter a broad range of physical and mental stimuli, and many of these stresses occur suddenly and unpredictably.

Ambulatory ECG studies of mental and physical activity

Evidence exists that mental stress and ischemia are associated, and that emotional states may account for some of the unexplained within-patient variability in the occurrence of transient ischemia over time.[112] A useful approach has been to correlate the results of ambulatory ECG ischemia monitoring with patient diary self-reports. In one of the earliest studies of ambulatory ischemia, conducted by Stern and Tzivoni,[12] patients maintained meticulous diary recordings during ambulant ECG monitoring of emotional changes, physical activity, mealtimes, and times of sleep and rising. Among the 37 patients with ST-T wave changes considered positive for ischemia, six had ischemia during emotional stress in the absence of physical exertion. Schang and Pepine[113] showed that most (75%) ischemia episodes were asymptomatic and occurred either at rest or with light physical activity such as slow walking or sitting. Only rarely was ischemia accompanied by strenuous physical exercise. Other studies[114] have since corroborated these findings.

The relationship between self-perceived level of physical and mental activity with the objective occurrence of ST-depression during daily life was investigated by Barry et al.[13] Patients maintained a diary in which segments of time were identified for various activities during the day. Study patients were taught to make an entry whenever their activities changed, to classify activities as either 'physical' or 'mental', and also to record the intensity of the activity as either 'rest', 'usual', or 'stress'. The majority of ischemic episodes occurred during daily activities involving low or moderate levels of physical activity. Examples of such activities include talking on the phone, doing clerical work, and conversing with a friend. Moreover, episodes of ST-segment depression also occurred during activities classified as 'usual' physical or 'usual' mental activity. Relatively

few ischemic events occurred during self-described stressful situations, or during sleep. Since activities described as 'usual' are, by nature, engaged in more frequently during daytime hours, the duration of ST-segment depression was divided by the total time spent in each category. When this correction was done, a graded relationship was found between ischemia and the intensity of both mental and physical activities. Hence, increasing intensity of both mental and physical activities is associated with greater transient ischemia during daily life. However, since high levels of exercise are infrequent, while mental activities are more frequent during daily life, usual mental activities may be a more common trigger of transient ischemia than intense exercise.

These findings were extended by work in the present authors' laboratory[14] which assessed the effects of specific emotions on ischemia using a rather detailed diary in 63 patients undergoing Holter ECG monitoring. ST depression (usually painless) occurred most frequently during physical and mental activities of moderate intensity. While patients spent the greatest proportion of time engaged in physical and mental activities of low intensity, the likelihood of ischemia was greatest during intense physical and stressful mental activities (Fig. 15.8). The proportion of ischemic time during high-intensity activity to the total time in that activity (5%) was approximately equivalent for high-intensity physical and mental activities, compared with 0.2% of the time when patients were engaged in low-intensity activities. Moderately strenuous physical activity (for example, walking) and intense anger were potent ischemic triggers. Among smokers, ischemia was more than five times more likely when patients smoked compared with periods where they did not smoke (27% versus 5% of diary entries). The association of coffee- and alcohol-drinking with ischemia disappeared after controlling for concurrent cigarette smoking.

Thus activities involving low physical exertion such as anger and smoking are important triggers of ischemia in daily life, and

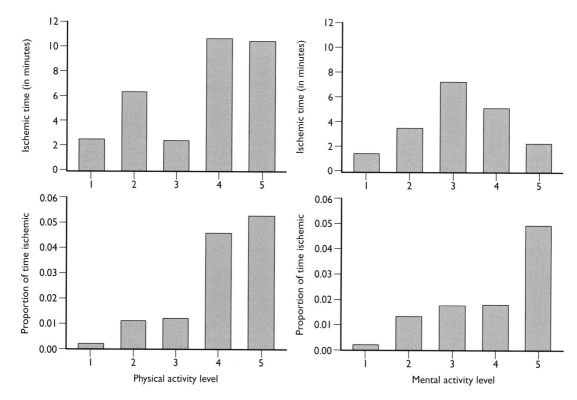

Figure 15.8 Total ischemic time by intensity of physical (left-hand panel) and mental (right-hand panel) activity during the period of Holter monitoring. Upper panel shows total ischemic time unadjusted for the time patients spent at each level of activity. To adjust for the time spent at each of the levels of physical and mental activity, ischemic time during each level of activity for each patient was expressed as a proportion of the time spent at that level of activity (bottom panel). (Adapted from Gabbay et al.[14])

mental activities appear to be as important as physical activities in triggering daily-life ischemia.

Circadian effects

Mental and physical activities may also contribute to the well established circadian rhythm (morning increase) in ischemia. In an elegantly designed study, Parker et al.[115] showed that the increase in activities upon awakening is important to the circadian pattern of ischemia. The effect of time of day on the potency of out-of-hospital mental and physical triggers of ischemia was recently studied in the present authors' laboratory.[15] Physical activity was most likely to trigger ECG ischemia on Holter monitoring in the morning. High levels of physical activity were associated with ischemia to a lesser, but still significant, extent in the afternoon, but not during the evening. Mental activity triggered ischemic events significantly during the morning and evening, but not in the afternoon. Hence, physical and mental activities appear to be most potent as triggers of ischemia during the morning hours. Nonetheless, there does appear to be an endogenous component to the circadian patterns of ischemia.

Summary of ambulatory ECG-diary findings

The results of ambulatory ECG monitoring studies indicate that a variety of physical and mental activities are associated with the occurrence of transient, asymptomatic ischemia during daily life. Moreover, a different profile of activities (more exercise-related; perhaps associated with greater anxiety) accompanies painful versus painless ischemic episodes. Additionally, circadian patterns of ischemia are in part accounted for by daily patterns of activity. Behavioral influences, including the stresses of daily life, have become increasingly apparent as important factors in the total ischemic burden.

LABORATORY STUDIES OF MENTAL STRESS AND MYOCARDIAL ISCHEMIA

Since field studies are correlational, causal relationships between mental stressors and ischemic episodes cannot be established. Moreover, evaluation of pathophysiologic mechanisms of stress–ischemia relationships becomes problematic. Laboratory studies employing standardized mental stress interventions have added substantially to our knowledge. While some laboratory studies have examined the effects of mental stress using only electrocardiographic changes to detect ischemia, the results of these studies[116,117] have been inconsistent at best. Specchia et al.[83] compared the mental arithmetic testing with exercise testing on the electrocardiographic markers of ischemia in 122 consecutive patients who had undergone coronary angiography. Although all patients had ECG ischemia on exercise testing, only 22 (18%) had ECG ischemia with mental stress, and chest pain was noted in only eight of these 22 patients.

The prevalence and biological characteristics of ischemia will depend on the method used for its detection. While, as a means to determine the prevalence of myocardial ischemia, angina pectoris represents only the 'tip of the iceberg', ECG detection of ischemia also occurs relatively late in the ischemic sequence. Other modalities which detect alterations of myocardial perfusion or contraction are in theory and in practice more sensitive means of detecting ischemia, particularly if transient or mild. In contrast to field studies of mental stress, which have been limited to ECG detection of ischemia, laboratory studies have benefited from the ability to use other techniques such as echocardiography, radionuclide ventriculography, PET scanning, and perfusion scintigraphy.

Nuclear cardiology studies

Using PET to measure diminished myocardial perfusion during mental arithmetic and separately with exercise, Deanfield et al.[20] reported that 12 of 16 patients evidenced diminished regional perfusion with arithmetic while only six of these patients showed ST-segment depression, and only four had angina. With exercise, all the patients showed abnormal regional perfusion in the same cardiac segments that evidenced ischemia with mental arithmetic.

Using radionuclide ventriculography, Rozanski et al.[26] studied the effects of a series of mental stressors on LV wall motion and ejection fraction and compared these with the effects of exercise. Of 29 of 39 CAD patients with exercise-induced wall motion abnormalities, 21(72%) also showed wall motion abnormalities to mental stress. The speech stressor was found to be the most potent of the mental tasks and was significantly different from the other mental tasks in the induced frequency and magnitude of wall motion abnormality. In several patients, the magnitude of wall motion abnormalities during the speech was comparable to those induced by exercise in the same patient. In patients without an exercise-induced wall motion abnormality, ischemic abnormalities induced by the mental stressors were infrequent. Another important finding within this study was that most of the mental-stress-induced ischemia was symptomatically silent and ECG abnormalities were observed only in a minority of these patients during mental stress. These findings have since been corroborated in several studies from other laboratories.[25,84,118–20]

Other studies have also found that decreases in ejection fraction can be greater with a mental stressor than with exercise testing at comparable rate–pressure products.[121,122] Furthermore, there are greater increases in systemic vascular resistance with ischemia induced by mental stress[122] than with ischemia induced by exercise stress. Moreover, in the study reported by Legault et al.[120] the 49% of patients in whom ischemia was induced with mental stress had greater severity of angiographic disease and ischemic functional severity on exercise thallium testing than coronary patients with negative mental stress tests. However, given the findings of the PIMI investigators,[44] that mental stress may produce decreases in ejection fraction and regional wall motion abnormality in normal subjects, care must be taken in utilizing these findings as evidence of mental-stress-induced ischemia.

Myocardial scintigraphy using sestamibi has also been used to demonstrate reversible perfusion defects during mental arithmetic in patients with recent MI and active ischemia.[123] Consistent with other studies, ischemia induced by mental stress was symptomatically silent, and ECG evidence of ischemia was absent. As shown in most studies, irrespective of imaging modality, mental stress is a weaker stimulus for ischemia than exercise.

Echocardiography

Since echocardiography permits beat-by-beat assessment of global and regional LV function, it is a potentially robust tool for assessment of transient ischemia, evidenced by new regional wall motion abnormality during mental stress.[124] Studying 45 patients with CAD, the present authors used two-dimensional echocardiography to show transient wall motion abnormalities occurring rapidly and asymptomatically in 24/45 patients (53%) during mental stress (Fig. 15.9).[25] Similarly to previous studies, few patients had ECG evidence of ischemia with mental stress, and chest pain was rare (1/24) during mental-stress-induced ischemia. The magnitude of stress-induced wall motion abnormalities and number

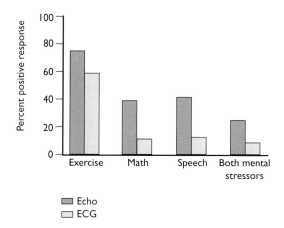

Figure 15.9 Proportion of coronary artery disease patients with inducible ischemia; comparison of upright bicycle exercise with two mental stressors, mental arithmetic (math) and a personally relevant speech task. Note relatively small proportion of individuals with ischemic responses to mental stress on echocardiogram who also had ischemic response on ECG, in contrast to findings with exercise stress. (Reproduced with permission from Gottdiener et al.[25])

of mental stressors capable of inducing ischemia were related to the functional severity of exercise-inducible ischemia in these patients, possibly reflecting a greater functional severity of coronary disease among those patients more susceptible to mental stress ischemia.

CLINICAL IMPLICATIONS OF MENTAL STRESS ISCHEMIA

Correspondence with ischemia during daily life

It is clear that mental stress can induce wall motion abnormalities and ejection fraction decreases in 40–70% of patients with coronary artery disease and active ischemia. However, the clinical significance of mental-stress-induced ischemia remains uncertain. Deedwania[125] has pointed out that mental-stress-induced ischemia is generally asymptomatic, brief in duration, and of lesser magnitude than ischemia induced by exercise. Correspondence between ischemia induced by mental stress and ambulatory ischemia assessed during daily life in the out-of-hospital setting has been shown in recent studies. In the authors' laboratory, it was found that ischemia, as determined by the presence of new regional wall motion on echocardiography during mental stress testing in the laboratory, was predictive of increased risk of ischemia during sedentary activities of daily life.[25] Two other studies have corroborated these findings by demonstrating that patients with mental-stress-inducible wall motion abnormalities[68] and transient ejection fraction decreases in response to mental stress[119] evidenced an overall greater likelihood of ischemia assessed during ambulatory ECG monitoring.

Prognostic significance of mental-stress-induced ischemia

The prognostic significance of exercise testing has been well established, and some,[110,126] but not all[127] ambulatory ECG studies have shown that patients with daily life ischemia have a worse prognosis when compared with those who do not manifest ischemia.[110,126] Now, recent studies suggest that the presence of mental-stress-induced myocardial ischemia may predict subsequent clinical events in patients with coronary artery disease. In a study reported by Jain et al.,[128] 10 of 15 patients who had decreases in ejection fraction of >5% with mental stress testing had adverse cardiac events (consisting of nonfatal MI or unstable angina) over a two-year follow-up compared with only four of 14 patients who did not evidence this dysfunction. Although highly suggestive, the small sample size and infrequent outcome events necessitate that these findings be interpreted with caution. However, two other research groups recently presented corroborating, but still not definitive, evidence for the clinical significance of mental stress ischemia among CAD patients with prior positive exercise tests. Over a period of three years, the authors followed up 79 patients with recent positive exercise stress tests who had been previously assessed for mental-stress-induced wall motion abnormalities with multiple stressors. New cardiac events (cardiac death, nonfatal MI, coronary artery bypass grafting (CABG), angioplasty) occurred in 28 (35%) of patients. New events occurred in 14/28 (50%) of patients with mental stress ischemia, compared with 16/51 patients (31%) without mental stress ischemia. However, the relative risk of 2.2 for the presence of mental stress ischemia did not reach levels of statistical significance in the relatively small sample size studied. Jiang et al.[95] prospectively followed 126 patients with stable angina of whom 28 (22%) had at least one clinical event (cardiac death, MI, CABG, angioplasty) over an average follow-up of 3.2 years. Mental stress ischemia, defined in terms of a transient decrease in ejection fraction on radionuclide ventriculography of >5% during mental stress testing, was associated with an increased risk of clinical events (odds ratio = 2.8, $P < 0.05$) (Fig. 15.10). This effect remained significant even after controlling for risk factors and for exercise ischemic response.

Despite the promising findings of the available prognostic studies, several limitations mandate caution in their interpretation. The sample sizes are relatively small and limited to CAD patients with prior positive exercise tests. Moreover, relatively few hard outcome events were available for cross-tabulation with predictor variables. Nevertheless, taken in combination, they suggest that myocardial ischemia triggered by mental stress is of clinical importance. Additional research using larger and more diverse patient groups should provide clarification. There are several possible mediators of the putative relationship between inducible mental stress ischemia and prognosis. Given the association between ischemia induced by mental stress in the laboratory and ischemia during the activities of daily life,[25,68,119] patients with 'positive' mental stress tests may be at increased risk simply by virtue of the presence of more ischemia during daily life. Mental stress ischemia is more likely in patients with more functionally severe disease; hence

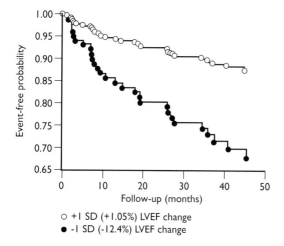

○ +1 SD (+1.05%) LVEF change
● -1 SD (-12.4%) LVEF change

Figure 15.10 Cox proportional hazards model of event-free survival (adjusted for baseline ejection fraction, history of myocardial infarction, and age) based on ejection fraction change during mental stress testing. Ejection fraction (LVEF) changes are plotted at two prototypical values, 1 sd below (LVEF change = 112.4%) and 1 sd above (LVEF change = +1.05%) the mean of the entire sample (LVEF change = –6.73%). The risk associated with a mental-stress-induced decrease in LVEF $</=-1$ sd is 2.40 ($P < 0.02$). (Reproduced with permission from Jiang et al.[95])

mental stress testing may serve to identify greater severity of disease in a manner that supplements the predictive value of conventional exercise stress testing. Additionally, it is possible that a positive mental stress test may indicate enhanced susceptibility to a variety of mental stress triggers of clinical events during daily life. Last, while mental stress in the laboratory is a weaker stimulus for ischemia than exercise testing performed using usual clinical protocols, the myocardial oxygen demand preceding ischemia more closely approximates that associated with ischemia during daily life. Thus while less sensitive than more severe forms of stress for detecting anatomic coronary disease, mental stress testing may more closely approximate the naturalistic clinical environment. Further investigation of

these considerations will lead to better understanding of the possible clinical relevance of mental stress testing.

Clinical management

It has been well documented that mental stress is a trigger of both myocardial ischemia and infarction. Despite the fact that mental stress is a weaker stimulus of ischemia than strenuous exercise, since patients with CAD engage in strenuous exercise only infrequently, mental stress may be comparable in importance to strenuous physical activities as a trigger for clinical events. Arguably, ischemia with mental stress may be more related to mechanisms associated with coronary vasoconstriction and a reduction in myocardial supply, than to increased oxygen demand. Since only about half of patients with exercise-inducible ischemia have ischemia induced by mental stress testing, it may be of importance to identify those patients who are susceptible to the pathophysiologic effects of mental stress and to assess pharmacologic and nonpharmacologic means for preventing the triggering of clinical events by mental stress. One preliminary study[129] has suggested that beta-adrenergic blockade may be only partially beneficial in preventing ischemia triggered by mental stress. Mental stress elicits relatively low heart rate increases, but substantial increases in blood pressure. However, beta-blockers are more effective in limiting heart rate responses to exercise stress than in moderating marked pressor responses to mental stress. Further research assessing the effects of calcium-channel blockers, alpha-adrenergic blockers and other pharmacologic agents is needed. Of interest, an epidemiologic study[100] observed that triggering of MI by mental stress was less evident in patients taking aspirin. This might suggest that the antiplatelet agents can diminish coronary thrombosis and/or vasoconstriction mediated by mental-stress-induced platelet activation.

Nonpharmacologic treatment approaches such as psychosocial treatment or behavior therapy may also prove useful as an alternative or adjunct

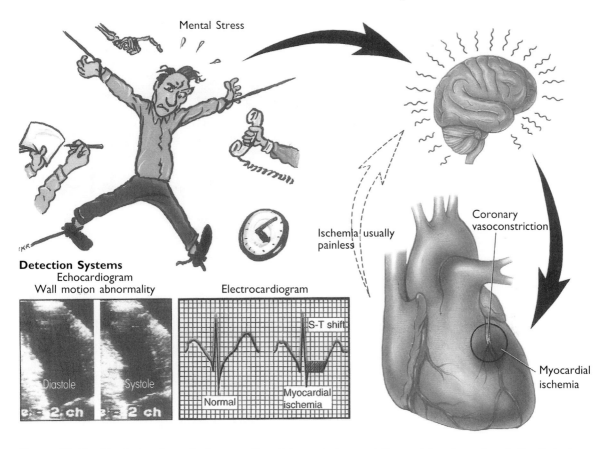

Figure 15.11   The ischemic cost of aggravation: linkages between daily mental and emotional stimuli, brain activity, coronary and myocardial physiology.

to drug treatment. Results from a randomized stress reduction trial in patients after myocardial infarction suggest that modification of environmental stress through psychosocial support may be beneficial in preventing morbidity and mortality. Frasure-Smith and Prince[130] reported a 51% reduction in post-MI deaths using a psychosocial intervention in which 453 post-MI patients reporting high levels of life stress were randomized to a simple counseling and social support intervention to help them deal with psychosocial stress. Moreover, evaluation of psychotropic agents to reduce stress may also be warranted in selected patient populations. Since psychosocial stress is pervasive and often unavoidable,

research on pathophysiological mechanisms mediating the associations between acute stress and cardiac pathology (Fig. 15.4) as well as on possible moderators of this association[100] must remain a priority.

The interplay of physical and psychological environments with the pathobiology of coronary disease is both immediate and complex (Fig. 15.11). Undoubtedly, much will be learned through the growth of interdisciplinary collaboration, utilizing an increasing array of techniques for detection of the presence as well as mechanisms of ischemia, characterization of the neurobiology of ischemia, and assessment of behavioral state and psychological triggers.

ACKNOWLEDGMENTS

Preparation of this chapter was assisted by grants from the NIH (HL47337) and USUHS (RO7233). The opinions and assertions expressed herein are those of the authors and are not to be construed as reflecting the views of the USUHS or the US Department of Defense.

REFERENCES

1. Williams J, Edwards G. The death of John Hunter. *JAMA* 1968; **204**: 806–9.
2. Angell M. Disease as a reflection of the psyche. *N Engl J Med* 12: 1570–72.
3. Hlatky MA, Lam LC, Lee KL et al. Job strain and the prevalence and outcome of coronary artery disease. *Circulation* 1995; **92**: 327–33.
4. Engel GL. Sudden and rapid death during psychological stress. *Ann Intern Med* 1971; **74**: 771–82.
5. Myers R, Dewar HA. Circumstances surrounding sudden deaths from coronary artery disease with coroners' necropsies. *Br Heart J* 1975; **37**: 1133–43.
6. Kamarck T, Jennings JR. Biobehavioral factors in sudden death. *Psychol Bull* 1991; **109**: 42–75.
7. Manuck SB, Marsland AL, Kaplan JR, Williams JK. The pathogenicity of behavior and its neuroendocrine mediation: an example from coronary artery disease. *Psychosom Med* 1995; **57**: 275–83.
8. Lazarus RS. *Psychological Stress and the Coping Process*. (New York: McGraw-Hill, 1966).
9. Mason JW. A historical view of the stress field. *J Hum Stress* 1975; **1**: 22–36.
10. Muller JE, Abela GS, Nesto RW, Tofler GH. Triggers, acute risk factors and vulnerable plaques: the lexicon of a new frontier. *J Am Coll Cardiol* 1994; **23**: 809–13.
11. Deanfield J, Shea M, Ribiero P et al. Transient ST-segment depression as a marker of myocardial ischemia during daily life. *Am J Cardiol* 1984; **54**: 1195–200.
12. Stern S, Tzivoni D. Early detection of silent ischemic heart disease by 24-hr electrocardiographic monitoring of active subjects. *Br Heart J* 1974; **36**: 481–6.
13. Barry J, Selwyn AP, Nabel EG et al. Frequency of ST-segment depression produced by mental stress in stable angina pectoris from coronary artery disease. *Am J Cardiol* 1988; **61**: 989–93.
14. Gabbay RH, Krantz DS, Kop WJ et al. Triggers of myocardial ischemia during daily life in patients with coronary artery disease: physical and mental activities, anger and smoking. *J Am Coll Cardiol* 1996; **27**: 585–92.
15. Krantz DS, Kop WJ, Gabbay FH et al. Circadian variation of ambulatory myocardial ischemia: triggering by daily activities and evidence for an endogenous circadian component. *Circulation* 1996; **93**: 1354–61.
16. Deanfield J, Selwyn A, Chierchia S et al. Myocardial ischemia during daily life in patients with stable angina: its relation to symptoms and heart rate changes. *Lancet* 1983; **ii**: 753–8.
17. Chierchia S, Gallino A, Smith G et al. Role of heart rate in the pathophysiology of chronic stable angina. *Lancet* 1984; **ii**: 1353–7.
18. Campbell S, Barry J, Rocco M et al. Features of the exercise test that reflect the activity of ischemic heart disease out of hospital. *Circulation* 1986; **74**: 72–80.
19. Cohn P, Lawson W. Characteristics of silent myocardial ischemia during out-of-hospital activities in asymptomatic angiographically documented coronary artery disease. *Am J Cardiol* 1987; **59**: 746–9.
20. Deanfield JE, Shea M, Kensett M. Silent ischemia due to mental stress. *Lancet* 1984; **ii**: 1001–5.
21. Yeung AC, Vekshtein VI, Krantz DS et al. The effect of atherosclerosis on the vasomotor response of coronary arteries to mental stress. *N Engl J Med* 1991; **325**: 1551–6.
22. Deedwania PC, Nelson JR. Pathophysiology of silent myocardial ischemia during daily life. Hemodynamic evaluation by simultaneous electrocardiographic and blood pressure monitoring. *Circulation* 1990; **82**: 1296–304.
23. Panza JA, Diodati JG, Callahan TS, Epstein SE, Quyyumi AA. Role of increases in heart rate in determining the occurrence and frequency of myocardial ischemia during daily life in patients with stable coronary artery disease. *J Am Coll Cardiol* 1992; **20**: 1092–8.
24. Deedwania PC, Carbajal EV. Silent myocardial ischemia. A clinical perspective. *Arch Intern Med* 1991; **151**: 2373–82.

25. Gottdiener JS, Krantz DS, Howell RH et al. Induction of silent myocardial ischemia with mental stress testing: relation to the triggers of ischemia during daily life activities and to ischemic functional severity. *J Am Coll Cardiol* 1994; **24**: 1645–51.

26. Rozanski A, Bairey CN, Krantz DS et al. Mental stress and the induction of silent myocardial ischemia in patients with coronary artery disease. *N Engl J Med* 1988; **318**: 1005–12.

27. Sheps DS, Ballenger MN, De Gent GE et al. Psychophysical responses to a speech stressor: correlation of plasma beta-endorphin levels at rest and after psychological stress with thermally measured pain threshold in patients with coronary artery disease. *J Am Coll Cardiol* 1995; **25**: 1499–503.

28. Cannon WB. *Bodily Changes in Pain, Hunger, Fear and Rage.* (New York: Appleton, 1929).

29. Selye H. *The Stress of Life.* (New York: McGraw-Hill, 1976).

30. Krantz DS, Manuck SB. Acute psychophysiologic reactivity and risk of cardiovascular disease: a review and methodologic critique. *Psychol Bull* 1984; **96**: 435–64.

31. Grignani G, Soffiantino F, Zucchella M et al. Platelet activation by emotional stress in patients with coronary artery disease. *Circulation* 1991; **83**: II128–II136.

32. Frankenhaeuser M, Rauste von Wright M, Collins A, von Wright J, Sedvall G, Swahn C. Sex differences in psychoneuroendocrine reactions to examination stress. *Psychosom Med* 1978; **40**: 334–43.

33. Dimsdale JE, Ziegler MG. What do plasma and urinary measures of catecholamines tell us about human response to stressors? *Circulation* 1991; **83 (suppl II)**: II-36–II-42.

34. Gottdiener JS, Hecht GM, Vargot SL, Patterson SM, Krantz DS. Physiologic effects of psychological activation on cardiac function. *Circulation* 1992; **82(4) (suppl I)**: I-866 (abst).

35. Krantz DS, Helmers KF, Bairey CN, Nebel LE, Hedges SM, Rozanski A. Cardiovascular reactivity and mental stress-induced myocardial ischemia in patients with coronary artery disease. *Psychosom Med* 1991; **53**: 1–12.

36. Brod J, Fencl V, Heil Z. Circulatory changes underlying blood pressure elevation during acute emotional stress (mental arithmetic) in normotensive and hypertensive subjects. *Clin Sci* 1959; **18**: 269–79.

37. Shapiro PA, Sloan RP, Bigger JT Jr, Bagiella E, Gorman JM. Cardiac denervation and cardiovascular reactivity to psychological stress. *Am J Psychiatry* 1994; **151**: 1140–7.

38. McKinney ME, Miner MH, Ruddel H et al. The standardized mental stress test protocol: test-retest reliability and comparison with ambulatory blood pressure monitoring. *Psychophysiology* 1985; **22**: 453–63.

39. Lindvall K, Kahan T, de Faire U, Ostergren J, Hjemdahl P. Stress-induced changes in blood pressure and left ventricular function in mild hypertension. *Clin Cardiol* 1991; **14**: 125–32.

40. Kaji Y, Ariyoshi K, Tsuda Y, Kanaya S, Fujino T, Kuwabara H. Quantitative correlation between cardiovascular and plasma epinephrine response to mental stress. *Eur J Appl Physiol* 1989; **59**: 221–6.

41. Kiess M, Dimsdale JE, Moore RH et al. The effects of stress on left ventricular ejection fraction. *Eur J Nucl Med* 1988; **14**: 12–16.

42. Rozanski A, Krantz DS, Bairey CN. Ventricular responses to mental stress testing in patients with coronary artery disease. Pathophysiological implications. *Circulation* 1991; **83**: II137–II144.

43. Hecht GM, Gottdiener JS, Patterson SM, Kovach JA, Vargot SL, Krantz DS. Dissociation of cardiac physiologic response from psychologic perception of mental stress. *Clin Res* 1992; **40**: 402A (abst).

44. Becker LC, Pepine CJ, Bonsall R et al. Left ventricular, peripheral vascular, and neurohumoral responses to mental stress in normal middle-aged men and women. Reference group for the Psychophysiological Investigations of Myocardial Ischemia (PIMI) study. *Circulation* 1996; **94**: 2768–77.

45. Musumeci V, Baroni S, Cardillo C et al. Cardiovascular reactivity, plasma markers of endothelial and platelet activity and plasma renin activity after mental stress in normals and hypertensives. *J Hypertens* 1987; **5 (suppl 5)**: S1–S4.

46. Andren L, Wadenvik H, Kutti J, Hansson L. Stress and platelet activation. *Acta Haematol* 1983; **70**: 302–6.

47. Haft JI, Fani K. Intravascular platelet aggregation in the heart induced by stress. *Circulation* 1973; **47**: 353–8.

48. Ushiyama K, Ogawa T, Ishii M, Ajisaka R, Sugishita Y, Ito I. Physiologic neuroendocrine arousal by mental arithmetic stress test in healthy subjects. *Am J Cardiol* 1991; **67**: 101–3.

49. De Simone G, Devereux RB, Chien S, Alderman MH, Atlas SA, Laragh JH. Relation of blood viscosity to demographic and physiologic variables and to cardiovascular risk factors in apparently normal adults. *Circulation* 1990; **81**: 107–17.

50. Ehrly AM, Landgraf H, Hessler J, Saeger-Lorenz K. Influence of videofilm-induced emotional stress on the flow properties of blood. *Angiology* 1988; **30(4)**: 341–4.

51. Muller JE, Tofler GH, Stone PH et al. Circadian variation and triggers of onset of acute cardiovascular disease. *Circulation* 1989; **79**: 733–43.

52. Patterson SM, Krantz DS, Gottdiener JS, Hecht G, Vargot S, Goldstein DS. Prothrombotic effects of environmental stress: changes in platelet function, hematocrit, and total plasma protein. *Psychosom Med* 1995; **6**: 592–9.

53. Tofler GH, Brezinski D, Schafer AI et al. Concurrent morning increase in platelet aggregability and the risk of myocardial infarction and sudden cardiac death. *N Engl J Med* 1987; **316**: 1514–18.

54. Malkoff SB, Muldoon MF, Zeigler ZR, Manuck SB. Blood platelet responsivity to acute mental stress. *Psychosom Med* 1993; **55**: 477–82.

55. Lowe GDO. Blood rheology in arterial disease. *Clin Sci* 1986; **71**: 137–46.

56. Fuchs J, Weinberger I, Tebovl A et al. Plasma viscosity and haematocrit in the course of acute myocardial infarction. *Eur Heart J* 1987; **8(11)**: 1195–2000.

57. Patterson SM, Gottdiener JS, Hecht G, Vargot S, Krantz DS. Effects of acute mental stress on serum lipids: mediating effects of plasma volume. *Psychosom Med* 1993; **55**: 525–32.

58. Kario K, Matsuo T, Kobayashi H, Yamamoto K, Shimada K. Earthquake-induced potentiation of acute risk factors in hypertensive elderly patients: possible triggering of cardiovascular events after a major earthquake. *J Am Coll Cardiol* 1997; **29**: 926–33.

59. McCraty R, Atkinson M, Tiller WA, Rein G, Watkins AD. The effects of emotions on short-term power spectrum analysis of heart rate variability. *Am J Cardiol* 1995; **76**: 1089–93.

60. Pagani M, Mazzuero G, Ferrari A et al. Sympathovagal interaction during mental stress. A study using spectral analysis of heart rate variability in healthy control subjects and patients with a prior myocardial infarction. *Circulation* 1991; **83**: II43–51.

61. Anderson EA, Sinkey CA, Mark AL. Mental stress increases sympathetic nerve activity during sustained baroreceptor stimulation in humans. *Hypertension* 1991; **17**: III43–9.

62. Langewitz W, Ruddel H, Schachinger H. Reduced parasympathetic cardiac control in patients with hypertension at rest and under mental stress. *Am Heart J* 1994; **127**: 122–8.

63. Noll G, Wenzel RR, Schneider M et al. Increased activation of sympathetic nervous system and endothelin by mental stress in normotensive offspring of hypertensive parents. *Circulation* 1996; **93**: 866–9.

64. Yand Z, Richard V, von Segesser L et al. Threshold concentrations of endothelin-1 potentiate contractions to norepinephrine and serotonin in human arteries: a new mechanism of vasospasm? *Circulation* 1990; **82**: 188–95.

65. Mosqueda-Garcia R, Inagami T, Appalsamy M, Sugiura M, Robertson RM. Endothelin as a neuropeptide: cardiovascular effects in the brainstem of normotensive rats. *Circ Res* 1993; **72**: 20–35.

66. Kovach JA, Gottdiener JS, Verrier RL. Vagal modulation of epicardial coronary artery size in dogs. A two-dimensional intravascular ultrasound study. *Circulation* 1995; **92**: 2291–8.

67. Kollai M, Kollai B. Cardiac vagal tone in generalised anxiety disorder. *Br J Psychiatry* 1992; **161**: 831–5.

68. Blumenthal JA, Jiang W, Waugh RA et al. Mental stress-induced ischemia in the laboratory and ambulatory ischemia during daily life. Association and hemodynamic features. *Circulation* 1995; **92**: 2102–8.

69. Manuck SB, Olsson G, Hjemdahl P, Rehnqvist N. Does cardiovascular reactivity to mental stress have prognostic value in postinfarction patients? A pilot study. *Psychosom Med* 1992; **54**: 102–8.

70. Jiang W, Hayano J, Coleman ER et al. Relation of cardiovascular responses to mental stress and cardiac vagal activity in coronary artery disease. *Am J Cardiol* 1993; **72**: 551–4.

71. Goseki Y, Matsubara T, Takahashi N, Takeuchi T, Ibukiyama C. Heart rate variability before the occurrence of silent myocardial ischemia during ambulatory monitoring. *Am J Cardiol* 1994; **73**: 845–9.

72. Kop WJ, Gottdiener JS, Verdino R, Howell RH, Haddad AH, Krantz DS. Relation of mental stress and vagal withdrawal to silent ischemia during the activities of daily life. *Circulation* 1995; **94**: I-676 (abst).

73. Muller JE, Ludmer PL, Willich SN et al. Circadian variation in the frequency of sudden cardiac death. *Circulation* 1987; **75**: 131–8.

74. Rosen S, Paulesu E, Nihoyannopoulos P et al. Silent ischemia as a central problem: regional brain activation compared in silent and painful myocardial ischemia. *Ann Intern Med* 1996; **124**: 939–49.

75. Davis TP, Alexander J, Lesch M. Electrocardiographic changes associated with acute cerebrovascular disease. *Prog Cardiovasc Dis* 1993; **36**: 245–60.

76. Kono T, Morita H, Kuroiwa T, Onaka H, Takatsuka H, Fujiwara A. Left ventricular wall motion abnormalities in patients with subarachnoid hemorrhage: neurogenic stunned myocardium. *J Am Coll Cardiol* 1994; **24**: 636–40.

77. Bittner HB, Chen EP, Craig D, Van Trigt P. Preload-recruitable stroke work relationships and diastolic dysfunction in the brain-dead organ donor. *Circulation* 1996; **94**: II-322–II-325.

78. Jern C, Eriksson E, Tengborn L, et al. Changes of plasma, coagulation and fibrinolysis in response to mental stress. *Thromb Haemost* 1989; **62**: 761–71.

79. Boltwood MD, Taylor CB, Burke MB, Grogin H, Giacomini J. Anger report predicts coronary artery vasomotor response to mental stress in atherosclerotic segments. *Am J Cardiol* 1993; **72**: 1361–5.

80. Gottdiener JS, Howell RH, Kop WJ et al. Serum lipids and hypertension potentiate coronary vasoconstriction with mental stress. *J Am Coll Cardiol* 1997; **29**: 524A(abst).

81. Papademetriu V, Gottdiener JS, Kop WJ et al. Transient coronary occlusion with mental stress. *Am Heart J* 1996; **132**: 1299–301.

82. Dakak N, Quyyumi AA, Eisenhofer G, Goldstein DS, Cannon RO III. Sympathetically mediated effects of mental stress on the cardiac microcirculation of patients with coronary artery disease. *Am J Cardiol* 1995; **76**: 125–30.

83. Specchia G, Falcone C, Traversi E et al. Mental stress as a provocative test in patients with various clinical syndromes of coronary heart disease. *Circulation* 1991; **83**: II108–II114.

84. Burg MM, Jain D, Soufer R, Kerns RD, Zaret BL. Role of behavioral and psychological factors in mental stress-induced silent left ventricular dysfunction in coronary artery disease. *J Am Coll Cardiol* 1993; **22**: 440–8.

85. Helmers KF, Krantz DS, Merz CN et al. Defensive hostility: relationship to multiple markers of cardiac ischemia in patients with coronary disease. *Health Psychol* 1995; **14**: 202–9.

86. Williams RB Jr, Haney TL, Lee KL, Kong YH, Blumenthal JA, Whalen RE. Type A behavior, hostility, and coronary atherosclerosis. *Psychosom Med* 1980; **42**: 539–49.

87. Willich SN, Maclure M, Mittleman M, Arntz HR, Muller JE. Sudden cardiac death. Support for a role of triggering in causation. *Circulation* 1993; **87**: 1442–50.

88. Howell RH, Krantz DS. The role of mental stress in the pathogenesis of coronary atherosclerosis and acute coronary events. *Med Exerc Nutr Health* 1994; **3**: 131–40.

89. Frasure-Smith N. In-hospital symptoms of psychological stress as predictors of long-term outcome after acute myocardial infarction in men. *Am J Cardiol* 1991; **67**: 121–7.

90. Ruberman W, Weinblatt E, Goldberg JD et al. Psychosocial influences on mortality after myocardial infarction. *N Engl J Med* 1984; **311**: 552–9.

91. Williams RB, Barefoot JC, Califf RM et al. Prognostic importance of social and economic resources among medically treated patients with angiographically documented coronary artery disease. *JAMA* 1992; **267**: 520–4.

92. Karasek RA, Theorell TG, Schwartz J et al. Job psychological factors and coronary heart disease: Swedish prospective findings and US prevalence findings using a new occupational inference method. *Adv Cardiol* 1982; **29**: 62–7.

93. Frasure-Smith N, Lesperance F, Juneau M. Differential long-term impact of in-hospital symptoms of psychological stress after non-Q-wave and Q-wave acute myocardial infarction. *Am J Cardiol* 1992; **69**: 1128–34.

94. Frasure-Smith N, Lesperance F, Talajic M. Depression and 18-month prognosis after myocardial infarction. *Circulation* 1995; **91**: 999–1005.

95. Jiang W, Babyak M, Krantz DS et al. Mental stress-induced myocardial ischemia and cardiac events. *JAMA* 1996; **275**: 1651–6.

96. Kuller LH. Prodromata of sudden death and myocardial infarction. *Adv Cardiol* 1978; **25**: 61–72.

97. Parkes CM, Benjamin B, Fitzgerald RG. Broken heart: a statistical study of increased mortality among widowers. *BMJ* 1969; **1**: 740–3.

98. Behar S, Halabi M, Reicher-Reiss H et al. Circadian variation and possible external triggers of onset of myocardial infarction. SPRINT Study Group. *Am J Med* 1993; **94**: 395–400.

99. Meisel SR, Kutz I, Dayan KI et al. Effect of Iraqi missile war on incidence of acute myocardial infarction and sudden death in Israeli civilians. *Lancet* 1991; **338**: 660–1.

100. Mittleman MA, Maclure M, Sherwood JB et al. Triggering of acute myocardial infarction onset by episodes of anger. Determinants of Myocardial Infarction Onset Study Investigators. *Circulation* 1995; **92**: 1720–5.

101. Jacobs SC, Friedman R, Mittleman M et al. Nine-fold increased risk of myocardial infarction following psychological stress as assessed by a case-controlled study. *Circulation* 1992; **86**: 1198 (abst).

102. Kark JD, Goldman S, Epstein L. Iraqi missile attacks on Israel. The association of mortality with a life-threatening stressor. *JAMA* 1995; **273**: 12.

103. Trichopoulos D, Katsouyanni K, Zavitsanos X et al. Psychological stress and fatal heart attack: the Athens (1981) earthquake natural experiment. *Lancet* 1983; **i**: 441–4.

104. Glass RI, Zack MMJ. Increase in deaths from ischemic heart disease after blizzards. *Lancet* 1979; **i**: 485–7.

105. Leor J, Kloner RA, Poole WK. The Northridge earthquake as a trigger for acute myocardial infarction. SO Sudden cardiac death triggered by an earthquake. *N Engl J Med* 1996; **334**: 413–19.

106. Cottington EM, Matthews KA, Talbot E et al. Environmental events proceeding sudden death in women. *Psychosom Med* 1980; **42**: 567–75.

107. Tofler GH, Stone PH, Maclure M et al. Analysis of possible triggers of acute myocardial infarction (the MILIS study). *Am J Cardiol* 1990; **66**: 22–7.

108. Mittleman M, Maclure M, Tofler G, Sherwood J, Goldberg R, Muller J. Triggering of acute myocardial infarction by heavy physical exertion. Protection against triggering by regular exertion. *N Engl J Med* 1993; **329**: 1677–83.

109. Mulcahy D, Keegan J, Cunningham J et al. Circadian variation of total ischemic burden and its alteration with anti-anginal agents. *Lancet* 1988; **ii**: 755–9.

110. Rocco MB, Barry J, Campbell S et al. Circadian variation of transient myocardial ischemia in patients with coronary artery disease. *Circulation* 1987; **75**: 395–400.

111. Nabel EG, Barry J, Rocco MB et al. Variability of transient myocardial ischemia in ambulatory patients with coronary artery disease. *Circulation* 1988; **78**: 60–7.

112. Freeman L, Nixon P, Sallabank P, Reavely D. Psychological stress and silent myocardial ischemia. *Am Heart J* 1987; **114**: 477–82.

113. Schang SJ, Pepine C. Transient asymptomatic ST-segment depression during daily activity. *Am J Cardiol* 1977; **39**: 396–402.

114. Cecchi A, Dovellini E, Marchi F, Pucci P, Santoro G, Fazzini P. Silent myocardial ischemia during ambulatory electrocardiographic monitoring in patients with effort angina. *J Am Coll Cardiol* 1983; **1**: 934–9.

115. Parker JD, Testa MA, Jimenez AH et al. Morning increase in ambulatory ischemia in patients with stable coronary artery disease. Importance of physical activity and increased cardiac demand. *Circulation* 1994; **89**: 604–14.

116. Schiffer F, Hartley LH, Schulman CL et al. The quiz electrocardiogram: a new diagnostic and research technique for evaluating the relationship between emotional stress and ischemic heart disease. *Am J Cardiol* 1976; **37**: 41–4.

117. DeBusk RF, Taylor CB, Agras WS. Comparison of treadmill testing and psychological stress testing soon after myocardial infarction. *Am J Cardiol* 1979; **43**: 907–9.

118. LaVeau PJ, Rozanski A, Krantz DS et al. Ischemic left ventricular performance during provocative mental stress testing. *Am Heart J* 1989; **118**: 1–8.

119. Breisblatt WM, Wolf CJ, McElhinny B, Salerni R, Smith VE. Comparison of ambulatory left ventricular ejection fraction and blood pressure in systemic hypertension in patients with and without increased left ventricular mass. *Am J Cardiol* 1991; **67**: 597–603.

120. Legault SE, Langer A, Armstrong PW, Freeman MR. Usefulness of ischemic response to mental stress in predicting silent myocardial ischemia during ambulatory monitoring. *Am J Cardiol* 1995; **75**: 1007–11.

121. Legault SE, Freeman MR, Langer A, Armstrong PW. Pathophysiology and time course of silent myocardial ischaemia during mental stress: clinical, anatomical, and physiological correlates. *Br Heart J* 1995; **73**: 242–9.

122. Goldberg AD, Becker LC, Bonsall R et al. Ischemic, hemodynamic, and neurohormonal responses to mental and exercise stress.

Experience from the Psychophysiological Investigations of Myocardial Ischemia Study (PIMI). *Circulation* 1996; **94**:

123. Giubbini R, Galli M, Campini R, Bosimini E, Bencivelli W, Tavazzi L. Effects of mental stress on myocardial perfusion in patients with ischemic heart disease. *Circulation* 1991; **83**: II100–II107.

124. Modena MG, Corghi F, Fantini G, Mattioli G. Echocardiographic monitoring of mental stress test in ischemic heart disease. *Clin Cardiol* 1989; **12**: 21–4.

125. Deedwania PC. Mental stress, pain perception and risk of silent ischemia (edit). *J Am Coll Cardiol* 1995; **25**: 1504–6.

126. Stern S, Cohn PF, Pepine CJ. Silent myocardial ischemia. *Curr Probl Cardiol* 1993; **18**: 301–59.

127. Quyyumi AA, Panza JA, Diodati JG, Callahan TS, Bonow RO, Epstein SE. Prognostic implications of myocardial ischemia during daily life in low risk patients with coronary artery disease. *J Am Coll Cardiol* 1993; **21**: 700–8.

128. Jain D, Burg M, Soufer R, Zaret BL. Prognostic implications of mental stress-induced silent left ventricular dysfunction in patients with stable angina pectoris. *Am J Cardiol* 1995; **76**: 31–5.

129. Bairey CN, Krantz DS, DeQuattro V, Berman DS, Rozanski A. Effect of beta-blockade on low heart rate-related ischemia during mental stress. *J Am Coll Cardiol* 1991; **17**: 1388–95.

130. Frasure-Smith N, Prince P. The ischemic heart disease lifestress monitoring program: impact on mortality. *Psychosom Med* 1985; **47**: 431–45.

131. Krantz DS, Kop WJ, Santiago HT, Gottdiener JS. Mental stress as a trigger of myocardial ischemia and infarction. In: Deedwania PC, Tofler GH, eds. *Triggers and Timing of Cardiac Events*, 2nd edn. (London: WB Saunders, 1996): 271–87.

Index